Clinical Management
of Mother and Newborn

Clinical Management of Mother and Newborn

Gertie F. Marx, Editor

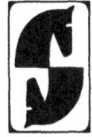

Springer-Verlag

New York   Heidelberg   Berlin

Gertie F. Marx, M.D.
Department of Anesthesiology
Albert Einstein College of Medicine
1300 Morris Park Avenue
Bronx, New York 10461

With 30 illustrations

Library of Congress Cataloging in Publication Data

Marx, Gertie F
  Clinical management of mother and newborn.

  Includes index.
  1. Infants (Newborn)—Diseases.   2. Puerperal
disorders. I. Title. [DNLM: 1. Infant, Newborn,
2. Infant, Newborn, Diseases. 3. Postnatal care.
WS420 C641]
RJ254.M37   618.9'201   79–12344

9 8 7 6 5 4 3 2 1

ISBN-13:978-1-4612-6175-9   e-ISBN-13:978-1-4612-6173-5
DOI: 10.1007/978-1-4612-6173-5

Preface

The birth of a baby is the culmination of months of anticipation and planning. Most often, mother and infant are healthy and readily able to establish close contact—a bond. However, in some situations either mother or baby or both present complications. The more prompt and rational the treatment, the sooner the normal parent–infant relationship will commence.

This book is devoted exclusively to the first days following birth. In its 15 chapters, postpartum and postnatal physiology and pathophysiology are reviewed by 18 specialists. Normal and abnormal development of mother and child is correlated with proven means of clinical management.

Chapters 1 through 3 cover maternal postpartum developments and complications. Chapter 4 stresses the importance of a normal parent–newborn relationship, a concept of increasing concern in modern society. The following ten chapters discuss neonatal physiology and pathophysiology; the effects of obstetric anesthesia on infant behavior, pulmonary function measurements in the postnatal period and treatment of the sick newborn are discussed in detail. The final chapter reviews maternal and perinatal mortality; the data, based on extensive surveys in New York City, indicate that current management is effecting an overall decline in mortality.

I wish to thank my collaborators and our publisher for their help in this endeavor to enhance the care given to mothers and their newly born infants —for the benefit both of the young family and of society in general.

Contents

7

Effects of Obstetric Analgesia-Anesthesia on Neonatal Neurobehavior   85

ROBERT HODGKINSON

8

Drug Sensitivity of the Neonate   101

SIMON HALEVY

9

Pulmonary Function in the Perinatal Period   109

EMILE M. SCARPELLI

10

The Meconium Aspiration Syndrome

137

JEAN F. HOBBS AND ARTHUR I. EIDELMAN

11

Treatment of Neonatal Metabolic Acidosis

153

ARTHUR I. EIDELMAN AND JEAN F. HOBBS

15

Maternal and Perinatal Mortality

241

JEAN PAKTER, MORTON A. SCHIFFER, AND FRIEDA NELSON

Contributors

GERARD M. BASSELL, M.B., B.S., Assistant Professor in Residence, Department of Anesthesiology, University of California at Irvine, Irvine, California 92717

PRASANTA CHANDRA, M.B., B.S., Assistant Professor of Obstetrics and Gynecology, Albert Einstein College of Medicine of Yeshiva University, Bronx, New York 10461

W. GODFREY COBLINER, Ph.D., Assistant Clinical Professor, Department of Obstetrics and Gynecology, Albert Einstein College of Medicine of Yeshiva University, Bronx, New York 10461

ERMELANDO V. COSMI, M.D., Professor and Chairman, Department of Prenatal Medicine, University of Chieta; *and* Professor of Anesthesiology and of Obstetrics, University of Rome, Rome, Italy

J. SELWYN CRAWFORD, M.B., Ch.B., Consultant Anaesthetist, Birmingham Maternity Hospital, Birmingham, Great Britain

ARTHUR I. EIDELMAN, M.D., Associate Professor of Pediatrics, Albert Einstein College of Medicine of Yeshiva University; *and* Director of Newborn Services and Assistant Director of Pediatrics at the Hospital of the Albert Einstein College of Medicine, Bronx, New York 10461

SIMON HALEVY, M.D., Professor of Anesthesiology, Health Sciences Center School of Medicine, State University of New York at Stony Brook; *and* Director of Obstetrical Anesthesiology, Nassau County Medical Center, East Meadow, New York 11554

JEAN F. HOBBS, M.D., Assistant Professor of Pediatrics, Albert Einstein College of Medicine of Yeshiva University; *and* Director of Newborn Services, Bronx Municipal Hospital Center, Bronx, New York 10461

ROBERT HODGKINSON, M.D., Associate Professor of Anesthesia, Obstetrics and Gynecology, The University of Texas, Health Science Center at San Antonio, Medical School, San Antonio, Texas 78284

STEPHEN R. KANDALL, M.D., Associate Professor of Pediatrics, Mount Sinai School of Medicine of the City University of New York; and Chief, Division of Neonatology, Beth Israel Medical Center, New York, New York 10003

GERTIE F. MARX, M.D., Professor of Anesthesiology, Director of Obstetric Anesthesia, Albert Einstein College of Medicine of Yeshiva University, Bronx, New York 10461

FRIEDA NELSON, B.A., Principal Statistician, New York City Department of Health, New York, New York 10013

GERARD W. OSTHEIMER, M.D., Assistant Professor of Anesthesia, Harvard Medical School, Boston Hospital for Women, Boston, Massachusetts 02115

JEAN PAKTER, M.D., M.P.H., Director, Bureau of Maternity Services and Family Planning, New York City Department of Health, New York, New York 10013

JOHN W. SCANLON, M.D., Associate Professor of Pediatrics, Georgetown University School of Medicine; and Director of Nurseries, Columbia Hospital for Women, Washington, D.C. 20037

EMILE M. SCARPELLI, M.D., Ph.D., Professor of Pediatrics, Associate Professor of Physiology, Director, Pediatric Pulmonary Division, Albert Einstein College of Medicine of Yeshiva University, Bronx, New York 10461

MORTON A. SCHIFFER, M.D., Chairman, Obstetric Advisory Committee to the Commissioner of Health, New York City Department of Health, New York, New York 10013

ELIZABETH D. STEIN, M.D., Assistant Professor of Anesthesiology, Director, Respiratory Therapy, Albert Einstein College of Medicine of Yeshiva University, Bronx, New York 10461

1
Postpartum Uterine Activity and Anesthesia

Gerard M. Bassell, Prasanta Chandra, and
Gertie F. Marx

Immediately following delivery of the placenta, uterine congestion decreases rapidly as the vigorous contractions of the uterine musculature squeeze blood out of the myometrium. The anterior and posterior walls come into apposition and the cavity becomes quite smooth except at the former site of placental attachment; the uterine cavity is then almost obliterated (28). Thus, the postpartum uterus is well suited for *in vivo* studies of the effect of anesthetic agents on activity of the term-pregnant uterus, as concern for fetal well-being is no longer present.

Uterine Muscle Physiology

Uterine musculature exhibits the same physiologic function as other smooth muscle or striated and cardiac muscle. Any differences occur mainly as a result of hormonal influences, but the cellular behavior of all muscles is similar.

The normal function of muscles is described by the term "contraction cycle" (2, 3, 4, 11, 17), during which the muscle undergoes various changes in tension and length enabling it to perform its required task efficiently. A "contracture," on the other hand, is a rare and unphysiologic state of sustained muscular activity, in which all cells are activated to contract tetanically, with profound loss of mechanical efficiency.

The two phases of the contraction cycle are the "isometric" and the "isotonic" periods. During the isometric portion of the cycle both ends of the muscle are fixed during the development of tension; no external shortening occurs. Once external shortening does occur, the muscle has entered

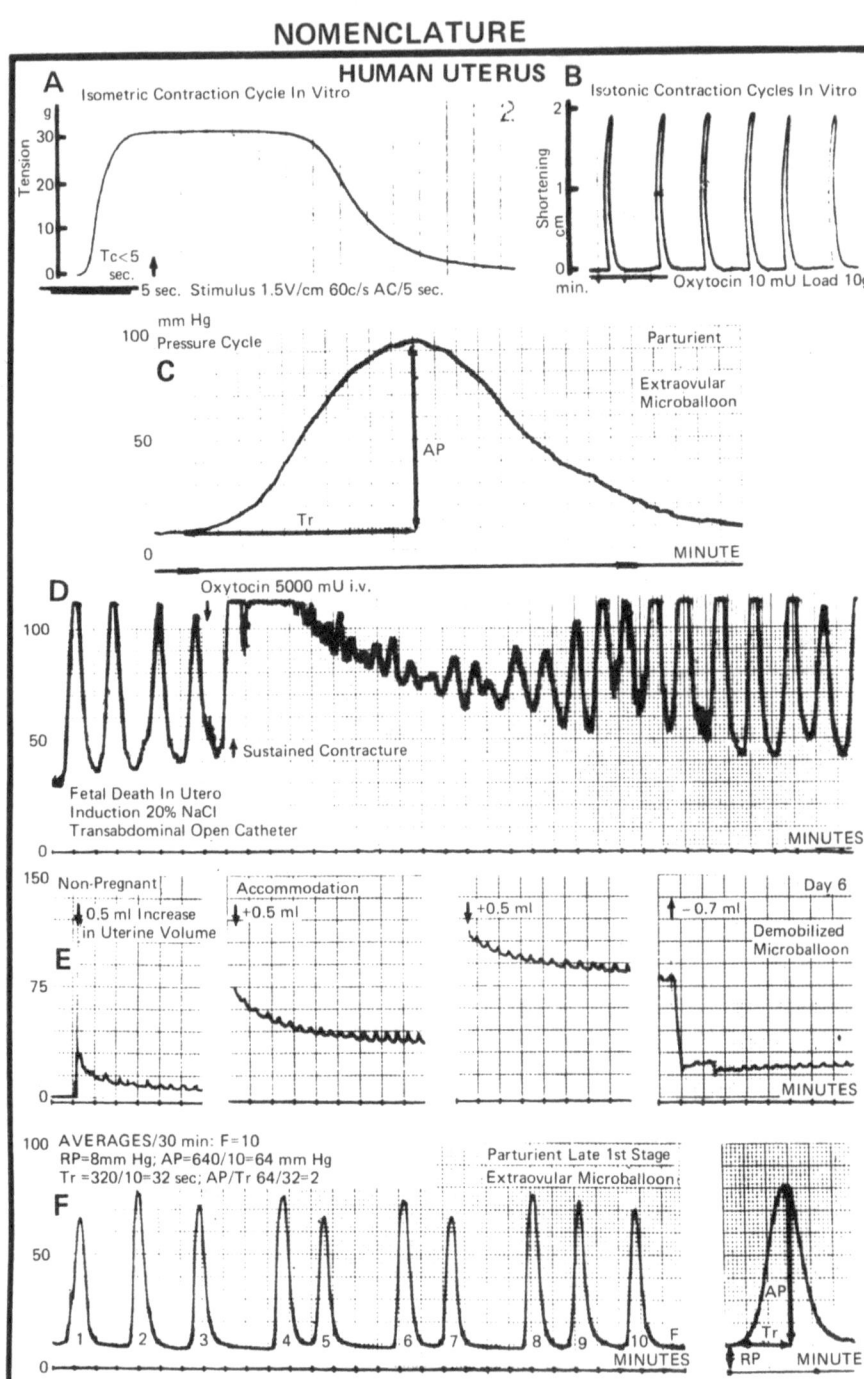

NOMENCLATURE
HUMAN UTERUS

the isotonic phase regardless of whether a load has been moved. The muscle can only move a load during the phase of isotonic shortening, and only a loaded muscle can perform external work (= load $\times$ distance). During the isometric period, if an unstimulated muscle undergoes a constant stretch, it develops a "resting tension" to which is added the "active tension" of the isotonic period of the contraction cycle. If moderate stretch is sustained for an appreciable length of time, the muscle "accommodates" by decreasing its resting tension.

These terms are used to describe the situation in the uterus as well as in other muscles. The resting uterus has a measureable "resting tension" (or "resting pressure") and undergoes both isometric and isotonic contraction cycles as well as pressure cycles (9) (Fig. 1.1). Thus, intrauterine pressure measurements reveal a resting pressure during the period between two contractions (pressure cycles), onto which is added the active pressure produced during the uterine contraction. As with other muscles, the uterus accommodates to sustained external stretch with a decrease in resting pressure. In a normal contraction cycle, only discrete areas of muscle cells are involved, with the resultant contractile rhythmicity ensuring that fatigue does not occur too readily and that a high level of efficiency is maintained over extended periods of time.

Methods of Intrauterine Pressure Measurement

For almost 80 years, investigators attempted to delineate uterine function by inserting various measuring devices into the human uterus. Reflecting

Fig. 1.1 Intrauterine pressure (original tracings, human uterus) for *in vitro* and *in vivo* experiments. **A.** Isometric tension in the electrically "tetanized" uterus, when all myometrial cells are simultaneously activated. Note that activity manifests after 1.5 seconds latency period and the contraction time (T_c) is less than 5 seconds. **B.** Isotonic shortening. Note the work performed in a "steady state." **C.** Pressure cycles during parturition. **D.** Contracture. Note the high resting pressure (over 30 mm Hg) sustained by the osmotic effect of intra-amniotic hypertonic saline in a patient with fetal death *in utero*. Note the "contracture," superimposed on the high resting pressure by an overdose of oxytocin. **E.** Accommodation of the nonpregnant human uterus to sustained stretch. Stretch is induced by stepwise increase in uterine (balloon) volume. Note the gradual decrease in resting pressure after the stretch-induced initial increase. Note the sudden drop in resting pressure after the reduction in uterine volume. **F.** The quantitation of the averages in frequency (F), resting pressure (RP), active pressure (AP), time of pressure rise (T_r) and AP/T_r of the parturient uterus in a 30-minute tracing. The "total averages" of clinical labor are measured by averaging the various parameters for the entire process. [From Csapo (9), with permission of the author.]

available technology, balloons connected to pressure-measuring instruments and filled with fluid or air have been inserted, x-ray with radiocontrast has been used, gas has been introduced into the uterine cavity, and open-ended catheter recordings of pressure waveform have been taken. In contrast to the nonpregnant uterus, the gravid uterus is closed and fluid filled, so that pressures are transmitted with minimal distortion to an internal pressure recording device, be it balloon or open-ended catheter, provided that insertion of the instrument does not create a large fluid leak. Open-ended catheters have been placed transabdominally into the amniotic sac, creating a bridge between the amniotic fluid and an external pressure transducer. Such procedures are not without hazard, however, and puncture of maternal blood vessels or fetal parts can occur during insertion of the pressure catheter.

Far safer is the use of the extraovular microballoon technique of Csapo (8, 12, 14), in which a catheter, closed by a microballoon of appropriate size and wall characteristics, is inserted transcervically into the extraovular space. This method can be used prior to rupture of membranes, as the balloon is placed without entering the amniotic sac. Provided that the volume of the balloon is between 0.5 to 0.8 ml, maximum pressure will be recorded during uterine activity. The problems associated with the transabdominal open catheter approach are thus circumvented and both methods have been shown to provide identical data (9). The recording system is air free and fluid filled, and has a short Teflon catheter, closed at one end by the microballoon and connected at the other end to a pressure transducer.

Among the advantages of the extraovular microballoon technique are lack of leakage from the amniotic cavity and absence of air introduction. As the microballoon is inserted per vaginam, puncture of maternal blood vessels or fetal parts cannot occur. Some inaccuracies can be introduced, however, if air is not properly purged from the catheter, if the balloon is over- or underdistended, or if the presenting fetal part is allowed to compress the balloon. Strict adherence to the recommended methods of insertion (30), together with careful removal of air from the system and filling the balloon to the correct volume, will ensure that pressure recordings will be accurate and reproducible. The presence of the microballoon within the uterine cavity has been shown not to affect normal uterine physiology (13). Therefore, the tracings obtained are an accurate representation of uterine activity during the period of measurement.

Although the extraovular microballoon method is used safely during labor, the effect of drugs and anesthetic agents on uterine function is studied more easily after expulsion of the products of conception. Consequently, the "demobilized microballoon technique," in which the lower portion of the recording catheter is fixed to the patient's thigh, is used following expulsion of the placenta, thereby preventing descent of the balloon toward the cervical canal. As the internal uterine walls are soon apposed after delivery of the placenta, and the uterine cavity is almost obliterated, transmission of pressure from the uterine wall to the microballoon is direct and unimpeded by any uterine contents. Although radius and tension have decreased, the uterus continues to behave like a sphere, and form and magnitude of contractions resemble those of the first and second stages of labor (6, 29). The hormonal milieu is unchanged over that of the term-pregnant state, and it is reasonable to extrapolate data obtained at this time to the uterus immediately prior to parturition. Measurements of uterine wall tension would be more accurate than measurements of intrauterine pressure, these variables are interdependent and intrauterine pressure reflects accurately the degree of tension in the uterine wall. This method offers definite advantages over investigations in nonpregnant women, pregnant animals, or isolated uterine muscle strips in that the study is undertaken in a human, term-pregnant uterus with normal blood supply, nervous control, and hormonal influences, but without the presence of the fetus.

Uterine Activity During Pregnancy

During the course of gestation, the muscle mass of the human uterus increases from a mean weight of 150 g at conception to 1100 g at term (18). The major growth occurs in the second half of pregnancy as the mean weight at the midpoint of gestation is 300 to 400 g. For this reason, studies of uterine activity during early pregnancy are not applicable to the term-pregnant situation where the width of the uterine wall and the radius of the uterus allow production of vastly different pressures according to the Law of Laplace.

$$\text{Pressure} = \frac{2 \times \text{wall thickness}}{\text{radius}} \times \text{tension}$$

At the mid-first trimester, when the corpus luteum is still active, the frequency of uterine contractions is high (66/30 minute), while active pressure (2.2 torr) and the oxytocin response are low (10). Toward the end of the first trimester, the placenta begins to become more important in the control of intrauterine pressure, and this function is maintained through the second and third trimesters. The placental secretion of progesterone prevents the uterus from realizing its full active pressure potential of 80 torr, and thus ensures that the fetoplacental unit is not subjected to intrauterine pressures high enough to produce abortion. After completion of the changeover from luteal to placental hormonal control during the second trimester, active pressure and oxytocin response begin a gradual rise.

At the 36th week, these increases accelerate dramatically; simultaneously, the cervix begins the changes that will ready it for parturition. It appears that plasma progesterone levels decrease close to term to allow the full potential of uterine activity to come into play during labor and parturition (10, 19). It has been shown that patients at term who undergo easy oxytocin inductions have low levels of plasma progesterone, while patients with difficult or failed inductions have correspondingly higher levels (19).

The uterus behaves like smooth muscle elsewhere, with changing rhythmicity and intensity of contractions and recruitment of different cell groups from contraction to contraction. Thus, the hallmark of uterine activity during early labor is its variability. In normal, non-oxytocin-induced labor, frequency, intensity, and duration of uterine contractions vary considerably. The measured active pressure changes from contraction to contraction and the period between contractions is not constant (27). Toward the end of the first stage of labor, however, contractions become more regular, probably because of oxytocin release. Nevertheless, in the assessment of drug effects, every patient has to serve as her own control. During oxytocin-induced labors, this individual variability is attenuated, with more constant frequencies and active pressures being recorded.

Analysis of Uterine Activity

Twenty years ago, Caldeyro-Barcia and co-workers suggested that the product of the intensity and frequency of uterine contractions could be used as an index of uterine activity (7). The resulting value is expressed in Montevideo Units (torr/10 minutes) and clinical labor usually starts when the cervix dilates more than 2 cm and uterine activity has attained values of 80 to 120 Montevideo Units (5). The intensity of uterine contractions is the active pressure, which Caldeyro-Barcia's group measured by the transabdominal open catheter method (1, 6). This method of measurement allowed the Montevideo researchers to study extensively the effects on normal uterine activity of a large number of hormonal and other agents, but the restrictions of this method preclude its use as a routine during labor and parturition.

Within the last 10 years, as a result of Csapo's work (9, 10), the microballoon technique has largely replaced open catheter methods as the means by which uterine function, and the effects of various drugs and procedures on uterine function, can be measured. Although uterine activity during labor is monitored clinically by noninvasive, surface methods, and Montevideo Units are rarely calculated, research methods demand the precision of Csapo's technique and results are expressed as the individual variables that make up Montevideo Units. Thus, modern methods of study incorporate the features of both Caldeyro-Barcia's and Csapo's work. It is important to realize that inaccuracies may be introduced if insufficient control periods are allowed prior to evaluation of the effects of the various agents under investigation, as the insertion of the microballoon may cause a temporary disruption of normal uterine activity. The small volume of the balloon has been shown not to affect the activity of the uterus while in situ (9).

Effects of Oxytocin and Anesthetic Agents

Oxytocin

During the latter part of the third trimester, infusion of oxytocin, at rates of 1 to 8 mU/minute causes large increases in the frequency and intensity of uterine contractions without increasing resting pressure (6). Studies in the postpartum uterus have shown a similar response when 10 mU of oxytocin is given as a bolus intravenously. Although a small increase in resting pressure may occur after the injection of the oxytocin, this effect is short lived and the uterus soon accommodates by reducing the resting pressure to preinjection levels. If oxytocin infusion is begun, uterine activity increases as an exponential function of the infusion rate, but this holds true only for rates within the physiologic range (less than 16 mU/minute). If the rate of infusion increases markedly, abnormal uterine activity will ensue, with unphysiologically high frequency and resting pressure (Fig. 1.2).

Ketamine

With low-dose ketamine finding increased use during obstetric procedures, it is important to ensure that this drug exhibits no major effect on normal uterine activity. Studies by Galloon (15, 16) during the first and second trimesters suggested that ketamine raised both resting pressure and intensity of contractions, and he postulated that hazardous increases in uterine base tone could develop. However, more recent data (20) of postpartum

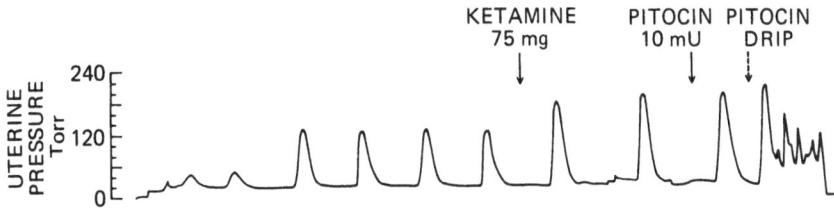

Fig. 1.2 The rise in intensity of contraction was similar following the intravenous injection of ketamine 75 mg and oxytocin (Pitocin) 10 mU. Note that resting uterine pressure did not change, in contrast to the effect of a 0.1 percent oxytocin infusion (30 drops per minute). (From Marx, Hwang, and Chandra: unpublished data.)

uterine pressures measured by the Csapo microballoon technique showed that the doses of ketamine presently employed in obstetrics (up to 1 mg/kg) are without deleterious effects on full-term uterine activity. The patients who received 25 mg of ketamine exhibited no change in the uterine contractile pattern, while those given 50 and 75 mg had an increase in intensity and duration of the first contraction following the injection, a response similar to that seen after the intravenous injection of 10 mU of oxytocin. On the other hand, ketamine in a dose of 100 mg led to an increase in the intensity and duration of the following two to three contractions, with the magnitude of the increases again being similar to that seen with 10 mU of oxytocin. None of the patients showed an increase in resting pressure following either ketamine or an oxytocin bolus injection of 10 mU, but all patients who received a 0.1% oxytocin infusion at a rate of 30 drops per minute showed an elevation of uterine resting pressure and an increase in the frequency and intensity of subsequent uterine contractions (Fig. 1.2).

Halogenated Anesthetic Agents

It has long been recognized that the halogenated anesthetics are potent depressors of uterine activity and that, clinically, this is a dose-related phenomenon. This anesthetic-induced uterine depression has been used during operative obstetrics where cessation of uterine activity has been indicated. Halothane, enflurane, and isoflurane have been shown to depress uterine activity in isolated pregnant and nonpregnant human myometrium (22, 23), while halothane has depressed activity in isolated pregnant rat myometrium (24, 25).

The effect of fluroxene on uterine activity has been studied in the human (31), and was found to depress the frequency, but not the intensity, of uterine contractions when blood levels exceeded the equivalent of 0.5 MAC* for a nonpregnant adult. The normal uterine response to oxytocin was maintained with fluroxene blood levels approaching one MAC at equilibrium. Halothane and enflurane show similar and dose-dependent effects on the postpartum uterus. Expressed in terms of MAC, depression of spontaneous uterine activity occurs at approximately 0.5 MAC of both agents, while the oxytocin response becomes suppressed at 0.8 to 0.9 MAC. Spontaneous uterine activity recovers rapidly when deep planes of halothane and enflurane anesthesia are lightened below these critical levels, and there is a corresponding reappearance of the usual response to oxytocin (21) (Figs. 1.3 and 1.4).

* MAC = minimum alveolar concentration of anesthetic that produces immobility in 50% of patients exposed to a noxious stimulus.

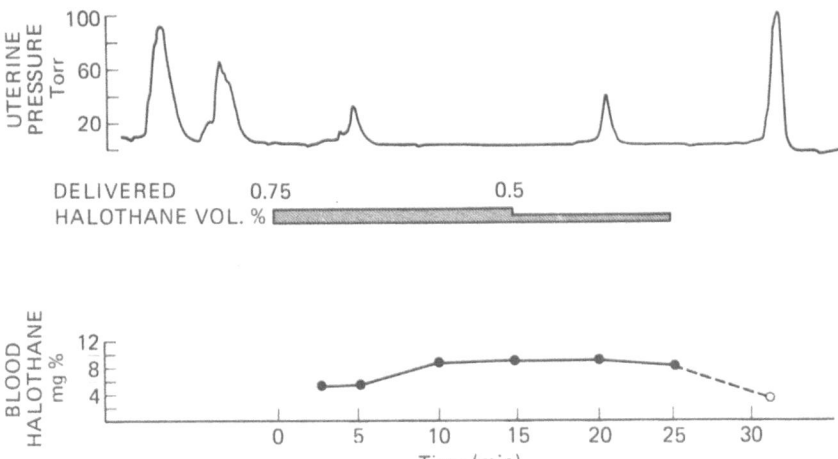

Fig. 1.3   Administration of 0.75 volume percent halothane led to a marked decrease in frequency and intensity of spontaneous uterine contractions. As the halothane concentration was decreased, uterine activity began to return. Blood halothane concentration is shown below the uterine pressure tracing. (From Marx, Kim, Lin, et al.: unpublished data.)

Conclusion

The postpartum uterus presents optimal conditions for evaluating the effects of anesthetic and adjuvant drugs on uterine activity. Muscle mass, resting pressure, as well as nervous control and hormonal milieu, are identical to those of the predelivery uterus, while concern for the fetus is no longer a limiting factor. The activity of the uterus during the immediate puerperium is unchanged, although the contractions become less frequent and less intense during the first four or five days after birth (26).

Oxytocin infusion of less than 16 mU/minute enhances uterine activity such that both frequency and intensity of contractions increases. Infusion of more than 16 mU/minute leads to a rise in resting pressure as well. A bolus of 10 mU oxytocin given intravenously increases both the intensity and duration of the first contraction following the injection, and this response is similarly seen after bolus injections of 50 or 75 mg of ketamine. The commonly used 25 mg dose of ketamine is without effect on uterine activity. The halogenated anesthetic agents, halothane and enflurane, depress uterine activity in a dose-related manner and suppress the response of the uterus to oxytocin infusion, but both effects disappear as soon as anesthesia is lightened.

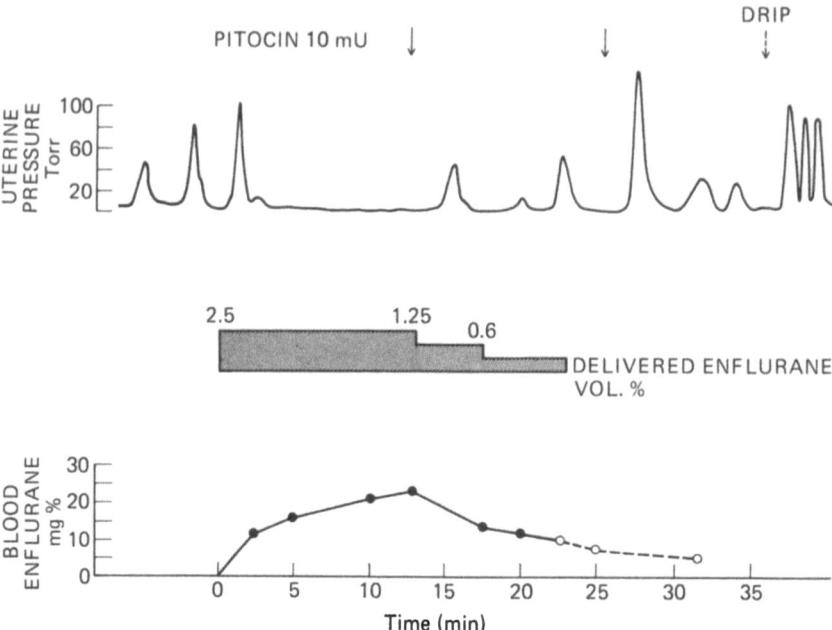

Fig. 1.4 Administration of 2.5 volume percent enflurane was associated with a decrease in spontaneous uterine activity and abolition of the response to 10 mU of oxytocin (Pitocin). As the concentration of enflurane was decreased, uterine activity began to return spontaneously, and the normal response to an oxytocin bolus and infusion was again apparent. (From Marx, Kim, Lin, et al.: unpublished data.)

References

1. Alvarez, H., Caldeyro-Barcia, R.: The normal and abnormal contractile waves of the uterus during labour. Gynaecologia **138**(2):190, 1954.
2. Bourne, G.H. (Ed.): Structure and Function of Muscle, Vols. I, II, and III. New York and London, Academic Press, 1960.
3. Bülbring, E.: Electrical activity in intestinal smooth muscle. Physiol. Rev. **42** (Suppl. 5):160, 1962.
4. Bülbring, E. (Ed.): Pharmacology of Smooth Muscle, Vol. 6. Proceedings of 2nd International Pharmacological Meeting. Oxford, Pergamon Press, 1964.
5. Caldeyro-Barcia, R., Poseiro, J.J.: Oxytocin and contractility of the pregnant human uterus. Ann. N.Y. Acad. Sci. **75**:813, 1959.
6. Caldeyro-Barcia, R., Poseiro, J.J.: Physiology of the uterine contraction. Clin. Obstet. Gynecol. **3**:386, 1960.
7. Caldeyro-Barcia, R., Sica-Blanco, Y., Poseiro, J.J., et al.: A quantitative study of the action of synthetic oxytocin on the pregnant human uterus. J. Pharmacol. Exp. Ther. **121**:18, 1957.

8. Csapo, A.: The theoretic, diagnostic and prognostic value of the intrauterine pressure. Bibl. Gynaec. **42**:93, 1966.
9. Csapo, A.: The diagnostic significance of the intrauterine pressure. Part I. Obstet. Gynecol. Surv. **25**:403, 1970.
10. Csapo, A.: The diagnostic significance of the intrauterine pressure. Part II. Obstet. Gynecol. Surv. **25**:515, 1970.
11. Csapo, A.I.: Smooth muscle as a contractile unit. Physiol. Rev. **42** (Suppl. 5):7, 1962.
12. Csapo, A.I.: Extraovular pressure—its diagnostic value. Am. J. Obstet. Gynecol. **90**:493, 1964.
13. Csapo, A., Pinto-Dantas, C.A., Kerenyi, T., et al.: Progesterone and myometrial activity, in Exerpta Medica International Congress Series No. 133. Proceedings of Fifth World Congress on Fertility and Sterility. Stockholm, 1966.
14. Csapo, A., Sauvage, J.: The evolution of uterine activity during human pregnancy. Acta Obstet. Gynecol. Scand. **47**:181, 1968.
15. Galloon, S.: Ketamine and the pregnant uterus. Can. Anaesth. Soc. J **20**: 141, 1973.
16. Galloon, S.: Ketamine for obstetric delivery. Anesthesiology **44**:522, 1976.
17. Hoffman, B.F., Cranefield, P.F.: Electrophysiology of the Heart. New York, McGraw-Hill, 1960.
18. Hytten, F.E., Cheyne, G.A.: The size and composition of the human pregnant uterus. J. Obstet. Gynaecol. Brit. Cwlth. **76**:400, 1969.
19. Johansson, E.D.B.: Progesterone level and response to oxytocin at term. Lancet **2**:570, 1968.
20. Marx, G.F., Hwang, H.S., Chandra, P.: Postpartum uterine pressures with different doses of ketamine. Anesthesiology **50**:163, 1979.
21. Marx, G.F., Kim, Y.I., Lin, C.C., et al.: Postpartum uterine pressures under halothane or enflurane anesthesia. Obstet. Gynecol. **51**:695, 1978.
22. Munson, E.S., Embro, W.J.: Enflurane, isoflurane, and halothane and isolated human uterine muscle. Anesthesiology **46**:11, 1977.
23. Naftalin, N.J., McKay, D.M., Phear, W.P.C., et al.: The effects of halothane on pregnant and nonpregnant human myometrium. Anesthesiology **46**:15, 1977.
24. Naftalin, N.J., Phear, W.P.C., Goldberg, A.H.: Halothane and isometric contractions of isolated pregnant rat myometrium. Anesthesiology **42**:458, 1975.
25. Naftalin, N. J., Phear, W.P.C., Goldberg, A.H.: Halothane and calcium interaction in isolated pregnant and postpartum rat myometrium. Anesthesiology **45**:31, 1976.
26. Reynolds, S.R.M., Harris, J.S., Kaiser, I.H.: Uterine contraction patterns during normal labor, in Clinical Measurement of Uterine Forces in Pregnancy and Labor. Springfield, Illinois, Charles C Thomas, 1954.
27. Schulman, H., Romney, S.L.: Variability of uterine contractions in normal human parturition. Obstet. Gynecol. **36**:215, 1970.
28. Taylor, E.S.: The puerperium, in Beck's Obstetrical Practice, 9th. Ed. Baltimore, The Williams and Wilkins Company, 1971.

29. Vasicka, A., Kretchmer, H.E.: Uterine dynamics. Clin. Obstet. Gynecol. 4:17, 1961.
30. Villaneuva, C., Sauvage, J.: Intrauterine pressure monitoring with a balloon-tipped catheter. Obstet. Gynecol. 45:287, 1974.
31. Zargham, I., Leviss, S.R., Marx, G.F.: Uterine pressures during fluroxene anesthesia. Anesth. Analg. 53:568, 1974.

2
Pathophysiology and Therapy of Postpartum Complications

Gertie F. Marx

The anesthesiologist is often called upon to aid in the diagnosis and treatment of postpartum complications regardless of the nature of the antecedent anesthetic management, i.e., whether regional, general or, indeed, none at all. Postpartum complications are most frequently obstetric or iatrogenic in origin and only rarely the result of a coincidental medical disease. They may affect one or multiple organ systems.

Obstetric Complications

Unsuspected Twin Gestation

Postpartum problems of a solely obstetric nature include unrecognized multiple pregnancy and failure of placental expulsion. Unsuspected twin gestation may require a rapid change in the conduct of anesthesia. If the second infant presents as a breech or is to be delivered by internal podalic version and extraction, prompt inhibition of uterine activity may be necessary. This is best accomplished by the administration of halothane (in concentrations exceeding 1 vol%) or enflurane (in concentrations exceeding 2 vol%) (30). Prior institution of a regional block is no contraindication to the use of halogenated agents for delivery; however, they should be "washed out" promptly thereafter to reduce the duration of any additive hypotensive effects. In contrast, intrauterine manipulations without adequate uterine "relaxation"* may be hazardous to both mother and infant (32). Therefore, continual preparedness for general anesthesia is essential for every delivery regardless of the planned method of pain relief.

Placental Expulsion Failure

Placental separation normally occurs during the first or second postdelivery uterine contraction. *Failure of placental detachment* may be caused by insufficient intensity of contractions (retained placenta) or by abnormal adherence of the placenta to the uterine wall (placenta accreta). *Placental retention* occurs in approximately 1% of vaginal deliveries. If it is impossible to express the placenta by downward pressure on the fundus within a reasonable period of time (10 to 20 minutes), manual removal is indicated. Although some patients are able to tolerate manual extraction of the placenta without anesthesia, most require general anesthesia or regional analgesia. However, inhibition of uterine activity is rarely necessary (5, 16, 21, 41).

Placenta accreta refers to adherence of part or all of the placenta to the myometrium with partial or complete absence of the decidua basalis. In placenta increta, there is, in addition, penetration of chorionic villi into the myometrium; in placenta percreta, the entire thickness of the myometrium is invaded. The etiology of placenta accreta appears to be endometrial injury by trauma, infection, associated gynecologic disorder, or endocrine imbalance. If the placenta is totally involved, symptoms are absent and bleeding is minimal; the diagnosis becomes evident with failure of attempts to manually separate and extract the placenta (5, 16, 21, 41). In a review of 200 cases of placenta accreta, only 10% of the patients were primiparae and 46% had had four or more pregnancies (13). The recommended treatment is abdominal hysterectomy. However, this is often preceded by a final attempt to manually detach the placenta under inhalation anesthesia with inhibition of uterine activity. Since bleeding may be profuse, operation and anesthesia should not commence until preparations for major surgery are complete; sufficient cross-matched blood and a blood-warmer must be available. For a vaginal trial at placental detachment, halothane-oxygen or enflurane-oxygen is the anesthetic of choice. Once laparotomy is decided upon, anesthesia should be managed in anticipation of hemorrhage, because the blood supply to the pelvis during pregnancy is increased, and friability of edematous tissue predisposes to poor hemostasis (4).

---

* In clinical concentrations, halothane and enflurane do not decrease the resting (base) tone of the uterus; however, they inhibit both the frequency and intensity of contractions in a dose-related manner (30).

Postpartum Bleeding

Postpartum *hemorrhage* is defined as abnormal blood loss during the first 24 hours after delivery. The average blood loss from an episiotomy has been reported as 253 ml (35), that from an uncomplicated single-fetus vaginal delivery as 500 ml, and that from twin vaginal delivery or elective cesarean section as 900 ml (37). The normal parturient responds to this loss of blood by elevating her cardiac output with an increased stroke volume and decreased heart rate; her postpartum hematocrit is usually maintained at the prepartum level (34, 37). The important causes of postpartum hemorrhage are (a) uterine atony, (b) retention of placental fragments, (c) lacerations of the birth canal, and (d) coagulation defects (5).

Uterine atony accounts for approximately 80% of all cases of postpartum bleeding (28). The condition is commonly associated with factors that interfere with the ability of the uterus to contract adequately such as prolonged labor, uterine overdistention from multiple pregnancy or hydramnios, and deep anesthesia with diethyl ether or halogenated agents. Treatment of atony consists of expression of blood clots, gentle massage of the uterus, oxytocics, and rapid removal by hyperventilation with oxygen of any anesthetic agent affecting uterine activity. If the uterus remains atonic despite these measures, it should be explored to rule out retained placental fragments or laceration of the uterine wall. If bleeding persists in the presence of a firmly contracted uterus or if the blood is arterial in color, a cervical tear should be suspected. Intra- or retraperitoneal bleeding may result from rupture of the veins of the broad ligament due to forceful forceps delivery; abdominal or back pain with signs of excessive blood loss will follow (5, 16, 28, 41).

At the first evidence of postpartum bleeding—before removal of placental fragments or repair of lacerations—blood should be cross-matched for possible transfusion, and the rate of infusion of a balanced salt solution should be increased. If the patient develops significant tachycardia and/or hypotension or if the blood loss exceeds 1000 ml and the situation has not been resolved, the first unit of packed cells (reconstituted with crystalloid solution) or fresh whole blood should be started (5). Excessive bleeding reduces the oxygen-carrying capacity of blood and is rationally treated by an increase in circulating red cell mass. If anesthesia is required, it should be a general endotracheal technique with low concentrations of inhalation agents, supplemented by a muscle relaxant. The inhalation agent should be rapid acting, permit administration of a high inspired oxygen fraction, and not depress uterine activity in the concentration used.

When postpartum hemorrhage is not caused by uterine atony, placental fragments, or lacerations, a coagulation disorder is probable. *Disseminated intravascular coagulation* (DIC) is an acquired syndrome in which the release into the circulation of tissue extracts or fluids rich in thromboplastin triggers both thrombotic and thrombolytic mechanisms leading simultaneously to intravascular clotting and a hemorrhagic diathesis. In pregnant women, the clotting process is almost always the primary response, with fibrinolysis developing secondarily (9, 23). Postpartum, the disorder is a complication of either amniotic fluid infusion or of conditions in which the triggering insult occurred before delivery, i.e., abruptio placentae, intra-auterine fetal death, or septicemia from amnionitis. The cardinal sign of DIC is abnormal bleeding from the vagina, venipuncture sites, gums, and incisional margins. The diagnosis is confirmed by blood coagulation studies. Bedside test-tube tests for clot formation and normal-clot lysis rapidly provide qualitative information regarding fibrinogen levels and the presence of fibrinolysins (28). A coagulation profile will show abnormally low levels for fibrinogen and plasminogen, the presence of fibrin degradation products, reductions in factors V, VIII, and XIII, decreased platelets, and prolonged thrombin and prothrombin times (10, 23). Management consists of replacing depleted clotting factors by infusion of fresh frozen plasma and platelet concentrates. If bleeding remains uncontrollable because of hypofibrinogenemia (levels below 100 mg/100 ml of plasma), an intravenous dose of 4 g of fibrinogen is indicated, although the risk of subsequent hepatitis is considerable. One gram of fibrinogen will increase the plasma level by 40 mg/100 ml in the average patient (33). In severe persistent cases, intravenous heparin (initial dose 50 units per kg followed by 1000 units per hour) may be used as a last resort in the attempt to block intravascular coagulation (26). Rarely is the infusion of an antifibrinolytic drug such as episilon-aminocaproic acid necessary.

Inversion of the Uterus

Inversion of the uterus is an obstetric complication associated with neurogenic shock. The most common causes are excessive traction on the umbilical cord or inordinately forceful fundal pressure. Occasionally the condition develops without any apparent reason, but only if the uterus is in a state of relaxation or atony. Therefore, "spontaneous" uterine inversion has occurred during prolonged halothane or methoxyflurane anesthesia (3, 20). The symptoms of vasomotor collapse (pallor, hypotension, tachycardia, etc.) are out of proportion to blood loss and are due to the constriction of blood vessels and compression of nerves when the uterus passes through the internal os along with the tubes and ovaries. Immediate treatment with intravenous fluids and manual reposition of the uterus is indicated. Since replacement of the uterus is painful, morphine analgesia or general anesthesia should be employed. If oxytocic drugs have already been administered, halothane or enflurane anesthesia may be necessary to inhibit uterine activity.

Amniotic Fluid Infusion

Two serious postdelivery complications affect multiple organ systems: amniotic fluid infusion and postpartum preeclampsia-eclampsia.

Amniotic fluid infusion (embolism), the sudden entry of amniotic fluid into the maternal circulation via endocervical veins or sinusoids at the uteroplacental site, is a rare but catastrophic situation. The typical patient is described as a multipara delivering a large infant following rupture of membranes and hypertonic labor. The essential physiopathology consists of cardiorespiratory changes, disseminated intravascular coagulation, and uterine hypotonia. A combination of chemical and mechanical processes, i.e., anaphylactoid reaction to components of the fluid and mechanical blockade of the pulmonary vessels by particulate matter, produces three main effects: (a) a sudden decrease in blood flow to the left heart; (b) pulmonary hypertension leading to cor pulmonale; and (c) marked ventilation-perfusion ratio aberrations (11, 18, 36). The increased amniotic fluid concentration of prostaglandin F during labor may contribute to the development of bronchoconstriction, that of prostaglandin E to peripheral vasodilation. The diagnosis is difficult; previously healthy parturients who suddenly manifest respiratory distress without chest pain, go into profound shock (particularly immediately following delivery), and exhibit signs of a coagulation disorder should be presumed to have amniotic fluid infusion. Over half of the patients die at the time of the original insult, and the diagnosis is confirmed by postmortem findings of fetal squames, meconium, and other debris plugging the pulmonary capillaries. In survivors, the diagnosis can be established by evidence of perfusion defects on pulmonary scanning together with the characteristic coagulation profile abnormalities. The treatment must have three objectives: (a) support of the cardiovascular system with provision of adequate oxygenation; (b) control of the coagulopathy; and (c) reestablishment of uterine tone. The following measures have been advocated: (1) oxygen with positive pressure ventilation via endotracheal tube, rotating tourniquets, digitalization, aminophylline, hydrocortisone in a large dose (2 g); (2) replacement of blood and clotting factors together with early heparinization (5000 units); (3) uterine packing followed by continued manual uterine stimulation and judiciously administered oxytocics (10, 11, 18, 36). At present, use of an autotransfuser is not recommended.

Preeclampsia and Eclampsia

Preeclampsia and eclampsia may arise during labor or postpartum. The basic pathologic mechanisms of this complication of human pregnancy are threefold: (a) widespread arteriolar spasm leading to varying degrees of tissue hypoxia; (b) retention of sodium and water far beyond that retained in normal gestation; and (c) slow intravascular coagulation causing fibrin deposits in the vessels of various organs, notably the placenta. Postpartum pre-eclampsia manifests as hypertensive crisis associated with oliguria or anuria, hyperreflexia, headache, nausea, visual disturbance, and the rapid develop-ment of edema about the face, especially the eyelids. Immediate antihyper-tensive therapy is indicated as 10% of maternal deaths from this disease are due to primary cerebral hemorrhage. If continuous extradural analgesia was instituted earlier, extension of sympathetic blockade may be utilized to decrease venous return to the heart and diminish the arterial pressure. Otherwise, hypotensive drugs with rapid, short action [such as trimetha-phan (Arfonad) or nitroprusside (Nipride) by continuous intravenous in-fusion or diazoxide (Hyperstat) by rapid intravenous injection] should be employed until definitive treatment with magnesium sulfate and longer act-ing hypotensive drugs [hydralazine (Apresoline) and methyldopa (Aldomet), singly or in combination] is effective. Chlorpromazine (Thorazine) is not a drug of choice because of its potential of enhancing liver damage (5, 6, 17, 25).

Postpartum eclampsia, i.e., convulsions with loss of consciousness, usually appears during the first 12 hours of the puerperium, but well-documented eclampsia has been reported up to five days postpartum. Dif-ferential diagnosis includes primarily epilepsy and water intoxication. Eclamptic convulsions are treated according to the same principles as con-vulsions from other causes, i.e.: (1) oxygenation (establishment of airway and intermittent positive pressure ventilation with 100% oxygen); (2) depression of cortical electrical seizure activity (ultrashort-acting barbitu-rate or diazepam (Valium); (3) control of muscular activity (succinyl-choline); and (4) reversal of metabolic acidosis (sodium bicarbonate). If not given already, magnesium sulfate should be administered to treat the underlying disease (6, 39).

Preeclamptic collapse implies shock at the time of delivery without ap-parent cause but with subsequent pathologic findings typical of preeclamp-sia. All such cases show glomerular lesions, and two-thirds have hepatic lesions; subendocardial hemorrhages are found if death was delayed at least two hours (25).

Iatrogenic Complications

Iatrogenic complications affect mainly the respiratory and circulatory sys-tems. While the pulmonary problems are commonly related to analgesia-anesthesia, the cardiovascular complications are due to oxytocic drugs.

Respiratory Depression

Pulmonary problems include respiratory depression and aspiration pneu-monitis. Respiratory depression following delivery is almost always caused by drugs, either narcotics or muscle relaxants, as postpartum pain does not produce splinting of the diaphragm, even after cesarean section. Narcotic-induced hypoventilation is usually antagonized by pain. This has been demonstrated in both conscious and anesthetized persons. Thus, patients who have severe pain due to injury or pathology breathe adequately after relatively large doses of narcotics as long as the pain is present. Once the stimulus of pain is removed, respiratory depression may rapidly ensue. Similarly, painful stimuli increase rate and depth of respiration in lightly anesthetized patients who have received narcotics, and respiration may become depressed in the postanesthetic period after the surgical stimulation has been abolished (12). When narcotic-induced hypoventilation is suspected postpartum, a small dose of intravenously injected antagonist may be therapeutic as well as diagnostic, if combined with pre- and postadministration measurements of the respiratory minute volume. Of the presently available narcotic antogonists, naloxone (Narcan) is best because it has no depressant properties of its own; however, its duration is shorter than that of most narcotic drugs, necessitating continued observation of the patient and possibly a second dose one hour after the first (42).

The response to muscle relaxants is, in the majority of gravidae, not altered notably. Although serum cholinesterase is commonly depressed some 30% in late pregnancy, succinylcholine metabolism is usually normal. There have been occasional reports of prolonged hypoventilation following clinical doses of succinylcholine; subsequent studies in these women disclosed qualitatively normal serum cholinesterase but abnormally, i.e., 50 to 60%, decreased activity (40). At times, reversal of a nondepolarizing relaxant is insufficient. Most frequently, the occurrence of prolonged postanesthetic muscular weakness results from potentiation of a muscle relaxant by magnesium sulfate used in the treatment of preeclampsia. Magnesium sulfate is a depressant of the neuromuscular junction and, as such, increases the effect of all muscle relaxants. In rat phrenic nerve-diaphragm preparations, the addition of 0.1 mg/ml of magnesium sulfate (a minimal dose) to muscle relaxant drugs produced a potentiation of 4.1 with *d*-tubocurarine, 3.7 with decamethonium, and 1.9 with succinylcholine (14). A peripheral nerve stimulator is helpful in confirming the diagnosis. If the muscle weakness is caused solely by a nondepolarizing relaxant, additional reversal is indicated; if due to succinylcholine or to the combination of relaxant and magnesium sulfate, ventilator therapy is best, although the effect of magnesium is reversible by the intravenous administration of a calcium salt.

Aspiration Pneumonitis

Aspiration pneumonitis has remained the leading cause of anesthesia-related maternal morbidity and mortality. Pulmonary aspiration of gastric contents may follow vomiting or regurgitation and may involve solid food particles, liquid gastric juice, or both. Aspiration of solid material produces a mechanical response (obstruction of the airways); aspiration of gastric juice of pH of 2.5 or less causes a chemical process (irritative reaction with transudation of a plasmalike fluid into alveoli and bronchi); associated with either is a reflex response (bronchospasm). The treatment of the former is directed toward removal of the foreign material, generally by bronchoscopy. The immediate therapy of the latter consists of suctioning aspirated liquid from mouth, pharynx, and trachea; insertion of a cuffed endotracheal tube; and intermittent positive pressure ventilation with 100% oxygen. The use of corticosteroids is controversial, but a single intravenous dose equivalent to 120 to 150 mg of methylprednisolone (Medrol) is frequently administered. Extended treatment includes continuous respiratory assistance with positive end-expiratory pressure and intermittent mandatory ventilation at a slow rate (aiming at maintaining the Pao_2 above 60 torr with an F_Io_2 of 0.5 or less), humidification and chest physiotherapy; intravenous fluid replacement utilizing both crystalloids and colloids or hyperalimentation; appropriate antibiotics; bronchodilators (aminophylline or nebulized isoproterenol); and digitalization if needed (15, 29).

Oxytocic Drugs

Both types of oxytocic drugs have pronounced cardiovascular effects. The ergot alkaloids cause a significant rise in blood pressure as a result of direct peripheral vasoconstriction; they increase the work of the heart and can produce coronary constriction (7). Persistent severe hypertension has been reported following the use of an ergot preparation in postpartum women who had received a vasopressor drug [ephedrine or methoxamine (Vasoxyl)] in conjunction with regional analgesia (27). In contrast, synthetic oxytocin has a marked but transient direct relaxing effect on vascular smooth muscle when large amounts are injected. A decrease in systolic and especially diastolic pressures ensues associated with flushing and an increase in limb blood flow. Reflexly induced tachycardia and elevated cardiac output accompany this depressor phase (7). Various cases of considerable hemodynamic instability following the use of oxytocin have been described. When 5 units of oxytocin were given intravenously to a healthy patient who was two hours postpartum, supine, and with her blood pressure stabilized at 115/60 torr, hypotension of 73/38 torr developed within 35 seconds while the heart rate rose from 70 to 110 per minute; recovery began three minutes later and was accompanied by a small overshoot (22). Therefore, oxytocins should not be administered in a bolus injection, but only in a dilute solution. Measurements of postpartum uterine activity have demonstrated that maximal contractions are elicited by as small a dose as 10 mU of oxytocin (31). It also must be remembered that synthetic oxytocin, although devoid of the coronary constricting action associated with the impurities of the natural drug, has the same antidiuretic properties. Administered by a constant intravenous infusion, oxytocin produces a decrease in urine flow in both pregnant and nonpregnant subjects. This decrease is dose dependent, is manifested within 15 minutes of the onset of the infusion, and lasts for a similar period of time following its discontinuation. The antidiuretic effect of oxytocin is of paramount importance because of the hazard of water intoxication. Diplopia, nausea, convulsions, and coma have been observed in postpartum women who had received an oxytocin infusion during labor or after parturition; serum sodium was low in all of these patients. Although the use of an isotonic salt solution reduces the danger of hyponatremia, it carries the risk of circulatory overload. Therefore, when oxytocin is to be given in larger amounts, the quantity of fluid may have to be restricted, and careful attention must be paid to the gravida's urine output and state of hydration (1, 8).

Complications from Coincidental Medical Disease

Of the medical diseases commonly associated with pregnancy, two are particularly liable to produce complications in the postpartum period: rheumatic heart disease and cerebral vascular anomaly.

Rheumatic Valvular Disease

Obstetric patients with rheumatic valvular disease, especially mitral stenosis, tend to develop cardiac failure during the early puerperium as a result of the strain placed on the heart by labor, parturition, and the postpartum circulatory adjustments. Stroke volume, cardiac output, and left ventricular work increase with each effective uterine contraction. Bearing-down efforts drive blood from the lungs into the left side of the heart, increasing cardiac work further. Following delivery, cardiac output is 30 to 50% elevated due to an additional increase in stroke volume accompanied by slowing of the heart rate (19). Left ventricular work was found to rise from an average of 8 kg meters/minute during the early first stage of labor to 9 kg meters/minute in the interval between contractions, and 12 kg meters/minute during the acme of contractions of the second stage, and to remain 11 kg meters/minute during the early puerperium (2).

Therapy of postpartum cardiac failure is the same as in nonpregnant patients. However, it is possible to minimize the risk of this complication by appropriate management of the gravida during labor and delivery: hydration should be by slow infusion of dextrose in water; stress and apprehension should be relieved early in labor by a "minor" tranquilizing drug [propriomazine (Largon), promethazine (Phenergan), hydroxyzine (Atarax, Vistaril)]; a segmental extradural block should be instituted to

Table 2.1   Common Causes of Postpartum Pulmonary Edema

1. Aspiration
2. Cardiac failure
3. Preeclampsia-eclampsia
4. Water intoxication

provide pain relief as well as to abolish bearing-down sensations; and oxygen should be administered by face-shield or nasal cannulae. A catheter extradural block offers the added advantage of permitting rapid extension of sympathetic blockade to reduce venous return to the heart should cardiac failure with pulmonary edema suddenly occur. Furthermore, sympathetic blockade may be continued after delivery to reduce the postpartum increase in cardiac work and can be tapered off slowly over the next 12 to 24 hours.

Cerebral Vascular Anomaly

In contrast to cerebral aneurysms, which rarely bleed during the period of parturition, hemorrhage from *arteriovenous anomaly* is not uncommon during labor and the early puerperium. It has been postulated that bleeds from vascular anomalies are related to periods of maximum cardiac output (38). The clinical picture of sudden severe headache, followed by semistupor, is suggestive of the complication and warrants specific neurologic work-up. Prevention of a postpartum cerebral hemorrhage in patients with known intracranial vascular anomaly entails avoidance of major rises in cerebrospinal, extradural, and blood pressures during labor and delivery. This is most rationally accomplished by the administration of continuous segmental extradural analgesia (24).

Conclusion

The foregoing review of postpartum complications serves to emphasize the potential difficulty in ascertaining the correct diagnosis. Thus, pulmonary edema (Table 2.1) or convulsions (Table 2.2) each may arise from four not unusual causes, while tachycardia (Table 2.3) may be due to any one

Table 2.2   Common Causes of Postpartum Convulsions

1. Eclampsia
2. Epilepsy
3. Intracranial hemorrhage
4. Water intoxication

Table 2.3 Common Causes of Postpartum Tachycardia

1. Anemia (chronic)
2. Aspiration
3. Blood loss
4. Cardiac failure
5. Hypoventilation
6. Infection
7. Opiate withdrawal
8. Preeclampsia
9. Pulmonary embolism

of at least nine etiologies. It becomes evident that diagnostic acumen is essential in order to successfully treat the mother who develops a complication in the postpartum period.

References

1. Abdul-Karim, R.W., Rizk, P.T.: The effect of oxytocin on renal hemo-dynamics, water, and electrolyte excretion. Obstet. Gynecol. Surv. **25**:805, 1970.
2. Adams, J.Q., Alexander, A.: Alteration in cardiovascular physiology during labor. Obstet. Gynecol. **12**:542, 1958.
3. BalaKrishna, H., Marx, G.F.: Inversion of the uterus during methoxy-flurane anaesthesia. Can. Anaesth. Soc. J. **15**:34, 1968.
4. Barclay, D.L.: Cesarean hysterectomy at the Charity Hospital in New Orleans—1000 consecutive operations. Clin. Obstet. Gynecol. **12**:635, 1969.
5. Barden, T.P.: Perinatal care, in Romney et al. (eds.): Gynecology and Obstetrics. New York, McGraw-Hill, 1975, pp. 657–712.
6. Bonica, J.J., Figge, D.C.: Toxemia, in Bonica, J.J. (ed.): Principles and Practices of Obstetric Analgesia and Anesthesia. Philadelphia, F.A. Davis, 1969, pp. 1127–47.
7. Brazeau, P.: Drugs affecting uterine motility, in Goodman, L.S., and Gilman, A.: The Pharmacological Basis of Therapeutics, 4th Ed. New York, Macmillan, 1970, pp. 893–907.
8. Burt, R.L., Oliver, K.L., Whitener, D.L.: Water intoxication complicating elective induction of labor at term. Obstet. Gynecol. **34**:212, 1969.
9. Cavanagh, D., Comas, M.R.: Shock, in Romney et al. (eds.): Gynecology and Obstetrics. New York, McGraw-Hill, 1975, pp. 241–67.
10. Chung, A.F., Merkatz, I.R.: Survival following amniotic fluid embolism with early heparinization. Obstet. Gynecol. **42**:809, 1973.
11. Courtney, L.D.: Amniotic fluid embolism. Obstet. Gynec. Surv. **29**:169, 1974.

12. Foldes, F.F., Swerdlow, M., Siker, E.S.: Narcotics and narcotic antagonists, in Pharmacology of Narcotics and Narcotic Antagonists. Springfield, Illinois, Charles C Thomas, 1964, pp. 37–112.
13. Gabriel, H., Ambré, C.: Le placenta accreta. Gynec. Obstet. **54**:345, 1955.
14. Ghoneim, M.M., Long, J.P.: The interaction between magnesium and other neuromuscular blocking agents. Anesthesiology **32**:23, 1970.
15. Gongawara, T.: Our approach to aspiration pneumonia and respiratory burns. Res. Staff Phys., April 1975, p. 66.
16. Greenhill, J.P., Friedman, E.A.: The third stage, in Biological Principles and Modern Practice of Obstetrics. Philadelphia, W.B. Saunders, 1974, pp. 296–303.
17. Greenhill, J.P., Friedman, E.A.: Hypertensive states of pregnancy, in Biological Principles and Modern Practice of Obstetrics. Philadelphia, W.B. Saunders, 1974, pp. 391–414.
18. Gregory, M.G., Clayton, E.M.: Amniotic fluid embolism. Obstet. Gynecol. **42**:236, 1973.
19. Hansen, J.M., Ueland, K.: Maternal cardiovascular dynamics during pregnancy and parturition, in Marx, G.F. (ed.): Parturition and Perinatology. Philadelphia, F.A. Davis, 1973, pp. 21–36.
20. Harris, R.E., Dunnihoo, D.R.: Inversion of the uterus in a patient under halothane anesthesia. Obstet. Gynecol. **27**:655, 1966.
21. Hellman, L.M., Pitchard, J.A. (eds.): Abnormalities of the third stage of labor, in Williams Obstetrics (14th ed.). New York, Appleton-Century-Crofts, 1971.
22. Hendricks, C.H., Brenner, W.E.: Cardiovascular effects of oxytocic drugs used postpartum. Am. J. Obstet. Gynecol. **108**:751, 1970.
23. Kleiner, G.J., Merskey, A.J., Johnson, A.J., et al: Defibrination in normal and abnormal parturition. Br. J. Haematol. **19**:159, 1970.
24. Laubstein, M.B., Kotz, H.L., Hehre, F.W.: Obstetric and anesthetic management following spontaneous subarachnoid hemorrhage. Obstet. Gynecol. **20**:661, 1962.
25. Levitt, M.F., Altchek, A.: Hypertension and toxemia of pregnancy, in Rovinsky, J.J., and Guttmacher, A.F. (eds.): Medical, Surgical, and Gynecologic Complications of Pregnancy (2nd ed.). Baltimore, Williams and Wilkins, 1965, pp. 76–110.
26. Marder, V.J.: Pathophysiology and therapy of disseminated intravascular coagulation. Ration. Drug Ther. **5**(12):1, 1971.
27. Marx, G.F.: Cerebrovascular accidents during anesthesia in obstetrics. Internat. Anesthiol. Clin. **1**:859, 1963.
28. Marx, G.F.: Shock in the obstetric patient. Anesthesiology **26**:423, 1965.
29. Marx, G.F.: Prevention and treatment of aspiration of gastric contents, in Shnider, S.M., and Moya, F. (eds.): The Anesthesiologist, Mother and Newborn. Baltimore, Williams and Wilkins, 1974, pp. 122–27.
30. Marx, G.F., Kim, Y.I., Lin, C.-C., et al: Postpartum uterine pressures under halothane or enflurane anesthesia. Obstet. Gynecol. **51**:695, 1978.
31. Marx, G.F., Lin, C.-C. Kim, Y.I.: Unpublished data.
32. McDonald, J.S.: Other operative obstetric procedures, in Bonica, J.J.

(eds.): Principles and Practice of Obstetric Analgesia and Anesthesia. Philadelphia, F.A. Davis, 1969, pp. 1366–75.

33. Messer, R.H.: Coagulation problems in obstetrics. Med. Clin. North Am. **53**:1085, 1969.

34. Niswonger, J.W., Langmade, C.F.: Cardiovascular changes in vaginal deliveries and cesarean sections. Am. J. Obstet. Gynecol. **107**:337, 1970.

35. Odell, L.D., Seski, A.: Episiotomy blood loss. Am. J. Obstet. Gynecol. **54**:51, 1947.

36. Peterson, E.P., Taylor, H.B.: Amniotic fluid embolism. An analysis of 40 cases. Obstet. Gynecol. **35**:787, 1970.

37. Pritchard, J.A., Baldwin, R.M., Dickey, J.C., et al. Blood volume changes in pregnancy and the puerperium. II. Red blood cell loss and changes in apparent blood volume during and following vaginal delivery, cesarean section, and cesarean section plus total hysterectomy. Am. J. Obstet. Gynecol. 84: 1271, 1962.

38. Robinson, J.L., Hall, C.J., Sedzimir, C.B.: Subarachnoid hemorrhage in pregnancy. J. Neurosurg. **36**:27, 1972.

39. Rubin, A. Erde, A.: Postpartum preeclampsia. Obstet. Gynecol. **24**:448, 1964.

40. Shnider, S.M.: Serum cholinesterase activity during pregnancy, labor and the puerperium. Anesthesiology **26**:335, 1965.

41. Taylor, E.S.: Retained and adherent placenta, in Beck's Obstetrical Practice, 9th Ed. Baltimore, Williams and Wilkins, 1971, pp. 449–502.

42. Way, E.L., Settle, A.A.: Uses of narcotic antagonists. Ration. Drug Ther. **9** (2):1, 1975.

3
Headache in the Postpartum Period

Gerard W. Ostheimer

The concept of postpartum headache usually brings two problems to the minds of those who care for the obstetric patient: the postdural puncture headache (PDPH) and the postpartum "blues." However, there are other less appreciated, but nevertheless important, causes of postpartum headache, related or unrelated to the administration of anesthesia.

This chapter will deal in depth with the postdural puncture headache and briefly review postpartum headaches of other etiologies.

Anesthesia-Related Headaches

Incidence

White and his associates (33) observed headaches during the postpartum period in 29 of 307 patients (9.6%) who had been given general anesthesia for delivery and in 32 of 54 (6.2%) who had received spinal block. Winkler et al. (34) also evaluated postpartum headaches in relation to different methods of anesthesia (Table 3.1). A "failed saddle" block was defined as failure to achieve relief of abdominal discomfort during contractions despite adequate perineal anesthesia. In their patients, headaches following inhalation anesthesia most often occurred on the first day after delivery and usually lasted only one day regardless of severity. Following spinal analgesia, the headaches commonly appeared on the second day and persisted from one to three days. In both groups, however, the headaches tended to be positional, i.e., aggravated while sitting or standing

Table 3.1   Incidence of Headache by Type of Anesthesia

Anesthesia	No. of Patients		Percent of Headaches	
Inhalation (Cyclopropane-O_2)	535		8.6	
"Failed saddle" block	32 ⎫		31.2 ⎫	
Low spinal block	411 ⎬ 464		20.0 ⎬ 21.3	
Spinal block for cesarean section	21 ⎭		33.3 ⎭	
Local infiltration	11		18.2	
None	9		11.1	

From Winkler et al. (34).

and relieved while lying down. Crawford (10) found a 19.4% occurrence of headaches in 923 patients after obstetric lumbar epidural analgesia; 5.9% followed inadvertent dural puncture and 13.5% followed uncomplicated performance of the epidural block.

Type of vaginal delivery does not appear to influence the incidence of postpartum headache. Grove (20) interviewed 187 puerperal women of whom 155 were delivered spontaneously and 32 by forceps or vacuum extraction; headaches developed in 22.3% of the former and in 25% of the latter.

The typical "spinal" headache, which will be discussed in detail, is due to sequelae of the dural puncture. "Nonspinal" types of headache are related to nonspecific etiologies. Proposed mechanisms include retention of carbon dioxide, slow elimination of anesthetic or sedative drugs, and cerebral vasodilation. In women with upper respiratory infections, headaches may develop as a consequence of thickened secretions and poor sinus drainage, secondary to the administration of scopolamine or other drying agents (33).

Postdural Puncture Headache

Historical Background

Bier, who introduced spinal anesthesia into clinical practice, was the first to develop a postdural puncture headache (PDPH). On August 24, 1898, he had his assistant, Dr. Hildebrandt, attempt a spinal anesthetic. It was never completed because the syringe and needle did not fit.

The following quotations are from Bier's original report:

> *After these experiments on our own bodies we both went to dinner without any physical complaints. We drank wine and smoked cigars. I went to bed at 11 o'clock and slept well throughout the night. I awoke feeling refreshed and well the next morning, and went for a walk for an hour. Toward the*

end of this walk, I noticed a slight headache, which increased during the course of the day while I did my usual work. Toward 3 P.M. my face turned pale, the pulse was rather faint but remained regular, and was about 70 beats per minute. Furthermore, I had the sensation of a very strong pressure in my head and felt slightly dizzy when I rose quickly from my chair. All these symptoms disappeared as soon as I lay down horizontally, but they returned when I arose. . . .

. . . I believe that the headaches and vomiting which we observed . . . in Dr. Hildebrandt and myself must be viewed as the results of circulatory disturbances (hyperemia or anemia in the central nervous system). Furthermore, the escape of a considerable amount of cerebrospinal fluid could bring about such effects. None of the others involved suffered as long as I did from the results of the puncture, although certainly only traces of cocaine, if any at all, reached the dural sac in my case. That some type of circulatory disturbance was present in my case is shown by the fact that I felt absolutely well in the supine position, and that disturbances appeared only if I sat up.

Etiology

Consensus of opinion holds that the etiology of PDPH is the leakage of cerebrospinal fluid (CSF) through the hole in the dura made by the needle with consequent decrease in CSF pressure (3). The loss of CSF permits displacement of the brain caudad causing traction on the lateral and sagittal venous sinuses, the basal dural cerebral arteries, and the supporting parts of the dura (falx and tentorium), all of which are sensitive to pain. Stimuli arising from the superior surface of the tentorium cerebelli and above are transmitted via the trigeminal nerve to the anterior half of the head. Pain from below the tentorium is transmitted via the glossopharyngeal, vagus, and upper three cervical nerves to the posterior part of the head. Brown and Jones (5) reported a patient with intractable PDPH in whom a dural fistula was sutured six months after the initial lumbar puncture, with immediate improvement. This case thus supports the "dural hole" etiology of PDPH. Furthermore, CSF leakage from a needle hole in the dural sac was demonstrated by Gass and his associates (17), who injected iodinated serum albumin ($^{131}I_2$) through a cisterna magna puncture and by Lieberman and his colleagues (23), who injected the same medium after dural tap at the L_{4-5} interspace.

Characteristics

1. *Postion:* The headache begins when the patient sits or stands upright. There is definite relief upon reclining, assuming the supine position, or with abdominal compression.

2. *Time Course:* Symptoms commence hours to days after lumbar puncture and may persist for hours to months. In a review of 185 cases sponsored by the Society for Obstetric Anesthesia and Perinatology (24), the average onset of headache occurred approximately 26 hours following dural puncture. Other studies (20, 29, 33, 34) found that PDPH usually started on the second day.
3. *Severity:* The headache may be mild to incapacitating. A patient once described her discomfort in the following manner: "When I sit up, the headache becomes so tense that I feel someone is grabbing my forehead in ice tongs and pulling me back down in bed."
4. *Type of Pain:* This is described most often as dull aching pressure.
5. *Localization:* The pain may be bifrontal, bitemporal, bioccipital, unilateral, or generalized. Classically, the headache begins in the occipital area, extends down the neck to between the scapulae, and then spreads to the top of the head, becoming most intense in the frontal areas behind the eyes.
6. *Associated Symptoms:* These include nausea, vomiting, dizziness, and visual or auditory changes. Visual complications consist of blurred vision, focusing difficulties, diplopia and, infrequently, abducens palsy. Auditory problems include tinnitus, stuffiness, and alterations in acuity; that is, normal sounds become distant or very close.

Occurrence

Tourtellotte and his associates (29) reviewed the world literature dealing with PDPH from Quincke's early report in 1891 through 1960. They studied a large series of patients who had either diagnostic lumbar puncture or spinal anesthesia to determine the incidence of PDPH. Their findings are summarized in Table 3.2. A decreased occurrence of PDPH was associated with the presence of one or more of the following factors: (1) increasing age, (2) male sex, (3) previous dural puncture without subsequent head-

Table 3.2 Incidence of PDPH in Large Groups of Patients

Group	Preventive Measures Yes	No	Average (%)	Range (%)
Diagnostic lumbar puncture		X	32	3–60
	X		6	0.5–18
Spinal anesthesia				
a. Nonobstetric		X	13.1	0–40
	X		5.5	0.4–16
b. Obstetric		X	18.4	7–33
	X		6.2	0–17

From Tourtellotte et al. (29).

Table 3.3   Incidence of PDPH According to Needle Size

Needle Gauge	No. of Patients	Percent of Headaches
22	2/21	9.5
25	10/195	5.1
26	20/298	6.7
	32/514 (Total)	6.2 (Total)

From White et al. (33).

ache, (4) lying down during the procedure, (5) use of small-diameter needles, (6) lying prone following the procedure, and (7) adequate hydration. The last four factors emerged as significant preventive measures. The benefit of small-gauge needles was noted also by White et al. (33) (Table 3.3).

The incidence of post-dural puncture headache is higher in the postpartum patient than in the female surgical postoperative patient. Various factors contribute to this predisposition, which results from a combination of reduced production of CSF (due to negative fluid balance) and enhanced loss of CSF (through the dural rent). Of importance are:

1. withholding of oral fluids and inadequate intravenous fluid therapy during labor,
2. diaphoresis during labor,
3. bearing-down efforts (Valsalva maneuver), causing temporary increases in CSF pressure,
4. vomiting during the peripartum period,
5. acute blood loss,
6. decrease in intraabdominal pressure subsequent to emptying of the uterus, and
7. postpartum diuresis during the second to fifth puerperal days.

Treatment

Until recently, therapy for PDPH had been symptomatic rather than directed at the cause of the headache and included:

1. Bedrest in either the supine or prone position for up to 48 hours.
2. Use of analgesics (from aspirin to narcotics).
3. Application of an abdominal binder to increase intraabdominal venous pressure which, transmitted via the lumbar veins, causes engorgement of the epidural venous plexus, thus reducing the size of the epidural space. This, in turn, results in "dural sac squeeze" with consequent rise in CSF pressure.
4. Forced fluid intake, either orally or intravenously, of up to 4 liters per

day in an attempt to increase the production of CSF. (Cerebrospinal fluid is produced at a rate of 20 ml/hour in normal man; the normal volume of CSF in the adult is 140 to 170 ml.)

The first specific approach to the problem of the low CSF pressure syndrome (PDPH) was the injection of saline intrathecally to increase CSF volume, or epidurally to increase CSF pressure (by dural sac squeeze). In 1949, Rice and Dabbs (26) injected an average of 82 ml of saline into the epidural space of patients with postlumbar puncture headache and obtained rapid relief in 99.5%; however, symptoms, usually mild, returned in 52.4%. Subsequently, Usubiaga and his associates (30) evaluated the effect of epidural saline injections on epidural and subarachnoid pressures. Ten or 20 ml of saline injected into the lumbar epidural space resulted in an immediate rise of 60 to 70 cm of water in both epidural and subarachnoid space pressures, lasting from 3 to 10 minutes. (Injection of the same volumes into the sacral epidural space was not accompanied by any change in CSF pressure.) In general, the larger the volume of saline, the higher the pressures, and the faster the injection, the steeper but more transient the peak. Because the rise in epidural space pressure following saline injection is only temporary, its beneficial therapeutic effect is difficult to explain. Usubiaga et al. (30) postulated initiation of the formation of a fibrin clot or prolapse of the arachnopia; on the other hand, a mere increase in pressure may suffice to produce apposition of the borders of the dural rent.

Permanent closure of the dural hole is the most effective means of relieving a post-dural puncture headache. This has been attempted by catgut suture, injection of methylprednisolone acetate, and, more recently, injection of autologous blood. Based on his observation of a lower than anticipated incidence of headache when the tap was bloody, Gormley (19) used autologous epidural blood patches (EBP) to cure seven spinal headaches, including one he experienced himself. Ozdil and Powell (25) described using a prophylactic EBP. They administered spinal anesthesia with a 20-gauge needle to two groups of 100 patients who were undergoing routine surgical or obstetric procedures. In one group, a small fresh clot of autologous blood (2.5 ml) was injected into the subdural and epidural spaces as the spinal needle was withdrawn. No PDPH occurred in this group. In the controls, PDPH developed in 15 patients, 4 male and 11 female; of the latter, 7 had obstetric procedures and 4 had surgical interventions. DiGiovanni and Dunbar (12) reported 45 patients in whom therapeutic EBP gave permanent relief of a post-dural puncture headache, in 41 immediately and in four within 24 hours. They described their technique as follows: "Following epidural needle placement, an assistant aseptically prepared the antecubital or other suitable skin area for venipuncture. Ten milliliters of blood withdrawn under aseptic conditions were injected into the epidural space. The patient was then placed supine; if he had not been on a forced fluid regimen, 500 to 1000 ml of lactated Ringer's solution were administered intravenously. After 30 minutes in the supine position, he was allowed to walk." The only problem they encountered was the occasional complaint of backache after injection of the blood.

Following continued success in the treatment of PDPH with EBP, DiGiovanni and his co-workers (13) investigated the fate of the autologous blood introduced into the epidural space of Angora goats. At 24 hours, the blood clot still contained a considerable population of intact red and white cells without fibrous reaction. Organization of the clot proceeded with disruption of the cellular elements and laking of the blood, which was noted by the fourth day. All evidence suggesting that blood was the instigating factor in the reaction had disappeared by the second week; many of the fibroblasts had reached maturity and the deposition of collagen tissue had begun. One week later, the fibroblastic reaction appeared to reach a peak. Thereafter, the fibroblasts tended to disappear as the collagen fibers shrank in size to the same thickness as the dura. The authors concluded that the resultant tissue reaction after various periods of time following the injection of autologous blood epidurally in their goats did not differ significantly from that following simple dural puncture in control animals.

The mechanism of action of the epidural blood patch is the formation of a gelatinous tamponade which prevents leakage of CSF and allows the dural rent to undergo normal healing. Blood confined in the epidural space is *not* an irritant; if blood enters the subarachnoid space, it tends to diffuse rapidly and to hemolyze readily (hemoxanthochromia clears by the sixth day). The only consideration is the prevention of infection introduced by the blood in the epidural or subarachnoid space; therefore, positive blood culture presents an absolute contraindication to EBP (see below). Table 3.4 summazies the known reports on EBP prior to 1977.

No *permanent* sequelae of EBP have been recorded. Transient problems have included: backache, neckache, abdominal cramps, fever, facial paralysis, vertigo, dizziness, tinnitus, ataxia, paresthesias in the back, buttocks, legs, and toes as well as radicular pain in one or both legs (possibly due to nerve root irritation or pressure). Subcutaneous hematoma at the site of injection and inadvertent dural puncture also have been reported.

Absolute contraindications to EBP are septicemia, local infection of skin, subcutaneous tissue or epidural area, and active neurologic disease. Regarding septicemia, the epidural space would be a perfect site for the incubation of bloodborne or local infection. With regard to neurologic disease, if exacerbation of a preexisting neurologic disease occurred, the blood patch could be implicated.

Other possible complications include adhesive arachnoiditis and radiculitis. There is also the possibility of obliterating the epidural space, which

Table 3.4   Reports on Epidural Blood Patch for the Treatment of Postdural
Puncture Headache

Author	Year	Cases	Successful*	Percent
Gormley (19)	1960	7	7	100
DiGiovanni and Dunbar (12)	1970	45	45	100
Glass and Dupont	1972	43	40	93
Glass and Kennedy	1972	50	47	94
Dupont and Sphire	1972	41	40	98
DiGiovanni et al. (13)	1972	63	61	97
Vondrell and Bernards	1973	60	58	97
Blok	1973	22	21	95
Cass and Edelist	1974	1	1	100
Balagot	1974	7	7	100
Ostheimer et al. (S.O.A.P.)	1974	185	182	98
Abouleish et al. (1)	1975	118	115	97
Ostheimer et al. (24)	1977	35	35	100
Total		677	659	97

* Headache relieved within 24 hours.

might prevent the future use of lumbar epidural, caudal, or spinal analgesia. However, Abouleish and his associates (2) have administered a spinal, lumbar epidural, or caudal block to three patients who previously had received an EBP; no alteration in onset, extent, or duration of the blocks was noted. I had the same experience with two patients, each of whose lumbar epidural block, some months after EBP, was entirely uncomplicated and successful. Thus, these possibilities are more theoretical than real.

Prophylaxis

Both epidural saline injection and epidural blood patch have been used in attempts to prevent the development of post-dural puncture headache. Craft and his colleagues (9) studied 33 obstetric patients who had an inadvertent dural puncture with a 16-gauge needle during attempted lumbar epidural analgesia for labor and delivery. In 16 of these, two prophylactic epidural injections of 60 ml each of saline were added to the standard treatment for spinal puncture (bedrest, forced fluids, and abdominal binder), while in 17, only the usual regimen was employed. The addition of the saline injections reduced the incidence of PDPH from 77 to 13%. Crawford (11) reported similar results with administration of a continuous epidural infusion of lactated Ringer's solution (1 to 1.5 liters) for 24 hours afted delivery in 16 women who accidentally had received a dural tap.

Prophylactic EBP, as mentioned earlier, was used orginally by Ozdil and Powell (25) after spinal analgesia. Recently, the method also has been employed after inadvertent dural puncture during attempted lumbar epidural analgesia. Doctor et al. (14) reported eight patients in whom the epidural needle was slowly withdrawn until CSF stopped dripping; 10 ml of autologous blood was then injected and the needle withdrawn. Pain relief for labor and delivery was provided by nonregional techniques, and only one of the eight women developed a headache, described as mild. In contrast, Walpole (31) failed to prevent the occurrence of PDPH in two patients in whom 10 ml of blood was injected through the epidural catheter. My own experience has been poor: three successes in eight attempts, and I believe that prophylactic blood patch is an unjustified procedure. The incident of PDPH following accidental dural puncture ranged from 16.6 to 45.8% in Hehre's series (21, 22) and was 39% in a recent review of our practice at the Boston Hospital for Women. However, in only 11% of these patients was the headache of such severity as to necessitate an EBP. If prophylactic EBP had been used, 89% of the women would have been subjected to an unnecessary procedure.

There may be two reasons for the failure of a prophylactic EBP. The clot may not be placed in the area of the dural hole, particularly if administered through the catheter. The CSF pressure may still be sufficiently high to prevent the formation of a fibrin clot across the dural defect.

My recommendation for the management of inadvertent dural puncture during attempted epidural block is as follows: The patient should be told what happened (a dural puncture), what may develop (a positional headache), and how this can be treated [conservative therapy versus epidural blood patch (or saline injection)]. She is instructed to keep well hydrated and take whatever analgesics have been ordered for her. If a PDPH should occur, she is placed on bedrest except for bathroom privileges, forced oral hydration (>3000 ml/day), and oral or parenteral analgesics. If no improvement occurs in 24 hours, EBP is discussed. The choice for this procedure remains with the patient; if she refuses, the previous treatment is continued.

EDITOR'S NOTE: I agree that prophylactic blood patching is not warranted. Effectiveness through the catheter is unpredictable, and injection through the initial needle entails abandonment of regional analgesia. The only remaining method is injection through an epidural needle placed after delivery, a procedure I consider excessive. However, I strongly favor one or two prophylactic injections, through the catheter, of physiologic saline (without preservative) in amounts of 60 to 80 ml, or until the patient starts complaining of pressure in the back.

An additional recommendation, following any lumbar puncture including spinal analgesia, is to refrain from the traditional "flat on back," a position that favors continued leakage of CSF. Instead, the patient should be encouraged to lie relaxed on either side with the usual pillow under the head.

Vasopressors

Although postregional block hypotension is preventable in most parturients by appropriate prehydration and adequate uterine displacement, prophylactic intramuscular administration of usual doses of vasopressors (e.g., 50 mg of ephedrine) is still being practiced. In contrast to therapeutic intravenous injections of small doses (e.g., 10 mg of ephedrine), the larger dosages may have a prolonged effect. Consequently, severe hypertension with incapacitating headache has been reported in postpartum patients following the use of ephedrine, methamphetamine, epinephrine, norepinephrine, phenylephrine, or methoxamine, given either alone or in combination with ergot preparations or natural oxytocin (7). The hypertension seems to be related to one or more of three factors: (1) the vasoconstrictive action of the drugs, possibly potentiated by oxytocic agents; (2) the rises in cardiac output and blood pressure associated with labor and delivery of infant and placenta; and (3) the progressive return of sympathetic control following discontinuance of the regional block.

The headache commonly is severe, throbbing, and most intense in the frontal or temporal areas. Nausea, vomiting, vertigo, tinnitus, visual disturbances, and auditory changes may also be present. Intensity and duration of the headache appear unrelated to the increase in systolic pressure, and the pain may persist even after the pressure has reverted to normal.

The headache may be ameliorated by the head-up position (reducing blood flow to the cranium) in conjunction with efforts to decrease the blood pressure (increase in sympathetic blockade where feasible, or rapid-acting vasodilator drugs).

Meningitis

Meningitis that occurs after dural puncture, spinal block, or epidural analgesia may be septic or aseptic (chemical) in origin. Both types present with general malaise, headache, fever, head retraction, and positive CSF findings. The headache is characteristically "bursting" in character and present in all positions.

Septic meningitis implies the presence of bacteria in the CSF. It is the result of contamination by infectious agents from blood (septicemia), skin, subcutaneous tissue, or epidural space. It is preventable by adhering to a strict aseptic technique and by *not* administering spinal or epidural analgesia to a patient with unexplained fever or areas of infection near the site of puncture by the needle. Treatment consists of intense antibiotic therapy.

Aseptic meningitis, which appears in clusters at varying time intervals, is a particularly vexing problem. Bacteria are not found in the smears or culture of CSF, but the cell content is high. Reports have incriminated either insertion of the spinal-epidural needle through skin wet with antiseptic solution or contamination of needles or syringes by detergents or disinfectants. Common to most of these reports were changes either in the personnel who prepared the trays or in the technique of preparation. Aseptic meningitis is self-limiting, and treatment is symptomatic.

Hopefully, reports of anesthesia-related meningitis will be eliminated by proper patient selection and the use of disposable trays prepared under rigid quality control. However, Weinstein and his associates (32) recently observed a cluster of five false-positive cerebrospinal fluid Gram stains due to the presence of nonviable bacterial contaminants in specimen tubes supplied in commercially prepared diagnostic dural puncture sets. In addition, the use of an introducer for spinal needles may diminish the chances for contamination by (1) not allowing the needle tip to come into contact with skin or subcutaneous tissue, and (2) decreasing the handling of the distal part of the needle.

Non-Anesthesia-Related Headaches

Obstetric Causes

Oxytocics, hormone imbalance, and psychogenic reactions may induce headaches in the puerperal patient.

Oxytocics

Ergot preparations (ergonovine maleate, methylergonovine) produce vasoconstriction by direct action on the muscular layer of the vessel wall. Severe sustained hypertension can occur from ergot preparations alone or from combination of these drugs with vasopressors or natural oxytocin. The first manifestation usually is an incapacitating headache.

Pituitrin, the extract of the posterior pituitary gland, is composed of pitocin, which is largely oxytocic in activity, and pitressin (vasopressin) which has pressor and antidiuretic properties. The use of the extract may cause severe cardiovascular reactions including hypertension and resultant headache. In 1955, a synthetic oxytocin free of vasopressor activity was formulated. This preparation, however, has antidiuretic effects and may cause water intoxication with headache, cerebral edema, convulsions, and coma (see Chapter 2).

Hormone Imbalance

The imbalance of estrogen and progesterone in the early postpartum period has been implicated in water retention with consequent cerebral edema and headache. An analogy has been made to the headache seen in nonpregnant women secondary to the use of combination oral contraceptives.

Psychogenic Postpartum Headache

The puerperal woman may develop emotional problems, usually of short duration. True mental illness rarely makes its first appearance in the postpartum period, and there is no difference between the puerperium and any other setting in the frequency of mental illness.

Transient depression, or the "postpartum blues," occurs in many new mothers. Ordinarily, this "blue" period begins 24 to 48 hours after delivery, lasts a few days, and subsides when the mother goes home with her child. "Loss" of the fetus from the uterus has been postulated to be an object of grief, necessitating transposition of the love for the fetus (an extension of self-love) to that of the newborn. Another theory holds that the mother may be fearful of her new responsibilities and the changes the baby will make in her life.

These feelings of grief, apprehension, anxiety and, on occasion, hostility, commonly are manifested as headache, generalized aches and pains, fatigue, and other symptoms referable to the labor and delivery process.

Coincidental Systemic Diseases

Hypertensive Disorders

Hypertensive crisis or encephalopathy (16) may develop in the postpartum patient as a complication of acute glomerulonephritis, preeclampsia (15), pheochromocytoma, and other hypertensive diseases. The sudden rise in arterial pressure is accompanied or preceded by severe headache. If untreated, transitory cerebral phenomena, convulsions, or coma may follow. The drugs recommended for immediate antihypertensive therapy are outlined in Chapter 2, as is the specific treatment of preeclampsia.

The diagnosis of pheochromocytoma is particularly difficult during pregnancy and the puerperium, as its cardiovascular manifestations may be masked by the normal physiologic alterations which occur during gestation. The most common symptoms are headache, nausea, vomiting, and sweating (4). Typically, headache and hypertension develop in the supine position and are relieved on standing. Maternal mortality is high; therefore, gravid and puerperal women with paroxysmal hypertension should be screened biologically for the possibility of pheochromocytoma (although misleading values can be obtained) (8). The definitive therapy of pheochromocytoma is surgical excision of the adrenal tumor; interim treatment consists of administration of alpha-adrenergic blocking agents.

Cerebrovascular Accident

Postpartum headache may be a prodrome of cerebrovascular accident as well. Cerebral hemorrhage is one of the major causes of death in severe preeclampsia but also occurs in vascular abnormalities (Berry aneurysm or arteriovenous malformation) and cerebral arterial or venous thrombosis (27). Gibbs (18) estimated that there are approximately 80 peripartum deaths from cerebrovascular accidents per year in the United States, with the majority happening during the postpartum period.

Migraine

In most female sufferers of migraine, the headaches are improved or remitted completely during pregnancy (6), although exacerbations have also been reported. In the early postpartum period, there is commonly a recurrence of a severe attack. This variable response remains an enigma. Migraine is frequently aggravated by the use of oral estrogen-progesterone combinations for contraception, but bioessays of estrogen, progesterone, or serotonin have not yielded conclusive information on any consistent biochemical alteration (28).

A history of migraine headache is not a contraindication to regional analgesia or the performance of an epidural blood patch. The potential advantage of the blood patch must be weighed against the possibility of initiation or exacerbation of a migraine attack. At the Boston Hospital for Women, we have observed two patients in whom an EBP completely relieved a typical postdural puncture headache; 24 hours later, both patients suffered a severe migraine onslaught, the symptoms of which were identical to those of previous migraines, i.e., unilateral and unimproved by the supine or prone position.

Conclusion

Postpartum headache is a vexing problem for the patient, the obstetrician, and the anesthesiologist. Comprehension of the possible etiologies is a major step in implementing the appropriate therapy to relieve the headache and distress of the patient.

References

1. Abouleish, E., de la Vega, S., Blendinger, I., and Tio, T.: Long-term follow-up of epidural blood patch. Anesth. Analg. **54**:459, 1975.
2. Abouleish, E., Wadhwa, R.K., de la Vega, S., et al.: Regional analgesia following epidural blood patch. Anesth. Analg. **54**:634, 1975.

3. Bonica, J.J.: Principles and Practice of Obstetric Analgesia and Anesthesia. Philadelphia, F. A. Davis Company, 1969.
4. Brown, A.A.: Maternal death associated with a phaeochromocytoma. J. Obstet. Gynaecol. Br. Commonw. 78:764, 1971.
5. Brown, B.A., Jones, O.W.: Prolonged headache following spinal puncture. Response to surgical treatment. J. Neurosurg. 19:349, 1962.
6. Callaghan, N.: The migraine syndrome in pregnancy. Neurology 18:197, 1968.
7. Casady, G.N., Moore, D.C., Bridenbaugh, L.D.: Postpartum hypertension after use of vasoconstrictor and oxytocic drugs. JAMA 172:1011, 1960.
8. Coombes, G.B.: Phaeochromocytoma presenting in pregnancy. Proc. R. Soc. Med. 69: 224, 1976.
9. Craft, J.B., Epstein, B.S., Coakley, C.S.: Prophylaxis of dural-puncture headache with epidural saline. Anesth. Analg. 52:228, 1973.
10. Crawford, J.S.: Lumbar epidural block in labour: a clinical analysis. Br. J. Anaesth. 44:66, 1972.
11. Crawford, J.S.: The prevention of headache consequent upon dural puncture. Br. J. Anaesth. 44:598, 1972.
12. DiGiovanni, A.J., Dunbar, B.S.: Epidural injections of autologous blood for postlumbar-puncture headache. Anesth. Analg. 49:268, 1970.
13. DiGiovanni, A.J., Galbert, M.W., Wahle, W.M.: Epidural injection of autologous blood for postlumbar-puncture headache. II. Additional clinical experiences and laboratory investigation. Anesth. Analg. 51:226, 1972.
14. Doctor, N., DeZoysa, S., Shah, R., et al: The use of the blood patch for post-spinal headaches. Anaesthesia 31:794, 1976.
15. Ferraz, E.M., Sherline, D.M.: Convulsive toxemia of pregnancy (eclampsia). South. Med. J. 69:152, 1976.
16. Finnerty, F.A.: Hypertensive encephalopathy. Am. J. Med. 52:672, 1972.
17. Gass, H., Goldstein, A.S., Ruskin, R., Leopold, N.A.: Chronic postmyelogram headache. Isotopic demonstration of dural leak and surgical cure. Arch. Neurol. 25:168, 1971.
18. Gibbs, C.E.: Maternal death due to stroke. Am. J. Obstet. Gynecol. 119:69, 1974.
19. Gormley, J.B.: Treatment of postspinal headache. Anesthesiology 21:565, 1960.
20. Grove L.H.: Backache, headache and bladder dysfunction after delivery. Br. J. Anaesth. 45:1147, 1973.
21. Hehre, F.W., Sayig, J.M.: Continuous lumbar epidural anesthesia in obstetrics. Am. J. Obstet. Gynecol. 80:1173, 1960.
22. Kalas, D.B., Hehre, F.W.: Continuous lumbar peridural anesthesia in obstetrics. VIII. Further observations on inadvertent lumbar puncture. Anesth. Analg. 51:192, 1972.
23. Lieberman, L.M., Tourtellotte, W.W., Newkirk, T.A.: Prolonged postlumbar puncture cerebrospinal fluid leakage from lumbar subarachnoid space demonstrated by radio-isotope myelography. Neurology 21:925, 1971.
24. Ostheimer, G.W., Palahniuk, R.J., Shnider, S.M.: Epidural blood patch for post-lumbar-puncture headache. Anesthesiology 41:307, 1974.

25. Ozdil, T., Powell, W.F.: Post lumbar puncture headache: an effective method of prevention. Anesth. Analg. 44:542, 1965.
26. Rice, G.G., Dabbs, H.C.: The use of peridural and subarachnoid injection of saline solution in the treatment of severe post spinal headaches. Anesthesiology 11:17, 1960.
27. Robinson, J.L., Hall, C.S., Sedzimir, C.B.: Arteriovenous malformations, aneurysms, and pregnancy. J. Neurosurg. 41:63, 1974.
28. Somerville, B.W.: The influence of hormonal changes upon migraine in women. Proc. Aust. Assoc. Neurol. 8:47, 1971.
29. Tourtellotte, W.W., Haerer, A.F., Heller, G.L., Somers, J.E.: Post-Lumbar puncture headaches. Springfield, Illinois, Charles C Thomas, 1964.
30. Usubiaga, J.E., Usubiaga, L.E., Brea, L.M., Goyena, R.: Effect of saline injections on epidural and subarachnoid space pressures and relation to postspinal anesthesia headache. Anesth. Analg. 46:293, 1967.
31. Walpole, J.B.: Blood patch for spinal headache. A recurrence and a complication. Anaesthesia 30:783, 1975.
32. Weinstein, R.A., Bauer, F.W., Hoffman, R.D., et al.: Factitious meningitis. Diagnostic error due to nonviable bacteria in commercial lumbar puncture trays. JAMA 233:878, 1975.
33. White, C.W., Weiss, J.B., Alver, E.C., Heerdegen, D.K.: Anesthesia and postpartum headache. Obstet. Gynecol. 20:734, 1962.
34. Winkler, W.P., Sherk, W.M., Hale, R.: Postpartum spinal headache. Am. J. Obstet. Gynecol. 85:500, 1963.

4
The Normal Parent-Newborn Relationship: *Its Importance for the Healthy Development of the Child*

W. Godfrey Cobliner

The purpose of this chapter is to describe and critically examine the variables that govern the parent (caretaker)-newborn relationship, to analyze the concepts that are being used to assess its nature, and to explore its impact on the child's cognitive and emotional developments.

Interest in this subject was sparked in the 1960s by two rapidly developing disciplines: neonatology and developmental psychology. The earlier findings that certain factors in the mother-child relationship affect not only the psychic but also the somatic health of the growing child provided the starting point for this new avenue of clinical and scientific endeavor.

Maternal Deprivation

Systematic studies in the 1940s on the role of maternal care in the well-being of the infant yielded the concept of "deprivation" of maternal care (2, 19–21). Bowlby, in his 1951 monograph, concluded that prolonged maternal deprivation of young children—especially if occurring during the second half of the first year of life—may be injurious to their character, thereby hurting them for their entire lives (2). Spitz had spelled out the noxious dimensions subsumed under the term "deprivation." He specified poor *quality* of maternal care and deficient *quantity* of maternal care in the critical period from age six months to one year. In a longitudinal study of a larger sample, he demonstrated that insufficient or absent care during longer periods resulted first in *infantile or anaclitic depression* and eventually, if the care were not restored in time, in marasmus and death. The wrong kind of mothering could result, among other problems, in the "three-month" colic or in infantile eczema (atopic dermatitis), provided there was simultaneous disposition to these symptoms in the particular child (19,20, 25).

The irreversible effect of maternal care deprivation was challenged in the 1950s in numerous papers written predominantly by academic psychologists, and even Bowlby retracted his original hypothesis. However, the issue was settled by way of reiteration of the original findings, albeit in modified form, in a series of texts by distinguished scientists. Some of these were published under the auspices of the World Health Organization in 1962 (5, 15, 30). The original findings and subsequent polemics led first to a more precise definition of the concept of mothering or maternal care, and then to a shift in attention to ever earlier periods in infancy, paralleling the development of sophisticated technical apparatus for the direct observation of mother-child interaction.

The exploration of earliest mother-infant interactions was given powerful impetus through the rapid flowering of the new discipline of ethology founded by Konrad Lorenz, Niko Tinbergen, and their associates. Their observations yielded the concept of "imprinting," which refers to the formation, in a critical early period, of a sudden and lasting attachment of the offspring to its mother. Harlow subsequently studied the perceptual and motor variables that occasion the attachment in monkeys by constructing, in an experimental setting, mechanical surrogate mothers. He supplied compelling evidence that monkeys that did not form an attachment to a "natural" mother never reached normal adulthood and failed to mate.

Systematic Studies on Large Samples

The Middlemore Studies

The first systematic study of the human mother-newborn relationship was carried out in Britain by Merell Middlemore, a pediatrician primarily interested in the variables governing breast feeding. She observed 46 mother-infant couples during the then prevailing lying-in period of eight to ten days on a maternity ward. She described and critically analyzed the series of variables in the interaction between mother and neonate, keeping in mind that the hospital setting limited the manifestation of natural tendencies of both partners during the feeding process (13). While her book was not "intended as a *vade mecum* for suckling mothers," she dealt with universal features of the mother-neonate situation so that her findings could also apply to contemporary bottle feeding mothers. She was not only concerned with the components of the mother-neonate relationship but also with the attitudes and latent or unconscious motives influencing the mother's skill or ability to acquire it. Beyond this she realized that the mother-neonate situation in the human species is "intricate because it consists of two groups of actions and interactions: those occurring between mother and child, and those other reactions of adaptation occurring between each member of the nursing couple and the 'outsider' who helps them—doctor or nurse" (13). She distinguished between babies who accept life from the onset and those who seem not ready to do so, a phenomenon that was apparent in the nursing situation. She dealt with the behavioral dimensions of activity and passivity, with the mental stress attendant upon frustration in the feeding situation. The mouth activities of babies and the process of sucking provide the first experience of pleasure and displeasure, of tension and tension relief; they shape the neonates' attitude towards food and eating as well as their emotional relationship to their mothers. These events can set the stage for future eating difficulties and for conflict between mother and child. In this connection, she distinguished between excited, ineffective, and inert sucklings; among the latter, she cited the simply inert, who were so from the beginning and the secondarily inert, in whom inertia set in after a few days due to an unsatisfactory mother-neonate relation.

The problem of whether breast feeding is essential for the well-being of the infant and for the development into a healthy, "normal" adult has as yet not been answered satisfactorily. However, it is a fact documented in surveys and systematic studies that the trend is away from breast feeding; its resurgence in isolated segments of the population in industrial societies is more of a fad. The most recent figures indicate that about 16 percent of women nurse their infants. Psychometric, longitudinal studies have failed to show whether breast or bottle feeding is more favorable for the child as measured in perceptual, cognitive, and social development.

Middlemore had the opportunity to observe the play at the breast before and after feeding and the great satisfaction that mothers derived from the experience. Naturally, a similar experience is absent in the bottle-feeding situation. However, before drawing conclusions too hastily, it should be realized that breast-feeding situations do not uniformly provide an optimal climate for the mother-neonate relation. I have observed more than half a dozen mothers who blocked their babies from playing at the breast; while fully aware of the babies' intentions, they did not comply because of pressures of time or privacy. They handled the babies roughly, grasping the heads as though they were basketballs and pushing them against their breasts. During feeding they would turn their heads toward their neighbors on the maternity ward and engage in conversation while pressing the babies' heads against their breasts. And yet these multiparous mothers had elected to breast feed their babies (6, 7).

Aspects of Infant Feeding

There are innumerable components incidental to the feeding situation which shape the mother-neonate relation. Among the important ones are holding and rocking the baby, face-to-face contact, eye-to-eye contact, harmony between the baby's feeding preferences and the mother's concerns and beliefs, which, apart from other factors, determine her intervention or lack of it. One of the most significant instances requiring the mother's intervention is the baby's need for burping. First there is its timing; second are the essential movements for picking up the neonate, and positioning him/her laterally or over the shoulder. It is one of the paramount measures for bringing timely and effective tension relief and implanting in the infant the notions that feeding can be pleasurable and that the mother's ministration brings relief and comfort.

Middlemore observed that the mother was responsible for certain instances of ineffective sucking: she could not tolerate her baby being excitable and, therefore, became clumsy in her handling. Occasionally, clumsiness was "strictly a psychological matter"; in other cases, it was "purely physical." Much significance has been attached to the parity of the mother. While it is an undeniable fact that a multiparous mother is less anxious and more skillful in handling her baby, I have seen many primiparae who showed an outstanding deftness in their ministrations. Upon inquiry, it turned out that these mothers had had prior experience in handling neonate siblings or had worked as mother's helpers for extensive periods (6).

Middlemore reported that mothers who were nervous after childbirth for whatever reason were apt to upset their infants by handling them badly and by having irrational fears regarding feeding. She drew the inference that "faults in handling were products of the mother's emotional disturbance" (13). She did not explore whether this emotional disturbance was a permanent feature of the respective mother or whether it was due to other circumstances. Spitz (21) observed in a large series of mother-infant couples that such emotional disturbance was occasioned "by the mother's unconscious attitudes towards *having* a child (in general) and toward her child's individuality."

We will return to Middlemore's conclusions concerning the mutual adaptation of the mother to her baby during the first days of life after describing some of the structural elements governing the mother-neonate situation. It is noteworthy that Middlemore's rich and pioneering data are rarely cited in the literature nor have they been duplicated in more recent studies. No existing textbook or pamphlet contains a fraction of her findings which are so vital to women who intend to breastfeed their children.

The Content of the Parent-Newborn Relationship

For all practical purposes, the parent-newborn relationship in the first few days of life is identical with that of the baby's caregiver, or the mother, since the father's direct contact is usually quite limited. The initiation of this interaction in most of the Western world occurs in the hospital. Longitudinal studies have provided evidence that the first two days prefigure, and in many instances are fateful, in that they determine the child's subsequent interaction with his/her parents and, by extension, with all future relationships.

The studies reviewed in this chapter, which more or less reflect our current knowledge and insights, refer to a number of structural elements that provide the setting for the initiation and evolution of the parent-newborn interaction. These structural elements are, so to speak, external or objective factors, while the mother's life experience and current life situation are the personal factors, and her conscious and unconscious attitudes are the immediate determinants shaping the caregiver-neonate interaction. As the title of this chapter indicates, we will consider mainly "normal" mothers and neonates, those free of gross physical or mental deviations. We will draw on deviations only to the extent that they help to understand and assess the normal situation. We also exclude the lying-in (rooming-in) arrangement provided in a few hospitals in the United States. Finally, no consideration will be given to prenatal phenomena.

The structural factors circumscribe the nature of the dyadic relationship between the caregiver and the neonate. It is a dynamic and ongoing process of an evolving give-and-take sustained by spatial-motor and rhythmic variables. In this system, the neonate is by no means as passive as his limited development may suggest. In fact, he is eliciting and regulating the behavior of the caregiver (6, 22–25).

Let us now look at some of these structural factors in a brief example

Table 4.1   Structural Elements Impinging on Caregiver-Newborn Relationship

Hospital setting	Feeding schedules; separation of caregiver-neonate couple; discontinuity of contact; extent of instruction and support
The caregiver (natural mother)	Parity or prior extensive contact with infants; relation to father; attitude toward motherhood; attitudes toward timing of pregnancy, toward this particular baby, toward sex of baby
Neonate	Impact of maternal medication incidental to delivery; state of initial and subsequent arousal; sex of child; activity and responsivity characteristics; reaction to proximal and distal stimulation

and learn how they separately and jointly affect the caregiver-neonate interaction.

In a cross-cultural study of mother-infant couples who had delivered in hospitals in the United States or Guatemala, as well as a third U.S. group whose delivery took place at home, it was observed that U.S. mothers had intense need for eye-to-eye contact with their offspring. Many mothers reported that "they did not feel the baby was theirs until they had looked into the eyes" (9). This being so, it is most important to recognize that certain drugs administered during labor may delay eye opening after delivery (10). In fact, very small doses of drugs can have drastic effects on the mother-neonate relationship (3). Kron explored the impact of obstetric sedation in a sample of 20 neonates by measuring sucking pressures and nutrient intake and observed significant differences between experimental and control babies. He stated that because of the fetus' dependence on maternal detoxification and excretion of drugs, barbiturates "may be stored in the infant's tissues for many days after delivery" (11).

According to our review of the literature just cited, both eye contact and proper sucking responses—insuring adequate food intake—are vital to the establishment of normal mother-neonate interaction. When the baby refuses or fails to look at the mother and additionally exhibits poor food intake, a mother may soon reject her infant; this, then, may trigger a vicious cycle that, other conditions being equal, may require intensive and prolonged pediatric care of the infant. It is an open question as to how many cases of "failure to thrive" seen in pediatric practice have their origin in this kind of circumstantial discord of the mother-neonate experience.

Returning now to the structural elements, the *traditional* hospital setting seems to be a significant inhibitor of the consolidation of an early caregiver-neonate relationship. A study of 52 home deliveries in California suggested that, in contrast to the hospital setting, the mother was "an active participant during labor and delivery rather than a passive patient. She immediately picked up the infant after birth" (10). The authors also reported that visual, tactile, and auditory interactions initiated "interlocking behavior patterns" within minutes after birth. They concluded that "shortly after delivery, these behavior patterns may mediate a special bond between mother and newborn which ensures immediate care of the young. These conclusions call attention to other factors inherent in many hospital settings, i.e., the discontinuity of contact between caregiver and neonate. While this may not be important when the mother is a primipara or when she ardently expected to have this particular child, the impairing feature of the old-fashioned hospital setting may have subsequent repercussions in other instances. Klaus et al. (10) pointed out that "in the U.S. most mothers first receive their baby several hours after birth when the infant is asleep and is not as easily aroused to the quite alert state" prevailing immediately after birth.

A comment was made earlier on the impact of some maternal attitudes concerning handling of the newborn. I have interviewed several hundred women on the maternity ward in Jersey City and subsequently observed their interactions with their baby. While most mothers welcomed their infants at birth, this was *not* the case at the time of conception. A certain ambivalence must have prevailed because these very mothers showed marked clumsiness in feeding their babies, particularly in regard to the timing of insertion of the bottle into the infant's mouth and to that of burping (7). Similar observations pertained to mothers who were disappointed in their baby's sex (6).

Based on a review of the literature as well as her many prior contributions, Korner (12) reported that "the infant's high arousal as expressed in wakefulness and restlessness . . . evokes more frequent interactions with the mother than quiet sleepiness." She observed that the sex of the child may trigger characteristic features of maternal ministrations: boys are apt to receive more proximal (tactile and kinesthetic) stimulation than girls, even though the latter have greater tactile sensitivity. She explained this paradox with the statement that "providing boys with more proximal, tactile stimulation may be, in part at least, an inadvertent, unconscious compensatory response to the male's lesser cutaneous sensitivity."

Another key factor is the responsibility or soothability of the baby. Korner and others have pointed out that, next to an infant's irritability, his/her responsiveness to maternal ministrations gives the mother a feeling of effectiveness and competence that cannot fail to determine her future relationship with the child (12). Thus, certain aspects of parental behavior are a function of the infant's characteristics, including his/her response to the caregiver's activity.

Theoretical Considerations

The neonate's behavior is phenotypic. To his genetic anlage at conception have been added intrauterine influences (4). From birth two fundamental principles ensure his/her survival. As Stierlin (27) put it: "All organisms must initiate *action* and actively impinge upon their environment, but . . . they must also make themselves accessible to being influenced; they must let their environment affect them." This formulation is in agreement with Piaget's (14) concepts of accommodation and assimilation, in that these two concepts specify what is meant by being influenced.

Alloplastic and Autoplastic Regulation

Some 50 years earlier, Stierlin's notion was contained in Freud's and Ferenczi's concepts of alloplastic and autoplastic regulation: the former produces changes in the organism's environment, the latter induces intra-individual changes (8). In the neonate, alloplastic alterations are brought about via social communication, or crying, and consist in the caretaker's ministration as described earlier (26). Sander (18) stated that "the allo-plastic mode operates in feedback transaction between the infant and the caregiver." A precondition of this successful transaction is the organism's ability to perceive the effect of the caregiver's ministrations. An appropriate balance or match must prevail between these two regulatory modes if the infant is to achieve eventual autonomy. It follows that the child represents a stimulus to his/her caregiver so that his/her communication, such as crying, elicits maternal attention (12). Thoman (28) has summarized the essence of the caregiver-neonate system in saying that the earliest organi-zation of the system "occurs as a function of . . . the infant's capabilities for indicating its status, signalling its needs and responding to maternal interventions, and the mother's ability to perceive clues provided by her infant and to respond appropriately to these cues. To the extent that they are mutually responsive, the relationship . . . should facilitate the infant's development." The mother-infant couple, thus, is a psychobiological sys-tem in which the partners undergo constant changes and in which the junior partner is propelled toward autonomy.

Affects

Missing in all these formulations, however, is the crucial role of affects. Spitz (22–24) examined this particular dimension of the caregiver-infant relationship and coined the term "dialogue" to encompass the reciprocity between mother and infant, which he conceived to be in the nature of a circular process within the dyadic relationship, a continuous, mutually stimulating feedback circuit, a stochastic process fueled by emotions. "The baby's initiatives provoke reverberations in the mother expressed in the form of behavior producing new constellations of increasing complexity" of the dyadic interchanges. "Each of these interchanges dispenses grati-fications and frustrations." Added to these evolving experiences is the in-fant's continuous and predetermined progress of maturation (24). Thus, the energizing elements in the dialogue, the caregiver-neonate system, are affects, and transformation is brought about by the infant's inevitable matu-ration. The mother or caregiver is guided by empathy in decoding the baby's signals; this empathy is in part conscious, to a greater extent unconscious, and both are crucial components of what we refer to as good or "normal" mother-child relationship. Thus, the dialogue acts as *vector* of the neonate's development.

It is obvious that poor caregiver-neonate interactions lead to a "derail-ment of the dialogue." It will then be marked by the caregiver's inappro-priate actions, those that do not serve the baby's needs. Ministrations will be interrupted suddenly; the caregiver will transmit contradictory cues; the infant will become restless and tense; progressive adaptation will cease,

resulting in desynchronization of exchanges, arrest of the baby's development and, in severe cases, regression (24). There is a tendency to link the
variations in caregivers' practices, those of competence and failure, to socioeconomic variables; such orientation ignores obvious and important intra-
class differences evident in larger samples and leads to a narrowing of
exploration and premature conclusions (7).

The Dimensions of the Caregiver-Neonate Relationship

From review of the current literature, we distinguish three levels of interchange in the caregiver-neonate system: the perceptual cognitive level, the
emotive-empathic level, and the interpersonal level. The first pertains to an
appropriate provision of stimuli (including provision of comfort) on the
part of the caregiver as well as the progressively sharpening recognition of
input qualities on behalf of the neonate. The emotive level relates to the
capacity by both partners to tolerate setbacks or frustrations or to enjoy
gratifications; this level also provides an incentive for the mother to maintain the interchange. On the interpersonal level, the mother is the focal
element, for even though we now concede an active, initiating role to the
neonate, the caregiver-newborn dyad is an asymmetric relationship in which
one of the partners is mature and maintains a multiplicity of connections
with the "outside," while the other maintains a single such connection.
Moreover, modifications, if any, undergone by the caregiver are solely
those of learning, whereas those by the neonate concern both learning and
maturing, a much more complex process. In order to discharge her proper
function, the caregiver must subordinate her needs to those of the infant.
   Our current knowledge provides no plausible link between these levels
within the caregiver-neonate system. We conceive of them, at this juncture,
as discrete factors entering the system just like tributaries flowing into a
river. Because of this state of our insight, certain contradictions obscure our
understanding. On the perceptual-cognitive level, the question is raised as
to whether the neonate perceives visual signals. Brazelton (5) argues that
babies see because they "fix and follow human faces immediately after
birth," that is, within the first few days (10). Yet, it is not clear whether
this behavior indicates vision as in the adult or rather in the manner of
"orienting" (21).
   Much less controversial is the neonate's ability to follow and discrimi-
nate acoustic signals. In several film records taken within 24 hours of
birth, neonates who were exposed, for a minute, to a number of voices,
to which they remained indifferent though fully alert, suddenly turned their
heads toward their mothers when she joined the conversation (7, 17). A
formulation to link the several dimensions of the caregiver-neonate relation
was offered by Wolf (29) in that the neonate is equipped with intrinsic

rhythmic patterns that are activated at birth through motor discharges mediated by the caregiver, and these motor discharges integrate the perceptual, cognitive, and emotive dimensions.

Conclusion

This review has depicted the caregiver-neonate relationship as a dynamic, evolving interaction engaging features biologically rooted in both partners. The interaction promotes the neonate's progress towards gradual autonomy, ultimately attained in adulthood. Circumstances and forces which promote or impair this interaction are to be found in institutional settings, in the provision of medication, in the caregiver's life experience, life situation, and attitudes regarding the neonate's somatic endowment, sex, birth order, and responsiveness to stimulation and ministrations. To this end, it is encouraging that modern hospital settings favor "family-oriented" perinatal conditions, while modern obstetric anesthesia practices favor the use of methods and drugs that have minimal depressant effects on both mother and neonate.

References

1. Ainsworth, M.D.: The effects of maternal deprivation: A review of findings and controversy of research strategy, in Deprivation of Maternal Care, A Reassessment of its Effects. Public Health Papers No. 14. Geneva, World Health Organization, 1962.
2. Bowlby, J.: Maternal care and mental health. World Health Organization, 1951.
3. Brazelton, T.B.: Effects of maternal medication on the neonate and his behavior. J. Pediatr. **58**:513, 1961.
4. Brazelton, B.: Neonatal Behavioral Scale. Spastics International Medical Publications. London, W. Heinemann Medical Books Ltd., 1973.
5. Brazelton, T.B., Tronick, E., Adamson, L., et al.: Early mother-infant reciprocity, in Parent-Infant Interaction, Ciba Foundation Series No. 33. North Holland, Elsevier, Excerpta Medica, 1975.
6. Cobliner, W.G.: Some maternal attitudes towards conception. Ment. Hygiene **49**, 1965.
7. Cobliner, W.G.: Observations, film records and interviews concerning 25 mother-neonate couples on the maternity ward. Unpublished, 1966.
8. Freud, S.: The loss of reality in neurosis and psychosis. Standard Edition of the Complete Psychological Works of Sigmund Freud, Vol. 19. London, Hogarth Press, 1961.
9. Klaus, M.H., Kennel, Y.H., Plumb, N., Zuehlke, S.: Human maternal behavior at the first contact with her young. Pediatrics **46**:187, 1970.

10. Klaus, M.H., Trause, M.A., Kennel, J.: Does human maternal behavior after delivery show a characteristic pattern? in Parent-Infant Interaction, Ciba Foundation Series No. 33. North Holland, Elsevier, 1975, p. 69.

11. Kron, R., Stein, M., Goddard, K.E.: Newborn sucking behavior affected by obstetric sedation. Pediatrics 37:1012, 1966.

12. Korner, A.: The effect of the infant's state, level of arousal, sex, and ontogenetic stage on the caregiver, in M. Lewis and L.A. Rosenblum (eds.): The Effect of the Infant on the Caregiver. New York, J. Wiley and Sons, 1974.

13. Middlemore, M.D.: The Nursing Couple. London, Hamish Hamilton Medical Books, 1941.

14. Piaget, J.: The Origins of Intelligence in Children. New York, International University Press, 1952.

15. Provence S., Lipton, R.C.: Infants in Institutions. New York, International University Press, 1962.

16. Prugh, D.G., Harlow, R.G.: Masked deprivation in infants and young children, in Deprivation of Maternal Care: A reassessment of its effects. Public Health Papers No. 14. Geneva, World Health Organization, 1962, p. 97.

17. Richards, M.P.M., Bernal, J.T.: Social interaction in the first days of life, in H.R. Schaeffer (ed.): The Origins of Human Social Relations. London, Academic Press, 1971.

18. Sander, L.W.: Adaptive relationship in early mother-child interaction. J. Child Psychiatry 3:231, 1964.

19. Spitz, R.A.: Hospitalism: An inquiry into the genesis of psychiatric conditions in early childhood; and Hospitalism: a follow-up report, New York, in The Psychoanalytic Study of the Child, Vols. 1 and 2. International University Press, 1945 and 1946.

20. Spitz, R.A.: The psychogenic diseases in infancy: An attempt at their etiological classification, in Psychoanalytic Study of the Child, Vol. 6. New York, International University Press, 1951, p. 255.

21. ——— No and Yes: On the Beginnings of Human Communication. New York, International University Press, 1957.

22. ——— Life and the dialogue, In H.S. Gaskill (ed.): Counterpoint. New York, International University Press, 1963.

23. ——— The derailment of the dialogue: stimulus overload, action cycles and the completion gradient. J. Am. Psychoanal. Assoc. 12:752, 1964.

24. The evolution of the dialogue, in M. Schur (ed.): Drives, Affects, Behavior. New York, International University Press, 1965.

25. ———, Cobliner, W.G.: The First Year of Life. New York, International University Press, 1965.

26. Stechler, G., Carpenter, G.: A viewpoint on early affective development, in J. Hellmuth (ed.): Exceptional Infant, Vol. 1, Normal Infant. New York, Brunner/Mazel, 1967.

27. Stierlin, H.: Conflict and Reconciliation. New York, Anchor Books, 1969.

28. Thoman, E.: How a rejecting baby may affect mother-infant synchrony, in Parent Infant Interaction. Ciba Foundation No. 133. North Holland, Elsevier, Excerpta Medica, 1975a, p. 192.

29. Wolff, P.H.: The causes, controls and organization of behavior in the neo-
    nate. Psychological Issues, Mongraph 17. New York, International Univer-
    sity Press, 1966, p. 5.
30. World Health Organization. Deprivation of Maternal Care: A Reassess-
    ment of Its Effects. Public Health Papers No. 14. Geneva, World Health
    Organization, 1962.

5
Reflections on the Apgar Scoring System

J. Selwyn Crawford

The introduction of the Apgar scoring system (1) was an outstanding milestone in the history of perinatology. Initially, its intended functions were twofold: to encourage clinicians to observe *all* newly born infants closely during the moments after delivery, and to provide a teaching aid in the practice of neonatal resuscitation. Subsequently, two additional advantages of the scoring system have become apparent: it can be used as a scale of measurement for comparatively evaluating therapeutic techniques (such as schemes of analgesia in labor, or of anesthesia for operative delivery), as well as how frequently and to what extent neonatal depression is related to categories of obstetric pathology. Secondly, it has been employed as an indicator of the likelihood of short- or long-term morbidity.

Of these four functions, the first, which is the impetus to attend to the newly born infant, has been amply fulfilled and requires little further emphasis. It is salutary to recall that no more than 20 years ago, even in the more advanced societies, the newly born, unless obviously in dire straits, was given little more than a passing glance during possibly the first 20 to 30 minutes of its extra-uterine existence, while the medical and nursing attendants were concerning themselves with the niceties of maternal care and comfort. If the infant was not lying in the bottom of a cot wrapped in wool or cotton, it was cocooned in swaddling clothes, close to its mother's shoulder, with only the tip of its nose visible. It is no exaggeration to say that the impact upon this pattern of behavior by the expanding interest in the Apgar scoring system was tremendous. It initiated the entire era of intense investigation, both clinical and scientific, within the field of neonatology.

Resuscitation

The relationship between the score and the matter of neonatal resuscitation is much more subtle. When the score was introduced, there was no intention that the choice of resuscitative maneuvers be predicated upon evaluation of the score. Although the topic of neonatal resuscitation was recently discussed from this viewpoint (10), we consider the matter to be not as straightforward. First, most authorities would insist that, should resuscitation be required, delaying its start simply in order to evaluate the one-minute score is unacceptable. Clinical assessment without specific reference to numerical evaluation of the various components of the score, or to the total, must provide the predominant impulse in making a decision. The ability to make such an assessment is the product of training, and it is here that the scoring system has proved of value by providing the structure upon which such an assessment is best based. In other words, it has indicated the way in which the infant's general condition may be most adroitly and relatively accurately assessed.

Once the resuscitator has gained experience in the application of the scoring system to a relatively small series of neonates, he or she will have the confidence and ability to assess the general condition of an infant rapidly (a 10-second exercise at most) and to gauge whether or not resuscitation is required, and, if so, how intensive it should be. Furthermore, he/she will with equal ease be able to define roughly the extent to which his/her efforts are meeting with success, by repetitive application of the same series of examinations. For recording purposes only, the score will be assessed at 60 seconds following completion of delivery, and at other previously defined times subsequent to one minute. These remarks, of course, apply particularly to those infants who require resuscitation urgently. Approximately 80% of infants will present with no such demand, and for them an assessment of the score is a formality, although in a small proportion of such cases a mild degree of depression, evidenced usually as a loss of a point for muscle tone, will be of interest in retrospective analyses.

It is appropriate here to insert some remarks regarding the actual application of the scoring system. It is amazing how few clinicians throughout the world know how most simply to count the pulse rate of a newly born infant. Too frequently one sees time-consuming attempts being made to palpate the apex beat, to feel a femoral pulse, or even to apply a stethoscope. Pulsation in the umbilical artery continues to be palpable, except in the moribund infant, for an average 15 to 20 minutes after delivery. The pulse rate can and should be assessed by gently grasping the base of the umbilical cord between finger and thumb.

Despite the fact that in the original account of the scoring system, it was advocated that "reflex irritability" be assessed on the basis of response to application of a catheter tip to a nostril, this procedure is now considered most inadvisable. Infants are obligatory nose breathers, and edema of the nasal mucosa, which can result from trauma, is an unacceptable hazard. The appropriate stimulus in this regard is a smart slap across the soles of the feet.

As has been suggested, repetitive application of the scoring system can be very helpful in determining the pattern of resuscitation. For example, if the infant were only moderately depressed (losing possibly one point each for respiratory effort, reflex irritability, and muscle tone), yet did not respond reasonably promptly to oxygen supplied via an endotracheal tube, plus skin stimulation, and if the mother had received a central-depressant drug during the final six hours of labor, it would be reasonable to assume that a component cause of the neonatal depression was the drug, and the appropriate antagonist should then be administered. Again, if the infant is severely depressed at one minute despite vigorous resuscitation applied immediately after delivery, and if the responsiveness to these measures continues to be poor for another minute, this is indicative (in the absence of gross congenital defect and of excessive trauma to the fetal skull) of severe metabolic acidosis, and should prompt the early administration of a solution of alkali plus glucose.

It will be observed that we have already shifted slightly from the limits of the scoring system as they were originally defined. Initially, it was proposed that the score be assessed once, 60 seconds after complete delivery of the infant. During the few years following general acceptance of the system, there gradually arose the tradition of applying the score at further successive intervals following delivery. The main foci of this growth, in geographic terms, is difficult to define, but the three major such addenda appear to be two minutes, five minutes, and 10 minutes. The scoring system, it is claimed, thus now provides the facility of a retrospective analysis not only of the condition of the infant at delivery, but also of the effectiveness of the resuscitative measures adopted. It is likely that this is to a considerable extent true, within the context of routine clinical practice, but there are limitations to the assumption, which will become apparent in discussion of the implications of the derived scores.

Individual Components of the Score

The original system involved the assessment of five attributes, each being given the same numerical "weighting." Uneasiness about the relative importance assigned to "color" was expressed several years ago (5). Recently, the reports of two investigators (6, 14) have substantiated these doubts. In contrast to the score ascribed to each of the other four attributes, the score given for color does not correlate well with the acid-base state of the infant as defined by analysis of a sample of umbilical artery blood obtained at the time of delivery. The extent of the discrepancy is such that inclusion of the points for color in the total score actually detracts from the level of significance with which the latter correlates with the acid-base values. Thus it is that, increasingly, reports in this field make reference to the "Apgar-minus-color" (A-C) score rather than to the Apgar score. This should occasion little surprise: the color of the skin is dependent upon several unrelated factors in addition to the effectiveness with which the vessels within the dermis are perfused with oxygenated blood. Skin thickness (the contrast, for example, between the immature infant and the mature infant), skin pigmentation, local vaso-activity (not infrequently, a bright pink line can be drawn on the blue trunk of an infant merely by finger pressure), and the quality of the lighting under which the infant is being observed, will each influence the allocation of points for "color."

The relationship of each of the other four components with the acid-base state was also examined (6) and it was observed that the points given for each attribute correlated well with the biochemical values. Thus, in theory, any one of the four components could provide an adequate measure of the condition of the infant. However, although the correlation coefficients relating the pairs of variables (points for component of score versus biochemical attribute) are in the main strong, they are by no means perfect, and thus it would seem to be advisable to retain all four components of the scoring system. A further point is worthy of emphasis. None of the patients in the study just referred to received a large dose of either systemic analgesia, tranquilizer, or anti-convulsants: the dose of meperidine did not exceed 150 mg in labor; promazine, if administered, was limited to a single dose of 50 mg, and diazepam to 10 mg. No patients in the series received chlormethiazole. Had the series included patients who received what would, in terms of current regimens, be viewed as heavy medication during labor, it is not at all unlikely that a much lower level of correlation between the biochemical values and the points allotted for "respiratory effort" (in respect to patients given narcotic analgesics), or for "muscle tone" (in respect specifically to patients who had received diazepam), would have resulted. Indeed, this is one feature of the scoring which offers the opportunity of investigating the effect on the fetus of transplacentally administered drugs. If two groups of patients are studied, all members of each group being free from obstetric pathology, and if the acid-base values derived from analyses of umbilical artery blood are not significantly different, then any difference in the Apgar scores is likely to reflect the differing effects upon the infant of drugs given during labor, or administered during the course of anesthesia for cesarean section.

The Time Factor

The choice of 60 seconds after complete delivery as the time at which the score should be assessed was undoubtedly an arbitrary one. It is a convenient interval in the context of clinical practice, and an easily recollected criterion. Similarly, the dictum that "the clock starts" at completion of delivery is based on convention rather than the particulars of delivery. It might have been more sensible to stipulate that completion of delivery of the fetal head should signal the start of the scoring period, for undoubtedly the time spent in completing the delivery of an infant who presented, either vaginally or at section, by the breech is of a different order of significance to fetal well-being than is the time spent in delivering a vertex-presenting infant. Again, however, the convention has been accepted on the grounds of convenience.

Consideration of these matters does serve to emphasize that the importance of time as a variable among the factors which determined the condition of the infant upon examination was somewhat neglected when the Apgar scoring system was originally introduced. It is true that, as an addendum to the score, it was suggested that note be made of the "time to sustained respiration" (TSR), and as has previously been suggested, in the era of heavy medication and far-from-light general anesthesia, this isolation of a single component of the score was understandable. The general adoption of the system of sequential assessment of the score, at two, five, or ten minutes, has served to relegate the importance briefly attached to precise evaluation of the TSR. At the same time, the introduction of these sequentially applied assessments reflects the appreciation among clinicians of the fact that the process of the neonate's adjustment to extra-uterine existence is of necessity dynamic, and the repetitive examinations can provide valuable information regarding, for example, the facility with which the infant spontaneously recovers from depression (and this observation can, in its turn, help in the assessment of the degree of severity of initial depression), or the effectiveness of resuscitative measures. In like manner, analysis of the recording of repeat scores can aid in the identification of factors which, occurring post delivery, are positively harmful to the infant. Two examples of the latter category will suffice as illustration.

Not infrequently, an infant delivered in excellent condition (A-C score 8 at one minute) by elective cesarean section, will have a considerable quantity of liquid bubbling up from its respiratory tract. It has been suggested that this condition reflects the absence of chest compression characteristic of delivery by section (13). Certainly the result is that the infant becomes increasingly depressed, and that active resuscitation is needed. The incidence and severity of the former consequence can be detailed by reference to notation of the Apgar score at two and possibly five minutes.

The second illustrative situation is of greater moment and occurs much more frequently. It is also entirely iatrogenic, and reflects the clumsy and uninformed attempts by the medical or nursing attendant to aspirate material from the oral pharynx by poking the tip of the aspiration catheter blindly over the back of the infant's tongue via either its mouth or its nose. The results of such stimulation in the neonate are laryngeal inhibition, apnea, cardiac arrhythmia and, in sum, an infant who desperately requires urgent resuscitation (4). The quantitative and qualitative aspects of this situation also can be detailed by reference to the Apgar scores repetitively calculated, and such data can carry considerable weight in the course of instructing potential "resuscitators" in the use of more appropriate instruments such as a bulb-syringe or a catheter with a protective guard (7).

Consideration of the time factor has further important implications in respect to the value of the score as an expression of the condition of the infant at birth. The acid-base status of the infant at delivery is of course only an isolated feature within a continuum of change. It is now well recognized that previous to vaginal delivery, and especially during the second stage, and the process of delivery itself, the fetus becomes increasingly acidotic (15, 17, 21). It is also well known that this progressive acidosis is continued after delivery even in the healthy infant. The duration of the apparent deterioration in respect to the vigorous neonate is a matter of some debate; probably the trend to increasing respiratory acidosis is reversed within half a minute (3), whereas evidence, derived from sequentially drawn blood samples, of increasing metabolic acidosis may be seen throughout the first 5 minutes after delivery (11). Thus, although it has been traditional to assert that the one-minute Apgar score is indicative of the condition of the infant "at birth," this can only be an approximation. The slope which represents the rate of change in the values of the acid-base parameters during the first minute is quite steep. Even among a group of vigorous infants it is far from constant; so that, if the Apgar score reflects the acid-base state of the infant pertaining to the time of assessment of the score, attempts to extrapolate back, by deriving correlations between the values of the score and the acid-base values pertaining to umbilical artery blood sampled at the time of delivery, are destined not to be fully successful. The fact that such correlations are of a reasonably high order (6) suggests that the scoring system itself offers a somewhat crude assessment of the condition of the infant.

Recently, Marx and her colleagues (14) have reported their interesting observation that the level of significance of correlation between the biochemical values and the Apgar score assessed at the time of delivery is higher than that between the biochemical values and the one-minute score. In light of the previous discussion, this makes good sense. Whether or not, in the context of clinical work, it is practicable to adopt the routine of assessing and noting the score immediately upon delivery (which, in effect, means during the first 10 seconds after completion of delivery), is a matter for discussion locally, but certainly Marx's report offers the prospect of a more refined tool for use in the field of investigation.

Prognostic Value

The score is of limited value in its facility as an indicator of both short- and long-term sequelae (8, 9). That it offers the opportunity of identifying the infant who is unlikely to survive the first 24 to 48 hours after birth is of little merit; a mere cursory examination of such an infant at the time of delivery will provide that information. However, the score can help to identify the infant who, in the special circumstance of low gestational age, is likely to develop the idiopathic respiratory distress syndrome (IRDS). As a result of an as yet unpublished survey (Crawford, Cross and Honour) we have established that when statistically appropriate standardization for gestational age and for the sex of the infant is made, the incidence of severe or moderate IRDS is significantly correlated with the A-C scores at one minute and at five minutes. Almost 25% of the infants who did not develop IRDS had an A-C one-minute score of less than 5, whereas almost 50% of those developing severe IRDS did so; 72% of the infants with no IRDS scored 8 at five minutes, compared with 57% and 39% of infants with mild and severe IRDS respectively. These findings, of course, reflect the important contribution which birth asphyxia makes to the estab- lishment of IRDS (12), and also the value of early and efficient resuscita- tion in helping to reduce the incidence of the condition (16).

The usefulness of the score as an indicator of the long-term prognosis of infants who survive the neonatal period is much less assured. It is prob- able that the one-minute score is of no value in this regard, and the five- minute score is only tenuously linked with the emergence of evidence of physical or mental handicap (9, 18). This, again, is hardly surprising, in view of the report (20) that even an infant who is so severely depressed that it exhibits cardiac arrest for up to five minutes after delivery, and does not achieve spontaneous respiratory activity until up to 30 minutes post delivery, has, all other things being equal, a good chance of surviving apparently without permanent damage. A further report (19) of a similar nature concerned the outcome of 48 cases in which the infant scored 0, 1, or 2 at one minute. Fifteen of these babies were apparently stillborn, and none of the remaining 23 achieved spontaneous respiration within 20 minutes of birth. Twenty-three of these infants survived the neonatal period; of these, 17 (74% of the survivors, 35% of the entire series) appeared to have sustained no permanent neurological damage. Six of them had cerebral palsy. Indeed, when one considers that so relatively crude a measure of neonatal well-being as the Apgar score cannot provide an indication of the potential developmental characteristics of the child, one is left to wonder how any more sophisticated analysis of the condition of the infant can possibly offer a guide to the quality of survival.

Summary

In sum, the current status of the Apgar scoring system appears to be as follows:

1. It is of outstanding merit, both historically and currently, for providing an impetus to the prompt and continuing observation of the newly born during the first several minutes after delivery.

2. It is excellent as a guide to resuscitation if used as the framework upon which formal (i.e., non-cotside) instruction in the elements of resuscitation is based. Experience in applying the scoring system improves the facility with which the degree of neonatal depression may be estimated. Repetitive scores provide a useful guide when prolonged resuscitation is required.

3. As a clinical interpretation of the extent of neonatal asphyxia it is very good, provided that the infant is not under the influence of large doses of placentally transmitted powerful depressants.

4. As an indicator of short-term prognosis, it is useful with respect to the preterm infant, in estimating the likelihood that it will develop IRDS.

5. As a prognostic index of long-term disability, it is poor.

References

1. Apgar, V.: Proposal for a new method of evaluation of the newborn. Anesth. Analg. **32**:160, 1953.
2. Apgar, V., James, L.S.: Further observations on the newborn scoring system. Am. J. Dis. Child. **104**:419, 1962.
3. Chou, P.J., Ullrich, J.R., Ackerman, B.D.: Time of onset of effective ventilation at birth. Biol. Neonate **24**:74, 1974.
4. Cordero, L., Hon, E.H.: Neonatal bradycardia following nasopharyngeal stimulation. J. Pediat. **78**:441, 1971.
5. Crawford, J.S.: Anaesthesia for Caesarean section: proposal for evaluation with analysis of a method. Br. J. Anaesth. **34**:179, 1962.
6. Crawford, J.S., Davies, P., Pearson, J.F.: Significance of the individual components of the Apgar score. Br. J. Anaesth. **45**:148, 1973.
7. Crawford, J.S., Walpole, J.B.: Mucus catheter with a protective guard. Lancet **2**:988, 1974.
8. Drage, J.S., Kennedy, C., Schwartz, B.K.: The Apgar score as an index of neonatal mortality. Obstet. Gynecol. **24**:222, 1965.
9. Drage, J.S., Kennedy, C., Schwartz, B.K., Weiss, W.: The Apgar score as an index of neonatal morbidity. Dev. Med. Child. Neurol. **8**:141, 1966.

10. Gregory, G.A.: Resuscitation of the newborn. Anesthesiology **43**:225, 1975.
11. James, L.S.: Acidosis of the newborn and its relation to birth asphyxia. Acta. Paediatr. Scand. **17**: Suppl. 122, 1960.
12. James, L.S.: Perinatal events and respiratory distress syndrome. N. Engl. J. Med. **292**:1291, 1975.
13. Klein, M.: Asphyxia neonatorum caused by foaming. Lancet **1**:1089, 1972.
14. Marx, G.F., Mahajan, S., Miclat, M.N.: Correlation of biochemical data with Apgar scores at birth and at one minute. Br. J. Anaesth. **49**:831, 1977.
15. Modanlou, H., Yeh, S-Y., Hon, E.H., Forsythe, A.: Fetal and neonatal biochemistry and Apgar scores. Am. J. Obstet. Gynecol. **117**:942, 1973.
16. Omer, M.I.A., Robson, E., Neligan, G.A.: Can initial resuscitation of preterm babies reduce the death-rate from hyaline membrane disease? Arch. Dis. Child. **49**:219, 1974.
17. Pearson, J.F., Davies, P.: The effect of continuous lumbar epidural analgesia upon fetal acid-base status during the second stage of labour. J. Obstet. Gynaecol. Br. Commonw. **81**:975, 1974.
18. Richards, F.M., Richards, I.D.G., Roberts, C.J.: Influence of low Apgar ratings on infant mortality and development, in McKeith, R. and Bax, M. (eds.): Clinics in Developmental Medicine, No. 27. Spastics International Medical Publications, 1968.
19. Scott, H.: Outcome of very severe birth asphyxia. Arch. Dis. Child. **51**:712, 1976.
20. Steiner, H., Neligan, G.: Perinatal cardiac arrest: quality of the survivors. Arch. Dis. Child. **50**:696, 1975.
21. Zilianti, M., Segura, C.L., Cabello, F., et al.: Studies on fetal bradycardia during birth process II. Obstet. Gynecol. **42**:840, 1973.

6
Clinical Neonatal Neurobehavioral Assessment: *Methods and Significance*

John W. Scanlon

At birth . . . Let her chant in a low voice, so that the infant's spirit,
rejoicing in harmony, may become cheerful. Let there be not noise
in the room or harsh voice or anything else which might frighten the infant.

Paulus Bagellardus, *On the Care of the Infant During the First Month*, 1494 (19)

That the human spirit or temperament might be active from, and influenced by, the natal event has been argued since antiquity. Only within the past decade has it become firmly established that the neonate uses complex integrative neurologic mechanisms to process stimuli and to respond, with remarkable appropriateness, to its environment (24). In modern times this general capacity has been described as "newborn behavior."

Despite this appreciation of the neonate's sophisticated capabilities, and the attendant growing body of literature which describes these functions, there has been, until recently, limited use made of these activities within the clinical setting to understand perinatal influences on the newly born human. Rather, there has been a pervasive and perpetuated notion that the human infant functions at a spinal reflex or, at most, brain stem level of neurologic organization. This led to a stereotyped evaluation of newborn performance, in which the presence, or absence, of simple reflexes was regarded as presumptive evidence for the presence, or absence, of a significant antecedent influence. Simply put, viability equalled normality.

Indeed, the single major outcome criterion most often employed in clinical perinatology has been the Apgar score. Sufficient studies have accumulated to indicate that intrauterine events, thought to have no consequence for the newborn when measured by the Apgar score, may have considerable impact when examined by other means (28). Some limitations in the use of the Apgar score in this regard can be seen in Table 6.1.

The five variables rated are essentially vital functions. What is scored is depression of these signs. A perinatal insult must be considerable to significantly lower the Apgar. That many infants with really low scores survive

Table 6.1   Some Limitations of the Apgar Score for Newborn Evaluation

Measures only depression of vital functions
Insensitive to subtle or delayed effects
Subjective and influenced by observer bias
Poor predictor of subsequent neurologic/intellectual outcome
Discontinuous and nonparametric scale

and "do well" is a testimony to the reserve physiological adaptability of the neonate, not to the sensitivity of the scale.

The Apgar score is subjective. This is at once a strength and a weakness: a strength because its simplicity allows easy training and rapid performance, and a weakness because it reduces the external applicability of derived data. Dr. Apgar admonished that scoring by an observer involved in the care of mother or infant greatly limits the validity of results (2). Its predictive ability for subsequent infant neurologic outcome has been overemphasized. It is true that neonates with low (0 to 3) five-minute Apgar scores have a statistically greatly increased risk for diminished neurologic performance (8). However, these same NIH Collaborative Study results indicate that 95% of surviving full-term neonates with such terribly low five-minute scores are *not* neurologically abnormal at age one year. Finally, the Apgar scale is discontinuous. That is, the biologic "distance" between an Apgar of 1 and 4 is larger than the difference between a score of 7 and 10. An Apgar of 1 defines flickering viability. The score of 4 describes a blue, floppy neonate with limited cardiorespiratory function. A 7 to 10 score is "within normal limits." Yet repeatedly one sees comparative observations based on parametric statistical analysis of "mean" or "average" Apgar scores. This is at best inappropriate and may be misleading.

Recently described clinically useful neurobehavioral techniques have quantitated the infant's remarkable plasticity in its response to external stimuli. For example, Prechtl and Beintema (22) called attention to the cycling of arousal states. These states, and their lability, provide the framework within which the neonate responds. Parmelee (17) also described activity level as an integral part of the neonate's neurologic assessment, particularly in its response to disturbing stimuli.

Brazelton (5) expanded this concept in clinically testing the infant's capacity to alter its initial reflexive responses, and thus provided a clinically useful measure of the infant's early attempts to control its environment. Sander's (25, 26) elegant studies of the infant's participation in the caretaking process and Klaus and Kennell's (13) cinematographic portrayal of the newborn's active participation in the mother-infant reciprocity underscore this previously underrated human neonatal ability. (See Chapter 4.)

Since the Brazelton Behavioral Assessment Scale (5) has become an accepted standard for clinical neonatal studies, a brief description might be useful.

There are 26 behavioral subtests on the Brazelton scale. These items assess the infant's organization of wake/sleep states, the ability to alter response to noxious or disturbing stimuli, to control activity or muscle tone over a variety of stimulatory events, and to integrate motor activity during the application of auditory, visual, and tactile "non-noxious" stimuli. Brazelton notes that the successful performance of these behaviors probably relies on a cortical level of CNS organization. He also feels that these activities occur routinely in the face of major physiologic demands from the fetal–neonatal transition (37). Testing takes 45 minutes to be performed by an experienced examiner, shows variable results during the first day of life, and requires considerable training to reach satisfactory reliability.

The Brazelton exam has been widely used to study a variety of perinatal influences on the newborn, including maternal medication (4, 11), the narcotic withdrawal syndrome (36), neonatal hyperbilirubinemia and phototherapy (6), intrauterine malnutrition (1), and subsequent neonatal performance after maternal oxytocin challenge testing (32). In these studies, the Brazelton score has been consistently demonstrated to be a sensitive and reliable outcome measure.

Data comparing the Brazelton score as predictor of one-year neurologic outcome with the standard NIH Collaborative Study Neurologic Examination has recently been reported (37). The Brazelton scale was equivalent in detecting neurologically impaired children and had far fewer "false" positives. That is, fewer subsequently normal children were thought suspect in the neonatal period.

The Brazelton scale has also been shown to correlate well with Bayley Mental Quotients at 10 weeks of age (35). Thus the Brazelton would seem to represent one early component of a continuum of testing modalities extending through the first year of life.

However, observing and quantitating neonatal behavior is not without its own problems. Limitations in behavioral studies which tend to reduce overall clinical utility include inadvertent or uncontrolled observer subjectivity, difficulties with quantitating the measures, difficulties in environmental control during the testing procedures, and biases in population selection and population comparability. Some ways to avoid these difficulties are to use objective, but cumbersome, recording equipment, rigid environmental controls and, most importantly, extremely careful research design and statistical analytic methods. Even considering these caveats, newborn behavior is measurable with accuracy, in the clinical setting, to provide a sensitive indicator of perinatal influence. Indeed, Quimby et al. (23) recently stated that newborn behavior is as sensitive as electron microscopy for detecting subtle effects from low-level exposure to anesthetic agents.

In an attempt to combine clinical behavioral techniques and standard neurologic testing into an early, rapid, short, simple and reproducible score, we developed the Early Neonatal Neurobehavioral Scale (ENNS) (29). Our initial goal was to provide tests of newborn response related to maternal *epidural* anesthesia. These tests were performed starting from birth during the blood halftime of the most frequently employed local anesthetic drugs for epidural anesthesia (8 to 12 hours of age).

The examination's elements (see Table 6.2) were adapted from the neonatal scales of Prechtl (22), Beintema (3) and Brazelton (5). We specifically chose items which were easy to elicit during the immediate postnatal period, were readily observable, and simple to score. Many of the subtests had been shown previously to be sensitive to perinatal influences.

We also employed response decrement as a measurement of behavioral integrity. The central concept embodied in response decrement is the demonstrated ability of neonates to modify their initial or reflexive response to repeated stimulation (16, 40). Another advantage of response decrement observation is its relative independence from the absolute magnitude of the infant's initial response and baseline activity. We have recently dem-

Table 6.2   The Components of the Early Neonatal Scale (ENNS) *

A. *Component Apgar Scoring*

B. *State Measurement Before Each of the Numbered Tests*
  1. Response to pin prick
     Response decrement to repeated pin prick
  2. Muscle tone evaluations
     Pull to sitting
     Arm recoil
     Truncal tone
     General body tone
  3. Rooting
  4. Sucking
  5. Response to Moro's maneuver
     Response decrement to repeated Moro
  6. Response decrement to light
  7. Response to sound
     Response decrement to sound

C. *General Scores*
     Alertness
     Overall assessment
     Predominant state
     Lability of state
     Comments

* See text for description.

onstrated that habituation of the limb withdrawal response to an air puff applied to the sole of the foot is independent of state (38). That is, infants regularly and reproducibly diminished, then lost, withdrawal on successive stimulus application while remaining within state as defined by physiologic and bioelectric criteria. Thus, this phenomenon is not one of fatigue.

Response decrement in the ENNS is scored following the infant's best or "maximal" response to various stimuli. The threshold, or number of stimulus applications, usually occurs within one to three trials. The repeat introduction of the stimulus is done after the response has abated (usually within 5 to 10 seconds). Twelve stimuli are the maximum number applied to avoid invoking fatigue as a mechanism for changing response.

In a general sense, the demonstration that the neonate's response alters with repeated application of a stimulus indicates not only that information has been gained from the event, but that this new information has been stored (memory function), and transformed into some functional capacity. This obviously implies a very sophisticated, complex and "high" level of central nervous system functioning.

Whether response decrement, or its more stringently defined analog, habituation, represents early "learning" is, at present, unresolved. The interested reader may wish to review the text by Peeke and Hertz (20), and especially the exemplary chapter by Petrinovich (21), by way of an introduction to this literature.

Scoring the Early Neonatal Neurobehavioral Scale

Testing is done in the sequence shown in Table 6.2. The sequence of testing was selected as an attempt to rouse the infant to maximal activity during the course of the examination. Therefore, tests involving physical manipulation or disturbing stimuli are performed prior to most of the measures of response decrement and integrative performance.

Component Apgar scoring is done at the start of each examination as a measure of vital signs. The components are summed for a total score.

The infant's state is recorded eight times during the examination, immediately prior to each specific test. Criteria for state assessment are as follows:

Awake States

A-1. The eyes may be opened or closed, the eyelids fluttering, the infant drowsy or semidozing. The activity level is variable with occasional mild startles. The infant may react to sensory stimuli, but delay in response is often seen. State change after stimulation is frequently noted.

A-2. The eyes are open, there is considerable motor activity with thrusting movements of extremities and an occasional spontaneous startle. The infant reacts to external stimulation with an increase in startles or motor activity, but discrete reactions are difficult to distinguish because of general high activity levels.

A-3. The infant looks bright and alert. Attention is focused on the source of stimulation. Impinging extrinsic stimuli may break through, usually with delay.

A-4. This state is characterized by intense crying which is difficult, or impossible, to break through with stimulation.

Sleep States

S-1. There is light sleep, the eyes are closed, the activity level is low. There are occasional random movements and startles. The infant's response to internal and external stimulation is by startle, often with a resulting change of state.

S-2. There is deep sleep with little or no spontaneous activity except for startles, usually at regular intervals. External stimuli produce delayed startles. Suppression of startles is rapid and state changes are less likely than in S-1.

Specific Tests

Response to Pin Prick

With the infant supine, the examiner pricks the sole of the subject's foot lightly with a blunt pin. This response has two components, local flexion (withdrawal) of the involved limb *plus* a more generalized response characterized by color change, crying, etc. The magnitude of the local withdrawal is scored from no response (zero) to vigorous, easily elicited, brisk response (three).

Response Decrement to Pin Prick

This is recorded as the number of stimuli required from the maximum response to alteration *either* of the local withdrawal response or the general response, whichever occurs first.

Muscle Tone Evaluations

Pull to Sitting. The infant is gently pulled by his hands to the sitting position and head control is scored. The score ranges from no evidence of head control (zero), through unable to maintain head erect (one), marked control (two), to head consistently held erect (three).

Arm Recoil. The infant's forearm is gently extended, then suddenly released by the examiner. Recoil is scored from absent (zero) to very strong, rapid recoil, usually with some overshoot (three).

Truncal Tone. The infant is suspended horizontally by the examiner's hand placed under the abdomen. Scoring ranges from complete hypotonia (zero) to the usual strong neck or hip extension with vigorous trunk straightening (two) through abnormal rigidity of neck, trunk and hips (three).

General Body Tone. This composite score is assigned for the evaluation of the infant's motor control from absent (zero) through weak (one), average (two) to rigid (three).

Rooting

The examiner gently strokes the skin of the cheek at the corner of the mouth. The infant, in the supine position, is observed for head turning and lip movements starting with the head in the midline position. Scoring ranges from no response (zero) through vigorous head turning and sucking lip movement (three).

Sucking

Again with the infant in the supine position, the examiner inserts the distal joint of the index finger into the infant's mouth. Sucking is scored from no response (zero) through three to ten sucks per group (two) through the optimal of vigorous, long periods of sucking (three).

Response to Moro's Maneuvers

The response is elicited by a rapid, short (25 degree) head drop with the infant in the supine position. Scoring of the infant's optimal moro response ranges from no response (zero) to rapid, complete flexion/extension of the arms, with encirclement (three).

Response Decrement to Repeated Moro's

Stimulus applications are repeated after the neonate completes each full response. The number of applications is counted. The response decrement, or habituation, number is the number of stimuli required until the maximal response is observably altered. No more than 12 applications are performed.

Response Decrement to Light

A bright light from a pocket flashlight is flashed briefly (one second) into the infant's eye. This is repeated after the infant's response has ceased. The response decrement number is that number of stimuli needed from the infant's maximal response until this is observably modified. The response may be a blink, a startle, or the typical eye widening reflex. Again, no more than 12 separate flashes are made.

Response to Sound

A bell is sounded sharply, but briefly, a few inches behind the infant's head in the midline, out of visual range. The response, usually observable movement or activity, is scored from no reaction (zero) to definite searching with almost immediate response to stimuli (three).

Response Decrement to Sound

The sound stimulus is repeated after the previous response has ended and the number of stimulus applications until change occurs are noted.

Placing

With the infant suspended in the upright position, the body is raised until the dorsum of the foot touches a protruding bassinet edge. Scoring is based on flexion then extension of the stimulated leg until placement of the ipsalateral foot on the edge is accomplished. Scores range from no response (zero) to easily and rapidly elicited full response.

General Observations

Alertness.   This is a composite score which includes observations of the infant's most alert period over the entire examination. The scoring takes into account head turning toward environmental stimuli, widening of eyes, "bright-looking" facies, shutting out extrinsic, interfering stimuli, etc. Scores range from dull or absent response for most stimuli (zero) to alert responses to almost all stimuli, either environmental or tester-applied (three).

Overall Assessment.   This score forces the examiner to judge the infant's overall performance on the entire examination. This is scored abnormal, borderline, normal, or superior. The reasons for so categorizing an infant are recorded.

Predominant State.   The predominant state score (the most frequently occurring state) is recorded.

Lability of State.   The number of individual changes in state occurring during the entire examination is recorded here.

Comments.   This space is used to describe any unusual aspect of the examination, any untoward events or interruptions occurring during testing, and such difficult-to-quantitate variables as significant body color changes and abnormal movements.

Methodologic Issues

Whether this scale is to be used for clinical appraisal, training purposes, or clinical investigation, it is important to measure the reproducibility of scores between observers. It has been our experience that reliability, or the overall ratio of agreements to total scores, averages 84% (29). When differences of only one state change between observers are excluded, the mean agreements to total scores percentage rises to 96.

When the ENNS is to be used as a research tool, there should be frequent (at least monthly) retesting of interobserver reliability. This retesting assures standardization of the method, its reproducibility of results, and provides further objectivity.

While individual users of this scale must define acceptable limits of normal for their subjects under evaluation, it might be useful to mention some general observations we have made during the past five years.

One of the most striking features is the lability of states in normal newborns. We consistently found a wide range in the number of state changes per examination and a tendency for the number of state changes per examination to increase with time after birth. These observations are consistent with those of Parmelee (18), who described discrete sleeping and waking state patterns during the first day of life. Furthermore, both Beintema (3) and Sander et al. (26) emphasize that state lability is a dominant behavioral feature of the first postnatal day.

In our evaluation of various measures of neuromuscular activity, all healthy, unaffected "control" infants demonstrated vigorous responses to pin prick and Moro's maneuver, had good muscle tone, and strong rooting and sucking behavior. That is, their median score for these tests was two. These infants demonstrated high scores throughout the first day of life and there appeared to be an increase in the quality of the response with the passage of time following birth. These observations are consistent with the report of Escardo and De Coriat (9) that infants born to mothers who are minimally, or not at all medicated, do not have a sustained period of hypotonia or reflex inhibition just after delivery. These findings are frequently noted in children born to sedated mothers and have been described as the "shock of birth."

Another observation is that the ability to respond to a repeated stimulus is pervasive in normal newborns. Despite the use of several different stimuli and different testing times after birth, the median number of stimulus applications required before response alteration occurred was usually between six and nine. This consistency occurred despite considerable variation in the absolute magnitude of response, suggesting that response decrement behavior was independent of neuromuscular strength and, further, can be tested as such.

Of interest is a notable sex difference in response seen in the early newborn period (14). In general, females are more alert and respond better to stimuli than males. These observations have included auditory, oral, and visual stimuli, and attendant responses such as cardiac acceleration, head turning, and attention time. While the mechanisms and clinical significance involved in this issue are fascinating to contemplate, the research methodologic implications are clear. Gender distribution must be equivalent for all groups compared.

Several other methodologic concerns must also be mentioned. First of all, when studying perinatal variables in an experimental setting, using the ENNS as an outcome measure, the examiner *must* consistently be unaware of the maternal history, particularly of those variables under investigation (e.g., maternal drug exposure). A useful research design technique is to require testing of some infants who will not be included in the ultimate data analysis.

As regards statistical analysis for the ENNS, it should be noted that none of the sub-items are continuous scales. For several scores (tone scores particularly), both extreme high and low scores might be abnormal. Therefore, a summation of "total" ENNS score can be misleading. Statistical technique should attempt to maximize beta error and measure differences in median scores. Several nonparametric tests are useful, such as Chi-square and Fisher Exact Test (34). F testing and matched-pair median subtest covariance analysis is also appropriate.

A frequent criticism is that there may be inherent, unidirectional selection prejudices operant in behavioral studies, especially when looking for the effects of maternal analgesia or anesthesia. It is often said that maternal temperamental characteristics, socioeconomic, education, and ethnic/racial biases operate to influence the choices of drug versus no drug, the use of specific drugs, their doses or frequency of administration, and subsequently, therefore, the behavior of the newborn. Recent studies do not support this critique. Yang et al. (41) found no relationship between maternal attitudinal factors and neonatal behavior. In this study there was a good inverse correlation between maternal drug administration and newborn behavior.

Zax et al. (42) investigated the influence of maternal anxiety, and its modification by childbirth education, for a number of perinatal factors, including whether or not drugs were used and, if so, their average doses. Only one maternal attitudinal variable (desire to participate in labor) correlated ($R = 0.26$) with anesthesia and this one not at all with analgesia. No other attitude variable was found so related.

In perhaps the most exhaustive study to date of the impact of ethnic and socioeconomic factors on newborn behavior, Brown et al. (7) investigated the effects of natal weight, birth order, and sex in a group of urban black mothers and their newborns. They emphasize that maternal medication consistently altered interactional behavior, even with respect to other confounding variables. They further noted that mothers who received *more* medication during labor spent *more* time trying to stimulate their babies, even though their infants were more passive and less responsive. This perhaps suggests that maternal drug selection biases, if present, would tend to favor more, not less, stimulating mothers and that this would act to improve, not impair, neonatal behavior. Therefore, the observed behavioral deviations in "medicated" neonates appear all the more striking!

Clinical Uses of the Early Neonatal Neurobehavioral Examination

As indicated earlier, we have used the ENNS to study full-term, normal infants delivered after continuous epidural lumbar anesthesia by means of lidocaine, bupivacaine, and mepivacaine (29, 30).

Representative results from these studies, showing significant differences between epidural and matched nonepidural newborns, can be seen in Figs. 6.1 and 6.2. Newborns whose mothers received lidocaine or mepivacaine

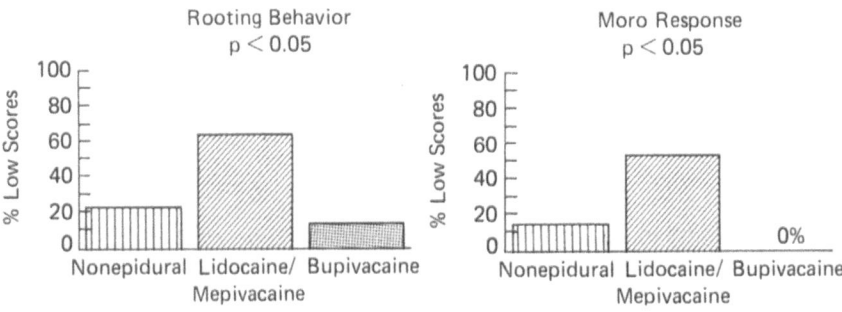

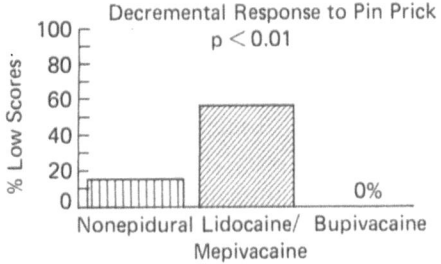

Fig. 6.1 Percentage of low scores on tests of adaptive capacity at 2 to 4 hours of age for infants whose mothers received epidural block with lidocaine, mepivacaine, bupivacaine, or no epidural anesthesia. Nonepidural, N = 13; lidocaine/ mepivacaine, N = 28; bupivacaine, N = 20. (Reproduced from the Bulletin of the New York Academy of Medicine (27), with permission.)

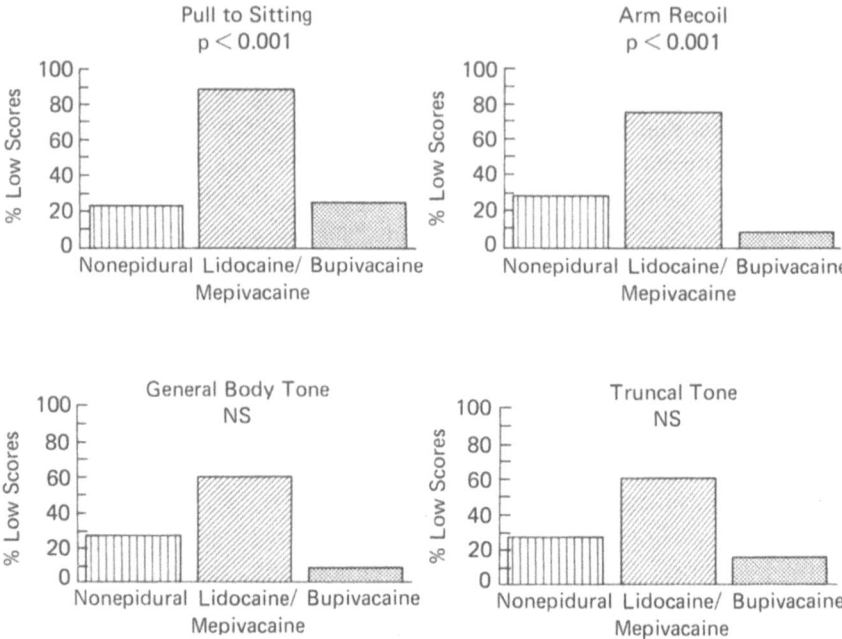

Fig. 6.2   Percentage of low scores on tests of muscle strength and tone at 2 to 4 hours of age for infants whose mothers received epidural with lidocaine, mepivacaine, bupivacaine, or no epidural anesthesia. Nonepidural, N = 13; lidocaine/mepivacaine, N = 28; bupivacaine, N = 20. (Reproduced from the Bulletin of the New York Academy of Medicine (27), with permission.)

had significantly lower median muscle tone scores, more absent decremental response to pin prick, lower median response, and less active rooting behavior. This was sufficiently characteristic to describe these babies as "floppy, but alert." These differences were not seen with bupivacaine.

Additional studies conducted during the first ten days of life in collaboration with Dr. Brazelton's group, confirmed these previously noted changes, and showed, as well, for a carefully defined "normal" population, that these differences tended to diminish with time (39).

We examined 54 newborns whose mothers had been carefully selected for uncomplicated obstetric history, labor, and delivery. These infants were carefully screened for pediatric and neurologic normality after delivery. They were then divided into eight groups on the basis of their maternal drug exposure (as shown in Table 6.3). The ENNS was performed during the first 12 hours of life; Brazelton exam was done on days 1 through 5, day 7, and day 10.

Table 6.4 shows the results, which compare minimal drug, analgesic, and epidural groups. As noted, motor organization was poorer early in life in the epidural group, but responsivity to external events was not af-

Table 6.3 Maternal Drug Experience of Infants Followed Over the First 10 Days of Life with Serial Behavioral Testing

Group	Medication	No. of Subjects	Mean Umbilical Cord Level	24-Hour Heel-Stick Level
Minimal Drug Groups				
1. No medication at all		6	—	—
2. Lidocaine spinal only (within 1 hr of delivery; no premedication)		4	0.10 μg/ml	0.04 μg/ml
3. Lidocaine local (just prior to delivery for episiotomy; no premedication)		10	0.00 μg/ml	0.04 μg/ml
Analgesic Groups				
4. Alphaprodine and/or promazine; 60 mg total		4	—	—
5. Alphaprodine and/or promazine; 60 mg total and lidocaine spinal as in group 2		7	0.04 μg/ml	0.00 μg/ml
6. Alphaprodine and/or promazine; 60 mg total and lidocaine local as in group 3		9	0.63 μg/ml	0.01 μg/ml
Epidural Groups				
7. Mepivicaine or lidocaine epidural within 4 hr of delivery		10	1.58 g/ml of mepivicaine; 0.55 μg/ml of lidocaine	0.46 g/ml of mepivicaine; 0.05 μg/ml of lidocaine
8. Mepivicaine or lidocaine epidural within 4 hr of delivery and alphaprodine and/or promazine as in group 4		4	—	—

Reproduced from Pediatrics (39), with permission.

Table 6.4   Early Neonatal Neurobehavioral Scores of Infants by Maternal Drug Experience

	Mean Scores for Different Groups			
Measures	Minimal Drug (1, 2, 3)	Analgesic (4, 5, 6)	Epidural (7 and 8)	
Motor Organization				
Pull-to-sit	2.0	2.0	1.0	6.68°
Arm recoil	2.0	2.0	1.4	8.02°
Truncal tone	1.7	2.0	1.4	2.68
Body tone	2.0	2.0	1.4	8.02°
Rooting	1.8	1.8	1.4	1.79
Sucking	2.0	2.0	2.2	0.38
Moro	2.0	1.8	3.2	1.11
Placing	2.1	1.7	2.0	1.67
Response to External Stimuli				
Response to pinprick	2.0	2.0	1.8	1.34
Decrement in response to repeated pinprick	7.2	6.0	7.0	0.48
Decrement in response to repeated light flashes (flashlight)	7.0	7.5	9.0	1.77
Response to sound (rattle)	1.7	2.0	1.8	0.51
Decrement in response to repeated sounds (rattle)	5.8	7.8	6.5	0.50
Decrement in Moro response with repeated elicitations	7.3	7.0	6.8	0.04
Alertness	2.0	2.3	2.0	2.23
$P < 0.01$				

Reproduced from Pediatrics (39), with permission.
* See Table 6.3 for groups.

fected. In addition, there were few significant effects over the subsequent ten days while the performance of all infants studied seemed to improve during this time. These observations should prove reassuring to physicians and mothers whose clinical situations *necessitate* the use of minimal doses of well-controlled analgesic premedication or epidural anesthesia. These results must *not* be used to justify the routine, ubiquitous administration of drugs to all laboring women under the circumstances. These data should also provide a normative reference for subsequent studies of different populations and for other perinatal factors.

We have also investigated, in a preliminary manner, the effects of spinal and general anesthesia for repeat, elective cesarean section (without labor) in a small group of healthy newborns delivered after uncomplicated pregnancies (31). These results suggest that general anesthesia for elective cesarean section is associated with a global depression of newborn neuro-behavioral performance, despite equal one- and five-minute Apgar scores (median 8 and 9) for both drug groups.

Scatliff and Palahniuk (33) have reported preliminary observations of newborn behavior using the ENNS for two groups of healthy women who underwent elective cesarean section near term. In one group, following standard thiopental/succinylcholine induction, mothers were maintained on 70% nitrous oxide/30% oxygen anesthesia. The second group, after a similar induction, was maintained on methoxyflurane (0.5% or lower)-oxygen. Induction to delivery intervals, umbilical blood gases, and Apgar scores were equivalent for both groups. There were decreased muscle tone scores, diminished rooting, sucking, and placing reflexes in the "nitrous" group of newborns. The neonate's response to several stimuli and its response decrement behavior showed no differences. This suggested to the authors that nitrous oxide anesthesia was more depressing to the newborn than methoxyflurane. However, it is more likely that the differences in neuro-behavioral scores were related to the difference in administered oxygen concentration. Higher inhaled oxygen fractions have been shown to produce better maternal and, consequently, better fetal oxygenation as well as improved neonatal clinical conditions. The essential factor in this study was that two comparable groups of infants, demonstrably different in be-havioral activity, were otherwise judged normal by the usual clinical and biochemical standards of wellbeing.

McDonald and Colli (15) have begun a random, double-blind study of naloxone's ability to reverse the action of maternal-administered meperi-dine. This investigation includes not only careful cardiovascular, acid-base, and bioelectric monitoring, but also the use of neurobehavioral evaluation (ENNS) from birth to four hours of age. Results from these studies have not yet been published. However, these efforts suggest that early neuro-behavioral testing might be useful to complement other modalities of new-born evaluation in the immediate postnatal period.

Finally, Hillman and others (10) have described a study investigating the use of mepivacaine and bupivacaine in paracervical block. They have combined bioelectric, acid-base, and pharmacokinetic data with outcome as measured by neurobehavioral scores. Again, while these investigations are preliminary and results unpublished, the integration of bioelectric, acid-base, drug level, and neurobehavioral data for clinical studies is most appropriate.

We are not suggesting that the ENNS provides anything more than a very early screening of newborn activity. Rather, this testing, modified to suit the investigator's needs, can and should be combined with other peri-natal data for a more balanced approach to outcome. In addition, this information may be used as part of a battery of evaluation techniques including the Brazelton examination, cinematographic observation of maternal–infant interaction, various maternal interviewing techniques, and quantifiable attitudinal questionnaires to provide a broad range of sophisticated, clinically useful measures for the perinatal investigator.

The bulk of these studies have started to define the impact of intrapartum iatrogenic maneuvers on the full-term, uncompromised fetus and neonate. They should provide, at least, some answers to questions about drug effects in the "normal" population of newborns. They might even provide a more comprehensive definition of normal.

A next major investigative step will be to examine similar measures in a high-risk obstetric population. Howard, Parmelee and their group have begun to do just this (12). Their studies show subtle, but real differences in prematures when examined by standard neurologic techniques at the date of their expected delivery (not their birth) when compared with term neonates so evaluated at birth. These differences were more striking in infants with evidence of intrauterine malnutrition. Als et al. (1) have also investigated the early behavior of infants suffering from intrauterine malnutrition. Using the Brazelton scale, these investigators were able to clearly differentiate the fetally malnourished infant because of altered passive motion of arms and legs, rooting, sucking and, most important, from certain subtests which seem important in the maternal–infant interaction. These Brazelton items are the infant's need for stimulation, its integrated motor activities, and attractiveness. When this group of infants was followed, it showed temperamental difficulties in neurologic organization, possibly related to maternal anxiety or perhaps to subtle cerebral dysfunction. These authors emphasize the difficulties in their work, and in that of others, in testing not only significant neonatal variables, such as hypoglycemia and low Apgar scores, from their data, but also in defining the psychologic impact on the mother of bearing a "high-risk" infant and its effect on their fragile, blossoming relationship.

In a similar fashion, we have begun a prospective study of the neurobehavioral performance of newborns whose mothers had oxytocin challenge testing (OCT) for clinical "high-risk" indications (32). Our preliminary data, looking only at normal Apgar, term infants, demonstrated both early and persistent behavioral differences in infants delivered after positive oxytocin challenge testing results. For example, infants with positive oxytocin challenge test results had significantly decreased passive muscle tone scores during the first 12 hours of life. This persisted for four days and seemed independent of the anesthesia used. Using the Brazelton scale, these positive OCT infants had diminished orientation to visual stimuli, decreased alertness, decreased motor maturity, and decreased evoked muscle tone on the fourth day of life. In addition, there was a significantly increased incidence of muscular tremulousness in this positive OCT group. While the etiology of these differences remains unexplained, as do the possible influences of other confounding variables such as the maternal condition prompting the "high-risk" assignment, and the management of her labor and delivery, our observations suggest that there are demonstrable differences quite early in the life of the "high-risk" infant. Quite obviously, much additional work is necessary to define these differences accurately, to understand their genesis and significance, and to discover the role of any therapeutic interventions which might provide ultimate successful outcomes.

The next chapter will describe, in considerable detail, further applications of these behavioral techniques in the clinical setting of obstetric anesthesia.

Acknowledgments

The author thanks T. Berry Brazelton, M.D., and Edward Tronick, Ph.D., for their help and expertise. The author also wishes to express his deep gratitude to Milton H. Alper, M.D., for his guidance and support during the work described herein.

References

1. Als, H., Tronick, E., Adamson, L., Brazelton, T.B.: The Behavior of the full-term yet underweight newborn infant. Unpublished manuscript, Harvard University, 1975.
2. Apgar, V., James, L.S.: Further observations on the newborn scoring system. Am. J. Dis. Child. 104:419, 1962.
3. Beintema, D.J.: A Neurological Study of Newborn Infants. London, W. Heinemann, Ltd., 1968.
4. Brackbill, Y., Kane, J., Maniello, R.L., Abramson, D.: Obstetric meperidine usage and assessment of neonatal status. Anesthesiology 40:116, 1970.
5. Brazelton, T.B.: Neonatal Behavioral Assessment Scale. Philadelphia, J.B. Lippincott, 1973.
6. Brazelton, T.B., Tronick, E.: Unpublished data.
7. Brown, J.V., Baheman, R., Snyder, P.A., et al.: Interactions of black inner-city mothers with their newborn infants. Child Dev. 46:677, 1975.
8. Drage, J.S., Berendes, H.: Apgar scores and outcome of the newborn. Pediatr. Clin. N. Am. 13:635, 1966.
9. Escardo, F., De Coriat, L.F.: Development of postural and tonic patterns in the newborn infant. Pediatr. Clin. W. Am. 7:511, 1960.
10. Hillman, L.W., Dodson, W.E., Hillman, R.E., et al.: The use of mepivacaine and bupivacaine in a double blind paracervical study. Annual Meeting, Society for Obstetric Anesthesia and Perinatology, 1976.
11. Horowitz, F.D., Ashton, J., Culp, R., Gaddis, E.: The effects of obstetrical medication on the behavior of Israeli newborn infants and some comparisons with other populations. Submitted for publication.

12. Howard, J., Parmelee, A.H., Kopp, C.B., Littman, B.: A neurologic comparison of pre-term and full-term infants at term conceptional age. J. Pediatr. **88**:995, 1976.
13. Klaus, M.H., Kennell, J.H.: Mothers separated from their newborn infants. Pediatric. Clin. N. Am. **17**:1015, 1970.
14. Korner, A.F.: Sex differences in newborns, with special reference to differences in the organization of oral behavior. J. Child Psychol. Psychiatry **14**:19, 1973.
15. McDonald, J.S., Colli, C.R.: Naloxone—fetal and neonatal response to meperidine reversal. Annual Meeting, Society for Obstetric Anesthesia and Perinatology, 1976.
16. Moreau, T., Birch, H.D., Turkewitz, G.: Ease of habituation to repeated auditory and somesthetic stimulation in the human newborn. J. Exp. Child psychol. **9**:193, 1970.
17. Parmelee, A.H., Michaelis, R.: Neurological examination of the newborn, in Hellmuth, J. (ed.): Exceptional Infant, II: Studies in Abnormalities. New York, Brunner/Mazel, 1971.
18. Parmalee, A.H., Schulz, H.R., Disbrow, M.A.: Sleep patterns of the newborn. J. Pediatr. **58**:241, 1961.
19. Bagellardus, Paulus: On the care of the infant during the first month, in Ruhrah, J. (ed.): Pediatrics of the Past. New York, Paul B. Hoeber, 1925, p. 34.
20. Peeke, H.V.S., Herz, M.J.: Habituation, Vol. I. New York, Academic Press, 1973.
21. Petrinovich, L.: A species-meaningful analysis of habituation, in Peeke, H.V.S. and Herz, M.J. (eds.): Habituation, Vol. I. New York, Academic Press, 1973.
22. Prechtl, H., Beintema, D.: The Neurological Examination of the Full-Term Newborn Infant. London, William Heinemann, 1964.
23. Quimby, K.L., Aschkenaze, C.J., Bowman, R.E., et al.: Enduring learning deficits and cerebral synaptic malformation from exposure to ten parts of halothane per million. Science **185**:625, 1974.
24. Robinson, R.J.: Cerebral hemisphere function in the newborn, in Robinson, R.J. (ed.): Brain and Early Behavior. New York, Academic Press, 1974, p. 343.
25. Sander, L.W., Julia, H.L., Stechler, G., Burns, P.: Continuous twenty-four-hour interactional monitoring in infants reared in two caretaking environments. Psychosom. Med. **34**:270, 1972.
26. Sander, L.W., Stechler, G., Burns, P., Julia, H.: Early mother-infant interactions and twenty-four-hour patterns of activity and sleep. J. Am. Acad. Child Psychiatry **9**:311, 1970.
27. Scanlon, J.W.: Effects of local anesthetics administered to parturient women on the neurological and behavioral performance of newborn children. Bull. N. Y. Acad. Med. **52**:231, 1976.
28. Scanlon, J.W.: How is the baby?: the Apgar score revisited. Clin. Pediatr. (Phila.) **12**:61, 1973.
29. Scanlon, J.W., Brown, W.U., Weiss, J.B., Alper, M.H.: Neurobehavioral

responses of newborn infants after maternal epidural anesthesia. Anesthesiology **40**:121, 1974.

30. Scanlon, J.W., Ostheimer, G.W., Brown, W.U., et al.: Neurobehavioral responses of newborns after epidural anesthesia with bupivacaine. Anesthesiology **45**:400, 1976.

31. Scanlon, J.W., Shae, E., Alper, M.H.: Neurobehavioral responses of newborn infants following general or spinal anesthesia for cesarian section. Abstracts of Scientific Papers, American Society of Anesthesiologists, 1975, p. 91.

32. Scanlon, J.W., Suzuki, K., Shea, E.: Neurobehavioral performance of newborns whose mothers had oxytocin challenge testing; a prospective study. Annual Meeting, Society for Obstetric Anesthesia and Perinatology, 1976.

33. Scatliff, J., Palahniuk, R.J.: Evaluation of cesarian section anesthesia. Annual Meeting, Society for Obstetric Anesthesia and Perinatology, 1975.

34. Siegal, S.: Nonparametric Statistics for the Behavioral Sciences. New York, McGraw-Hill, 1956.

35. Sostek, A.M., Anders, T.F.: Relationships between the Brazelton neonatal scale, Bayley infant scales and early temperament. Submitted for publication.

36. Soule, A.B., Standley, K., Copans, S., Davis, M.: Clinical uses of the Brazelton neonatal scale. Pediatrics **54**:583, 1974.

37. Tronick, E., Brazelton, T.B.: Clinical uses of the Brazelton neonatal behavioral assessment scale, in Friedlander, B.Z., et al (eds.): Exceptional Infant, III: Assessment and Intervention. New York, Brunner/Mazel, 1975.

38. Tronick, E., Scanlon, J.W.: The habituation of an avoidance reaction in human neonates: independence of state as a variable. Unpublished study, Harvard University.

39. Tronick, E., Wise, S., Ab, H., et al.: Regional obstetric anesthesia and newborn behavior; effect over the first ten days of life. Pediatrics **58**:94, 1976.

40. Turkewitz, G., Moreau, T., Birch, H.D.: Relation between birth condition and neurobehavioral organization in the neonate. Pediatr. Res. **2**:243, 1968.

41. Yang, R.K., Zweig, A.R., Douthitt, T.C., Federman, E.J.: Successive relationships between attitudes during pregnancy, maternal analgesic medication during labor and delivery and newborn behavior. Develop. Psychol., in press.

42. Zax, M., Sameroff, A.J., Farnum, J.E.: Childbirth education, maternal attitudes and delivery. Am. J. Obstet. Gynecol. **123**:186, 1975.

7
Effects of Obstetric Analgesia–Anesthesia on Neonatal Neurobehavior

Robert Hodgkinson

A clear understanding of the effect of drugs on the neonate can be obscured by the concept of the placental "barrier," by uncritical reliance on the Apgar score, and by unjustified extrapolation from our limited knowledge of pharmacodynamics. Most drugs pass easily from mother to fetus through the placental interchange. The few exceptions include highly ionized drugs such as succinylcholine and curare, and very rapidly destroyed drugs such as chloroprocaine. Analgesics, tranquilizers, and other drugs affecting the central nervous system pass rapidly because the blood-brain interchange possesses the same characteristics as the placental interchange; it allows the free transfer of unionized, lipid soluble, non-protein-bound drugs. In effect, the physiochemical properties of drugs modifying pain and fear at the cerebral level are exactly the properties needed for free passage to the fetus.

The Apgar score and other evaluations of the neonate made in the delivery room may blind us to the delayed effect of drugs. For the Apgar score to be depressed by maternally-administered drugs, the dosage must have been grossly excessive, the time elapsing between administration and delivery too short, or the infant unduly sensitive. The neonate just subjected to the intense stimulation of birth may be compared to an inebriated man thrown out of a bar into the cold air. For both the drunk and the neonate, the effect of drugs is temporarily hidden. Their condition can be more meaningfully assessed later.

Pharmacodynamics may confuse the issue further by concentrating on fetal and umbilical serum levels and by emphasizing the protective effect of the liver and the effect of protein binding on placental transmission. The liver may protect the brain from the initial onslaught of the drug, but redistribution almost certainly takes place later. Finster (11) has shown high tissue levels of bupivacaine despite a high degree of protein binding in the maternal blood. A more relevant measure would be cerebral tissue concentration, especially in the midbrain where high levels of many drugs such as barbiturates are found. Even more relevant is the effect of cerebral drug concentration on the baby's cerebral functioning. This is what neurobehavioral tests are designed to assess.

Neurobehavioral tests performed after the neonate has been transferred to the nursery and on the following days are an accurate index of the effect of drugs. Quimby (25) describes them "as sensitive as electronmicroscopy for detecting damage from exposure to a trace level of toxicant." Before describing the effects of drugs on the broadly based neurobehavioral scales associated with the names of Brazelton, Prechtl, Beintema, and Scanlon, and the various modifications of these tests, some of the individual tests will be discussed.

Wakefulness

Sleep/wakefulness was studied on 20 normal neonates left undisturbed for 10 hours after birth (10). Minute-by-minute judgments of the behavioral state were made by five observers whose interobserver agreement was 93%. The five behavioral states were alert and crying; alert but inactive; drowsy; rapid eye movement (REM) sleep; and quiet, non-REM sleep. In the 10 infants of mothers who had received meperidine (50 to 75 mg) and/or tranquilizers, the duration of wakefulness was less than half in both the first two hours and the subsequent eight hours after birth. Non-REM sleep was increased by 400% in the first two hours and by 50% in the subsequent eight hours in the medicated group. The author's comment was, "Wakefulness is the behavioral state of the newborn during which most information processing takes place. There is no reason to believe it does not have developmental continuity with later wakefulness and self-awareness." Increased sleepiness and lack of alertness have also been noted by a number of other authors following secobarbital (6, 18), vinbarbital (19), meperidine (2, 19), and morphine (19) during the study of other aspects of neurobehavior.

Electroencephalography

The EEGs of 20 normal neonates whose mothers received secobarbital during labor were compared with those of neonates whose mothers had no medication (18). The neonates exposed to secobarbital showed marked electrical cortical depression "characterized by a pronounced decrease in slow waves of moderate amplitude and some increase in fast waves of low amplitude." The changes were followed and persisted for three days even after drowsiness had disappeared. In a further study (19) meperidine (100 to 300 mg) was administered to 31 mothers, vinbarbital (325 to 520 mg) to 29, and morphine (10 to 15 mg) to 36. The majority of neonates showed EEG changes consisting of decrease in amplitude of brain potentials. Many babies showed bursts of slow waves of high microvoltage. Changes persisted for three days. Some babies showed changes on the second and third day, but did not show changes on the first. Clinical drowsiness on the first day correlated well with drug dosage. Borgstedt and Rosen (2) also found fast low voltage activity, particularly in the front cortical tracings, associated with meperidine, promethazine, and phenobarbital in combination. They correlated these with impairment of waking states, arousal activity, and muscle tone. The abnormal activity had disappeared by four days of age.

Attentiveness

Attentiveness and visual scanning were evaluated between the second and fourth day of life in 20 full-term infants (35). During a nine-minute session, three visual stimuli were presented to the infant for one minute. The stimuli consisted of identical size pieces of paper. One was blank, one had a simple face, and one had a dye showing three dots. The neonates were graded for total looking or scanning time. There were two analyses of the data on the effect of drugs. In the first analysis, neonates whose mothers had received medication within one and a-half hours of delivery were compared with those whose mothers had received no medication. In the first group the mean looking time was 195 seconds and in the second group, 287 seconds ($p < .025$). In the second analysis, the dosage of drug was weighted for the effect of time. Each administration of drug was described as high ($++$) or low ($+$) and this was multiplied by four if the drug was given within one and a-half hours of delivery; multiplied by three if given between one and a half and two hours; and multiplied by two if given between four to eight hours, and by one if it was given more than eight hours after delivery. The total looking time of the baby showed an inverse relationship with the weighted total dosage of medication given to the mothers ($r = .55; p < .01$).

Sucking

From a study of 41 multiparous women, Brazelton (6) concluded that there was a 24 to 48 hour lag in the neonates' ability to breast feed as a result of the administration of barbiturates one to six hours prior to delivery. The percentage of responsive feeding of the neonate whose mothers had received barbiturates only became equal to the control neonates on the fifth and sixth day.

Kron et al. (21) found that infants born to mothers given 200 mg of secobarbital intravenously 10 to 180 minutes prior to delivery had only slightly lower Apgar scores, but they exhibited markedly reduced sucking rates and pressures and consumed less nutrients than the infants from nonmedicated mothers. These effects lasted for at least five days, the time the infants remained in the nursery. Sucking rates as well as average pressures developed during sucking were found to be significantly reduced in infants born to mothers addicted to heroin or methadone compared with a control group born to normal mothers and a second control group born to toxemic mothers (22). The subgroup of infants born to methadone-addicted mothers was significantly more depressed with regard to sucking behavior than those born to heroin-addicted mothers.

Sucking time, count, and rate, as well as feed intake were studied in 210 neonates for the first four days of life by Dubignon et al. (9). One-third of the babies had one or more nonoptimal factors (pre- and postmaturity, long labors, breech deliveries, etc.). In this heterogenous and unselected group of babies nutritive sucking scores were influenced by the length of labor, the type of delivery, and by anesthesia. Food intake over four days was influenced by length of labor, sedation, birthweight, gestational age, Apgar rating, and parity of mothers. Neither the identity, amount, or time of administration of sedatives, nor the identity of the anesthetic agents was given. Kraemer et al. (20) studied the first postnatal feeding at 12 hours of age of 124 term, normal infants. An Esterline Angus event recorder measured the number of feeding intervals and the duration of both the feeding and nonfeeding intervals. The "length of labor, parity, and drugs are all shown to affect behavior, with length of labor exerting the strongest influence on the particular types of behavior studied." It should be noted that the most frequent analgesics used were alphaprodine (29.8%) and meperidine (22.7%). In their largest subgroup of patients, these two drugs were given 4.79 ($\pm$2.37) hours before delivery. Caudal anesthesia, using an unidentified local anesthetic, was used for 64% of deliveries. The length of the first and second stages of labor was not stated.

Habituation

Sixty term, normal, female infants were classified into two groups according to whether or not a general anesthetic had been administered (23). There was "no evidence of differential distribution of either type or dosage of analgesic agents in the two anesthesia groups." At a mean age of 41 hours ($\pm$11.13), each infant was exposed to 40 presentations of either 90 dB auditory stimulus or somesthetic stimulation with a paint brush. Cardiac acceleration response and ipsilateral eye movements were scored by two independent observers from a polygraph recording. Habituation to the auditory stimulation, measured by eye movements, occurred on the fifth exposure in those infants whose mothers received a general anesthetic and on the eighth exposure in those not exposed to general anesthesia ($p <$ .03), but there was no difference in habituation measured by cardiac acceleration. On somesthetic stimulation, habituation occurred on the seventh exposure in the nongeneral anesthesia group and fourteenth in the general anesthesia group ($p <$ .03).

Brackbill et al. (3, 4) studied 25 neonates. They compared the effect of maternal administration of meperidine with lack of exposure to meperidine on habituation to noise. Babies in the meperidine group took twice as long to habituate ($p <$ .0001). Habituation to the orientating reflex was negatively correlated with meperidine dosage ($r = .852, p <$ .001). In another study (37), auditory habituation of 24 newborns aged between 46 and 66 hours was studied. The stimulus was a two-second burst of white noise presented at random intervals of 5 to 15 seconds. The response (a startle) was measured on a four-point scale ranging from no response to a full Moro-like reflex. The absence of response to five consecutive exposures was defined as habituation. The amount, time of administration, and identity of anesthetic and analgesic agents were not given, but the authors found "a significant linear increment in trials to criterion as a function of medication level."

Brazelton Neurobehavioral Scale

Brackbill et al. (3, 4) compared the effect on the baby of the administration of meperidine with the absence of maternal meperidine. The assessment criteria was a modified Brazelton Neurobehavioral Scale. Neonates were tested at a mean age of 28.4 hours. All were delivered by uncomplicated epidural anesthesia using 2% prilocaine. The babies, labor, and the mothers were all completely normal. Eleven mothers received no meperidine, four mothers received 50 mg, five mothers 75 mg, four mothers 100 mg, and one mother 150 mg. The Brazelton Scale, defense to air block, interest in the tester's voice, consolability, cuddliness, number of states entered, number of startles, and the total score were all depressed at a statistically significant level ($p <$ .05 to <.001). This study concluded that "the greater the environmental demands on the infant and the more complex the action required of him to cope with these demands, the greater the difference in quality of performance among infants in terms of their perinatal premedication history."

In a further study, neonatal neurobehavioral patterns, using the Brazelton Scale, were studied in the first month of life (1). Each neonate was examined on each of the first five days of life and then on days 7, 10, and 28. Drug administration was expressed in multiples of a basic dose (e.g., meperdine 50 mg, morphine 10 mg, or alphaprodine 30 mg). "A high drug score could be obtained with a high dosage of one drug, with many drugs, or with a combination of a relatively high dosage and relatively many drugs." The items of the Brazelton Score with the largest relationship to drugs were habituation, orientation, responsiveness, smiles, and cuddliness.

Standley et al. (34) studied the possible effect of local anesthetics and analgesics given to the mother on 60 first-born infants age 48 to 72 hours. The Brazelton Score was divided into three cluster scores: alertness, irritability, and motor maturity. The administration of local anesthetics was correlated with decreased motor maturity and greater irritability. Analgesics were correlated with lower scores on motor maturity. This study was criticized (12) in that the authors combined all forms of local and regional techniques (42 of the 52 patients receiving regional anesthesia had saddle block, spinal anesthesia with minimal dosage of tetracaine); they did not differentiate between ester (tetracaine, chloroprocaine) and amide (lidocaine, mepivacaine and bupivacaine) type local anesthetics; they did not consider that 39 babies were delivered by forceps and that the control group, receiving no anesthesia or analgesia, consisted of only seven babies.

Tronick et al. (36) examined 54 normal infants within 12 hours of delivery by means of the Scanlon Early Neonatal Neurobehavioral Test on days 1, 2, 3, 4, 5, 7; and 10 by means of the Brazelton Scale. The babies were classified in three groups: a minimal drug group, an analgesic group, and an epidural group. Twenty babies were in a minimal drug group whose mothers received no medication, a lidocaine spinal, or lidocaine local infiltration just prior to delivery. The analgesic group consisted of 20 infants whose mothers received alphaprodine (less than or equal to 60 mg) and/or promazine, alone or with a spinal or local infiltration. The epidural group consisted of 14 neonates. Ten mothers in the epidural group received either mepivacaine or lidocaine alone, while four received them with alphaprodine and promazine. The epidural group of infants had diminished tone in the first 12 hours. The authors concluded: "The results of this study demonstrate that low dosages of certain medications administered to women during labor and delivery have minimal effects on the behavior of their newborn infants. Local anesthesia and analgesic premedication produced few significant behavioral changes." The amount of alphaprodine used was approximately equal to 100 mg of meperidine and the time of administration was not given.

Scanlon's Early Neonatal Neurobehavioral Scale

The Early Neonatal Neurobehavioral Scale (31) was used to assess 28 infants whose mothers had received continuous lumbar epidural blocks with either lidocaine or mepivacaine, and 13 infants whose mothers did not receive epidural blocks. The babies exposed to lidocaine or mepivacaine showed decreased muscle power and tone and a reduced decremental response to pinprick at two, four, and six hours. A further study by the same group (28) evaluated 20 neonates, two to four hours of age, whose mothers had received epidural anesthesia with bupivacaine. The mean dose was 112 mg ($\pm$7) and the mean time elapsing between the first dose and delivery was 177 minutes ($\pm$22). No demonstrable difference was found from control infants and they did not show the decreased muscle tone and strength observed following lidocaine and mepivacaine.

Scanlon (29) also evaluated neurobehavioral function at four to six hours after birth of 14 infants delivered by cesarean section under tetracaine spinal anesthesia and this was compared with that of eight infants delivered under thiopental general anesthesia. Preanesthetic medication was considerably greater in the spinal group. Only three patients in the general anesthetic group received pentobarbital (75 to 100 mg), whereas seven patients in the spinal group received 100 mg pentobarbital and nine received 50 mg meperidine. Gravidity, gestational age, maternal age, mean birth weight and Apgar scores did not differ significantly. Despite the small number of cases there was a significant ($p < .05$) depression of pinprick response, habituation to pinprick, tone, rooting, and response to sound. In no test did the general anesthesia group outperform the spinal group.

The ENNS was used in a series of trials by Hodgkinson et al. to assess the effect of drugs on the neonate on the first and second day after birth (13–17). All mothers were free of complicating diseases and their ages ranged between 18 and 35 years. All babies were more than 2500 g in weight, normal, term, and had Apgar scores of 7 or above at one minute and 10 at five minutes. The evaluator was unaware of the anesthetic management, the method of delivery, or the perinatal risk factors.

In a group of 88 babies delivered by elective cesarean section (14) 31 received tetracaine spinal anesthesia, 26 had been induced into general anesthesia with less than 1 mg/kg of ketamine and 31 with less than 3 mg/kg of thiopental. Infants delivered under spinal anesthesia had a greater percentage of high scores on the following neurobehavioral tests: overall score, pinprick response, tone, rooting, Moro response, placing, and habituation to pinprick on day 1. Thiopental anesthesia gave the lowest neurobehavioral scores; ketamine gave intermediate scores. On day 2, the differences were less marked, but scores for overall response, rooting, and placing showed a statistically significant difference between the spinal and thiopental groups. In a further group of 274 neonates delivered vaginally, ketamine-nitrous oxide anesthesia was given to 45 mothers, thiopental-nitrous oxide to 52, and a chloroprocaine epidural block to 177 (16). Chloroprocaine epidural block was associated with the greatest percentage of high scores on both the first and second day for overall assessment, tone, rooting, sucking, Moro response, placing, alertness, and habituation to pinprick. No relationship was found between neurobehavior and low forceps extraction, oxytocin augmentation, parity, or duration of labor.

The ENNS was used to evaluate changes in neurobehavior of 920 babies on the first and second day of life that were associated with maternal administration of 0 mg, 50 mg, and 75 to 150 mg of meperidine intravenously in the four hours before delivery (17). The anesthetic given to the mothers was chloroprocaine epidural block for 280 mothers, lidocaine pudendal block for 280, thiopental-nitrous oxide anesthesia for 180, and ketamine-nitrous oxide anesthesia for 180. Neurobehavioral test scores were lower on both the first and second day in babies whose mothers had received meperidine, and the effect was greater at high than at low dosage. A significant difference was found in the percentage of high scores for overall effect, tone, rooting, sucking, Moro response, placing, alertness, and decremental score to pinprick ($p < .05$ to .001). Depression was present regardless of the type of anesthetic given, but was more marked following thiopental and ketamine general anesthesia. For most tests, there was a 10 to 20% reduction in the number of babies showing high scores following the maternal administration of 50 mg of meperidine and 10 to 40% in those exposed to 75 mg or more.

Clark et al. (7) compared the effect of intravenous naloxone, given to the mother 15 minutes prior to delivery, on the neurobehavior of babies whose mothers had received moderately large doses of meperidine (150 to 500 mg) with babies whose mothers had received no meperidine. The mean interval of the last dose of meperidine to delivery was 55 minutes. The neurobehavioral scores of the meperidine/naloxone group was depressed markedly at birth compared with the no meperidine group.

Wiener et al. (38) compared the effects of neonatal intravenous administration of 40 μg of naloxone with normal saline and the effects of an intramuscular injection of 200 μg of naloxone with normal saline. Following intramuscular, but not intravenous, injection of naloxone, the following neurobehavioral parameters were improved for up to 48 hours: response to light, rooting, sucking, Moro response, and defensive movements to an obstructed airway. In a further study (13) the administration of 40 μg of naloxone intravenously, 15 minutes before delivery, was used to counteract the effects of meperidine. There were three groups of neonates. Twenty-eight were delivered to mothers receiving neither meperidine nor naloxone, 33 to mothers receiving meperidine (50 to 200 mg), and 40 to mothers receiving meperidine (50 to 200 mg) and naloxone (400 μg). At two hours, there was no statistical difference in overall score, tone, rooting, sucking, Moro response, response to sound, placing, alertness, and decremental score to pinprick between the no narcotic group and the meperidine-naloxone group. However, there was a statistical difference in all these parameters, except response to sound, at four and thirty hours. Comparing the meperidine and the no-meperidine groups, there was a significant difference in all the above parameters at two and four hours and in all, except tone and Moro response, at 24 hours. It was concluded that intravenous naloxone given to the mother 15 minutes before delivery counteracted the effects of mepridine for approximately two hours.

Other Neurobehavioral Scales

Three behavioral tests were used by Conway and Brackbill (8) in 1970 to follow 23 infants for four weeks after birth. The Graham Scale Test was originally designed to assess behavioral deficit in the neonate. It consists of an assessment of muscle tension, of the extent to which the infant visually follows an object, and a maturation subscale. The orientation test is a measure of ability to inhibit response to a two-second burst of white noise presented at a mean interval of 10 seconds (range 5 to 15 seconds). Five successive no responses is the criterion of extinction. The Bayley Scale Test was designed for infants up to three years of age and was used for the assessment at four weeks. The potency of medication, summarizing the agent, the dosage, and the timing was defined for the study "as the mean score derived from the independent rankings of two experienced obstetricians." On testing at two and five days, the potency of medication was inversely related to muscle tension on the Graham Scale ($p < .001$), and orientation ($p < .005$). At four weeks of age the total Bayley Scale was also inversely related to medication potency ($p < .02$), as was orientation ($p < .01$). Comparing the babies from mothers who had received no anesthetic with those mothers receiving local anesthetic or general anesthetic, the general anesthetic group was most depressed in terms of muscle tension and visual response at two and five days.

   In a study by Yang et al. (39) 85 neonates from primiparous mothers were tested at a mean age of 58 hours (± 8.41). Six sleep variables were measured to sample basal level functioning under conditions of minimal external stimulation. The six assessments consisted of the percentage and duration of, and the autonomic variability during both the second active and the second quiet period of sleep. The total number of sucks were counted and discriminative sucking measured to represent behavior under moderate stimulation. Discriminative sucking was the difference between the "total amount of sucking on the nipple and the total amount of sucking on a tube." The five cry variables represented the infant's behavior under conditions of aversive stimulation. The cry measurements were cry latency measured by the time elapsing between the withdrawing of a standard rubber nipple and the first cry; the total number of cries; the total number of cries in 60 seconds in response to a rubber band snapped against the instep of the left foot; the rate of recovery from this aversive stimulation and the reaction to aversive stimulation with intervention (counting the number of cries occurring in the 60 seconds following completion of swaddling after aversion stimulation). The drugs used in this study included meperidine, scopolamine, promethazine, pentobarbital, promazine, hydroxyzine, and secobarbital. The mean number of drugs given was 3.33 ($\pm$2.32) and the time elapsing between the estimated point of maximal effect and delivery was 168 minutes ($\pm$132). Thirteen mothers did not receive analgesics. The authors found that there was a negative correlation between the total number of drugs administered to the mother and the Apgar score. The relationship between the maternal medication variables and newborn behaviors were minimal and of low magnitude in most cases. The authors pointed out that the lack of effect may have been due to the long duration of time elapsing between the time of maximal drug effect and delivery.

Parental-Neonate Interaction

The effect of obstetric medication on mother-infant interaction has recently received increasing attention (26). The early relationship may have a significant role on the later development of the infant. In modifying neonatal neurobehavior, medication may in turn have an effect on the behavior of both the mother and father. In a study of parental-child behavior 6 to 48 hours after delivery, Parke et al. (24) found a positive correlation between medication and maternal vocalization and rocking and a negative correlation between medication and paternal vocalization and rocking. As medication increases maternal interaction increases and paternal interaction decreases, possible because the mother becomes more eager for the child to respond and the father becomes disinterested.

Discussion

Differences in designing and describing clinical trials on neonatal neurobehavioral testing can lead to differences in results between investigators (Table 7.1). The effect of a maternally administered drug on the neonate depends on the drug's identity, dosage, route of administration, and the time elapsing between administration and delivery. Other drugs, including anes-

Table 7.1   Difficulties in Neurobehavioral Clinical Trials

1. Independent variable: drug, dosage, route, time of delivery, other drugs
2. Dependent variable: ranking scale
3. Age of neonate
4. Inter- and intraobserver errors
5. Echo results and prior test bias
6. Minor variation in technique

thetic agents, may modify its action. Unfortunately, many papers fail to give these data and become difficult to evaluate. Obstetricians use a variety of analgesics and tranquilizers in different combinations and dosages at various times before delivery. Unless a standardized protocol can be accepted by the obstetrician, one solution to this dilemma rests in having a second observer assign for evaluation all cases receiving the medication under review, and all cases meeting rigidly defined criteria for the control series.

A number of papers, however, use a modification of the rating scale of Sostek et al. (33), which describes drug administration as 1 = none, 2 = local anesthetic only, 3 = analgesic only, 4 = local anesthesia + analgesic, 5 = spinal, caudal, and pudendal block, and 6 = general anesthesia. Intrinsic in this scale is just sufficient hint of increasing usage of drugs with increasing numerical order to make the scale a trap for the unwary who analyze it as if it were a ranking or ratio scale. The minute dosage of local anesthetic used for spinal anesthesia is lumped with the relatively huge dose used for caudal block and separated from the considerable dose used for local infiltration. Fragmented information, apparently designed for a computer rather than for a clinician, is used particularly in one paper in which exposure to drugs is described by number of drug administrations per patient, time of effective administration of first and last drug, and time of maximal effect. One of the better methods (8) is a scheme where "potency of labor-delivery medication was defined as a mean score derived from the independent rankings of two experienced obstetricians." However, the question then becomes how do obstetricians rank potency: by pain relief or liability to produce neonatal depression? Several papers (34, 35) give a weighted drug dosage depending on time of administration relative to delivery. The principle is sound, but the weighting given can only be described as an intelligent guess.

If authors encountered a major difficulty in describing the independent variables (i.e., identity of the drug, the dosage, the route, and time of drug administration), this is compounded by difficulty with the dependent variables. All neurobehavioral tests are on ranking scales; $4 > 3 > 2 > 1$ but

4 does not equal 2×2. The familiar Apgar score is also assessed on a ranking scale and this may be used to demonstrate possible errors. Assign different numbers to the Apgar score, weighting it so that greater emphasis is given to heart rate and respiration and less to color, and call it the "Century Apgar Score" (Table 7.2). This is a perfectly permissible maneuver with a ranking scale if the "better" value has a higher number than that given to the "poorer" value. Using the "Century Apgar Score," the two babies A and B, which had both a conventional Apgar score of 6, now have scores of 4.6 and 8.0.

In analyzing data on a ranking scale, arithmetic processes such as means and standard deviations should not be used without careful consideration, and preference given to the employment of nonparametric statistics [e.g., chi square]. If parametric statistics (including means, standard deviations, t-tests, analysis of variance, etc.) are to be employed, they should be used with caution and checked whenever possible against a nonparametric test. For the same reason, the practice of giving the results of neurobehavioral tests, as cluster scores, is suspect.

A number of investigators have assessed babies at widely different times after birth (e.g., 48 hours $\pm$ 25). Presumably, the effect of the drug on the neonate wears off with time and those examined at an excessively long time after delivery will show no drug effects. This may dilute the positive data obtained at an earlier time.

Interobserver variations in testing can be eliminated by using only one evaluator, or defined, but not corrected, by giving a statistical measure of the variability between the investigators. The effects of day-to-day intra-

Table 7.2   Ranking Scales: Two Babies with Apgar Score of 6

Conventional Apgar Scoring	0	1	2
"Century" apgar score			
Heart rate	0	25 A	50 B
Respiratory effort	0 A	18	20 B
Response	0 B	2	10 A
Tone	0	9 A B	18
Color	0	1 B	2 A

Baby	Total Score	
	Conventional Apgar	"Century" Apgar
Baby A	6	46
Baby B	6	80

observer variation can be minimized by evaluating an approximately equal number of patients from each treatment group each day. Repeated "quality checks" on evaluators are mandatory.

Echo results (repeat examinations on the same baby producing similar results) are probably a limited source of error unless earlier findings are available to the evaluator. However, there is no obvious answer to prior test bias (obtaining a low score on the earlier items on the ENNS or Brazelton scale and then producing a low score on later items). Apart from these scores of error, discrepancies between investigators are frequently due to variations in testing techniques.

Despite these difficulties, certain conclusions seem to be warranted about particular drugs. From the many papers that described the effect of several drugs acting together (e.g., compare a heavily medicated group with a non-medicated group), the general summary may be made that most analgesics, anesthetics, and tranquilizers depress most neurobehavioral tests for at least 48 hours.

Local anesthetics have not so far been shown to have a potent effect on neurobehavioral studies. Lidocaine and mepivacaine appear to affect the muscle tone and produce an "alert but floppy baby." This does not appear to be the case with bupivacaine and chloroprocaine.

Meperidine has been the most fully investigated analgesic. Blood levels show that it freely passes through the placental interchange and that fetal levels may be considerable (32). Maternal intravenous administration produces an immediate effect on the fetal electroencephalogram and changes persist for at least three days (27). The duration of sleep, especially non-REM sleep, is increased. Newborn attention is decreased. The neonate takes twice as long to habituate to auditory stimulus and these changes persist for at least three days. The Scanlon tests for at least the first 48 hours are decreased, as are many of the Brazelton scores.

The barbiturates have been demonstrated to depress the electroencephalogram as well as the sucking reflex; the latter may persist for several days. Little is known regarding the effect of tranquilizers. However, diazepam has been shown to depress thermoregulation and muscular tone.

References

1. Aleksandrowicz, M.K., Aleksandrowicz, D.R.: Obstetrical pain-relieving drugs as predictors of infant behavior variability. Child. Dev. **45**:935, 1974.
2. Borgstedt, A.D., Rosen, M.G.: Medication during labor correlated with behavior and EEG of the newborn. Am. J. Dis. Child. **115**:21, 1968.
3. Brackbill, Y., Kane, J., Manniello, R.L., Abramson, D.: Obstetrical meperidine usage and assessment of neonatal status. Anesthesiology **40**:116, 1974a.

4. Brackbill, Y., Kane, J., Manniello, R.L., Abramson, D.: Obstetrical pre-medication and infant outcome. Am. J. Obstet. Gynecol. **118**:337, 1974b.

5. Brackbill, Y.: Psychophysiological measures of pharmacological toxicity in infants: perinatal and post natal effects, in Morselli, P.L. et al. (eds.): Basic and Therapeutic Aspects of Perinatal Pharmacology. New York, Raven Press, 1975.

6. Brazelton, T.B.: Psychologic reaction in the neonate, II: Effects of maternal medication on the neonate and his behavior. J. Pediatr. **58**:513, 1961.

7. Clark, R.B., Beard, A.G., Greifenstein, F.E., Barclay, D.L.: Naloxone in the parturient and her infant. South. Med. J. **69**:570, 1976.

8. Conway, E., Brackbill, Y.: Delivery medication and infant outcome: an empirical study, in Bowes, W.A. et al. (eds.): The Effects of Obstetrical Medication on the Fetus and Infant. Monogr. Soc. Res, Child. Dev. **35**:24, 1970.

9. Dubignon, J., Campbell, D., Curtis, M., Partington, M.W.: The relation between laboratory measures of sucking, food intake, and perinatal factors during the newborn period. Child. Dev. **40**:1107, 1969.

10. Emde, R.N., Swedberg, J., Suzuki, B.: Human wakefulness and biological rhythms after birth. Arch. Gen. Psychiatry **32**:780, 1975.

11. Finster, M.: Toxicity of local anesthetics in the fetus and newborn. Bull. N.Y. Acad. Med. **52**:222, 1976.

12. Hodgkinson, R., Marx, G.F., Kaiser, I.H.: Local-regional anesthesia during childbirth and newborn behavior. Science 189:571.

13. Hodgkinson, R., Bhatt, M., Grewal, G., Marx, G.F.: Neonatal neurobehavior in the first 48 hours of life. Effect of meperidine with, and without naloxone on the Scanlon Neonatal Neurobehavioral Test. Pediatrics **62**:294, 1978.

14. Hodgkinson, R., Bhatt, M., Kim, S.S., Grewal, G., Marx, G.F.: Neonatal neurobehavioral tests following cesarean delivery under general and spinal anesthesia. Am. J. Obstet. Gynecol. **132**(6)670, 1978.

15. Hodgkinson, R., Wang, C.N., Marx, G.F.: Evaluation of the effects of general anesthesia and pethidine on neurobehavioral tests during the first 2 days of life. Paper presented at Obstetrical Anaesthetists Assoc. West Yorkshire Meeting, Bradford, England, September 1975.

16. Hodgkinson, R., Marx, G.F., Kim, S.S., Miclat, N.M.: Neonatal neurobehavioral tests following vaginal delivery under ketamine, thiopental and extradural anesthesia. Anesth. Analg. **56**(4):548, 1977.

17. Hodgkinson, R., Bhatt, M., Kim, S.S., Wang, C.N.: Double blind comparison of the neurobehavior of different doses of meperidine to the mother. Canad. Anaesth. Soc. J. **25**(5), 1978.

18. Hughes, J.G., Ehemann, B., Brown, U.A.: Electroencephalography of the newborn: III. Brain potentials of babies born of mothers given "Seconal Sodium." Am. J. Dis. Child. **76**:626, 1948.

19. Hughes, J.G., Hill, F.S., Green, C.R., Davis, B.C.: Electroencephalography of the newborn: V: Brain potentials of the babies born of mothers given meperidine hydrochloride (Demerol hydrochloride), vinbarbital sodium (Delvinal sodium) or morphine. Am. J. Dis. Child, **79**:996, 1950.

20. Kraemer, H., Korner, A., Thoman, E.: Methodological considerations in

evaluating the influence of drugs used during labor and delivery on the behavior of the newborn. Dev. Psychol. 6:128, 1972.

21. Kron, R.E., Stein, M., Goddard, K.E.: Newborn sucking behavior affected by obstetric sedation. Am. J. Psychiatry 37:1012, 1966.

22. Kron, R.E., Litt, M., Finnegan, L.P.: Narcotic addiction in the newborn: Differences in behavior generated by methadone and heroin. Clin. Pharmacol. Ther. 12:63, 1975.

23. Moreau, T., Birch, H.G.: Relationship between obstetrical general anesthesia and rate of neonatal habituation to repeated stimulation. Dev. Med. Child. Neurol. 16:612, 1974.

24. Parke, R.D., O'Leary, S.E., West, S.: Mother-father-newborn interaction: effects of maternal medication, labor and sex of infant. Proc. Annu. Meet. Am. Psychopathol. Assoc., 1972.

25. Quimby, K.L., Aschkenase, L.J., Bowman, R.E., et al. Enduring learning deficits and cerebral synaptic malformation from exposure to 10 parts of halothane per million. Science 185:625, 1974.

26. Richards, M.P.M., Bernal, J.F.: Effects of obstetric medication on mother-infant interaction and infant development. Presented at the Third International Congress of Psychomatic Medicine in Obstetrics and Gynaecology, London, April 1971.

27. Rosen, M.G., Scibetta, J.J., Hochberg, C.J.: Human fetal electroencephalogram: III. Pattern changes in presence of fetal heart rate alterations and after use of maternal medications. Obstet. Gynecol. 36:132.

28. Scanlon, J.W., Ostheimer, G.W., Lurie, A.O., et al.: Neurobehavioral responses and drug concentrations in newborn after maternal epidural anesthesia with bupivacaine. Anesthesiology 45:400, 1976.

29. Scanlon, J.W., Shea, E., Alper, M.H.: Neurobehavioral responses of newborn infants following general or spinal anesthesia for cesarean section. Paper read at ASA Meeting, Chicago, October 1975.

30. Scanlon, J.W.: Effects of local anesthetics administered to parturient women on the neurological and behavioral performance of newborn children. Bull. N.Y. Acad. Med. 52:231, 1976.

31. Scanlon, J.W., Brown, W.U., Weiss, J.B., Alper, M.H.: Neurobehavioral responses of newborn infants after maternal epidural anesthesia. Anesthesiology 40:121, 1974.

32. Shier, R.W., Sprague, A.D., Dilts, P.V.: Placental transfer of meperidine HC1. Am. J. Obstet. Gynecol. 115:556, 1974.

33. Sostek, A.M., Sameroff, A.J., Sostek, A.J.: Evidence for the unconditionability of the Babkin Reflex in newborns. Child. Dev. 45:509, 1972.

34. Standley, .K., Soule, A.B. III, Copans, S.A., Duchowny, M.S.: Local-regional anesthesia during childbirth: Effect on newborn behaviors. Science 186:634, 1974.

35. Stechler, G.: Newborn attention as affected by medication during labor. Science 144:315, 1964.

36. Tronick, E., Wise, S., Als, H., et al.: Regional obstetric anesthesia and newborn behavior: Effect over the first ten days of life. Pediatrics 58:94, 1976.

37. Vander Maelon, A.L., Strauss, M.E., Starr, R.H.: Influence of obstetric medication on auditory habituation in the newborn. Dev. Psychol. 11:711, 1975.
38. Wiener, P.C., Hogg, M.I., Rosen, M.: Paper U.K. Obstetric Anesthetists Assoc., September 1976.
39. Yang, R.K., Zweig, A.R., Douthitt, T.C., Federman, E.J.: Successive relationships between maternal attitudes during pregnancy, analgesic medication during labor and delivery, and newborn behavior. Dev. Psychol. 12:6, 1976.

8
Drug Sensitivity of the Neonate

Simon Halevy

Neonatal pharmacology is a developing, and fascinating, branch of modern pharmacology. A number of reviews have been published recently (31, 46–48), but many questions remain unanswered. Sensitivity to drugs, including anesthetics, is greater in the neonatal period than at any other time of life. This increased susceptibility may occur as a consequence of certain prenatal conditions, e.g., presence of maternal inhibitory factors such as female gonadal hormones, influence of growth hormone (47), or inadequacy of some hepatic functions (48); it may result from perinatal drug exposure (including drug ingestion through breast milk), or may constitute a specific drug sensitivity. Predisposing factors of special interest to the anesthesiologist concern hepatic microsomal and other enzyme induction or depression, maternal drug dependence, and various genetic conditions (11, 13, 14, 18, 29, 35, 47). The genetic factors act either by altering the action of the drug on the organism (e.g., malignant hyperthermia; hemolysis due to glucose-6-phosphate dehydrogenase deficiency; drug-sensitive hemoglobins), or by altering the body's response to the drug (e.g., abnormal succinylcholine hydrolysis; methemoglobinemia due to defective hydroxylation of phenacetin) (20, 25, 29, 42).

Mechanisms of the altered reaction to drugs in the newborn infant may reside in drug absorption, distribution, metabolism, elimination, as well as in receptor responsiveness. Each of these factors is subject to genetic and environmental influences.

Drug Absorption

Drug absorption in the neonate has not been systematically investigated. However, there are data showing special effects following oral as well as parenteral administration (2, 17, 23, 26, 38, 39, 48). Gastric pH is generally higher in the newborn infant than in the adult; this facilitates absorption of weaker basic drugs which are less ionized in an alkaline medium (37). Similarly, long-acting sulfonamides and ampicillin showed a greater absorption in newborns than in adults (46, 47). The intestinal activity of beta-glucuronidase is increased; this tends to enhance the reabsorption of glucuronides, which are excreted through bile into the intestine (47, 48).

Regional vasomotor instability in a hypoxic infant, or one exposed to cold, may lead to irregular absorption from intramuscular or subcutaneous routes of injection (47). Hypothermia has also been noted to impair perfusion in localized regions such as the splanchnic bed, resulting in decreased hepatic blood flow and, consequently, delayed drug absorption and retarded detoxification.

Drug Distribution

In contrast to absorption, drug distribution has been extensively investigated. Anesthetics, sedatives, and tranquilizers are primarily lipophilic drugs, and the high water content of the developing brain might be expected to limit their uptake (17). This, however, is counteracted by a higher proportion of lipid mass in the central nervous system than in other tissues. In addition, drug entry into the brain nerve tissue is facilitated by temporary, but incomplete, myelinization. Consequently, the cerebral concentration of these drugs tends to be increased and their pharmacologic action may be pronounced. Thus, narcotics given to the mother in clinical doses during labor have depressant effects on the neonate's respiration at birth.

Serum protein binding is limited in the newborn, accounting for alterations in bilirubin metabolism as well as drug interactions due to binding displacement (12, 28, 36). Because of high protein binding properties, drugs such as sulfisoxazole, diazepam, and caffeine sodium benzoate tend to displace bilirubin from binding sites, thus favoring the development of hyperbilirubinemia and kernicterus. In contrast, phenobarbital, diphenylhydantoin, and certain antibiotics possess less protein binding capacity than bilirubin; this leaves more free drug in the serum, thus enhancing their pharmacologic action. Most of the present work in this area is related to the distribution of antibiotics, the most commonly used drugs in the neonate, but similar effects may be anticipated from other medications, including anesthetics.

Drug Metabolism

Neonatal drug metabolism has undergone intensive investigation over the past 20 years (8). An early study revealed the absence of side-chain oxidation of hexobarbital in rabbits less than two weeks of age as well as lack of N-dealkylation of aminopyrine, of sulfur oxidation of chlorpromazine, nitro-reduction of p-nitrobenzoic acid and aromatic hydroxylation of acetanilid (15). Despite considerable variations between strains and, at times, sexes, most investigators have demonstrated prolonged sleeping times secondary to decreased hexobarbital enzymatic metabolism by hepatic microsomes in newborn mice (21, 24), rabbits, rats, and guinea-pigs (15, 16, 24, 34). Thus, drug metabolism is temporarily decreased in the newborns of most mammalian species studied.

These findings also apply to the human neonate. Glucuronidation and other conjugative processes, as well as oxidative metabolism, are decreased in the early postnatal period. Inefficient glucuronidation accounts for the prolonged half-lives of p-aminobenzoic acid, p-aminophenol, derivatives of acetanilid (a compound related to local anesthetics), salicylamide, and chloramphenicol, while diminished oxidative processes are responsible for the protracted effects of diazepam and aminopyrine. Reduced bilirubin conjugation results in neonatal hyperbilirubinemia, as mentioned earlier. The half-lives of ethanol, nortriptyline, and diphenylhydantoin were noted to be prolonged following maternal administration (and placental transfer) of these drugs. Interestingly, when diphenylhydantoin was given to the newborns themselves for the treatment of convulsive disorders, the half-life of the drug appeared to be "normal" (13, 47).

Different enzymatic metabolic processes do not develop at the same rate, at least with respect to the human fetus. For instance, the microsomal cytochrome P-450 system and the uridine diphosphate (UDP) glucuronyl transferase system both depend on the development of liver smooth endoplasmic reticulum, which can be identified in the third month of gestation. However, the cytochrome P-450 system becomes active earlier than UDP-glucuronyl transferase. At birth, this is reflected in a relatively fast metabolism of drugs such as chlorpromazine, meperidine, or hexobarbital, and relatively slow breakdown of drugs such as diazepam or p-nitrophenol derivatives (10, 18). As a consequence of the more rapid enzymatic development, various metabolites of chlorpromazine and of meperidine have been identified in the infant's tissues as early as 24 hours after delivery (33).

Neonatal drug metabolism and disposition may also be influenced by external factors. One of these is hypothermia, which can alter both the enzymatic activity and the splanchnic and hepatic perfusion with resultant delay in drug metabolism. This has been demonstrated in newborn puppies following intravenous lidocaine administration as well as in other species with different drugs (32). Nutritional status and housing are other environmental conditions that may affect drug metabolism in the newborn, as they do in adults (40, 41). For instance, weaning of mice is associated with reduced sleeping time and increased *in vivo* hexobarbital oxidation (47).

In addition to species variations, there is considerable individual variability within the same species, making it difficult to establish a "normal" range of time for a newborn's increased sensitivity to drugs. These individual variations, which depend on genetic, hormonal and environmental factors, have been altered experimentally as well as therapeutically (13, 21, 35). A representative example of "manipulation" of the neonate's response to drugs is the prophylactic administration (via placental transfer) of phenobarbital to induce hepatic microsomal activity of glucuronyl transferase. This enzyme induction facilitates conjugation of bilirubin, thus decreasing the amount of circulating free bilirubin with resultant reduction in the degree of hyperbilirubinemia and the risk of kernicterus (6, 13, 48). However, enzyme induction is nonspecific and may, therefore, involve other enzymes as well. Such additional activity may lead to the production of toxic metabolites of certain drugs including anesthetics (19), or to enhanced hormonal metabolism with endocrine changes (e.g., testosterone deficiency in phenobarbital pretreated infants).

Enzyme inhibition has also been suggested to occur in neonates. For instance, the presence of pregnanediol in the maternal milk tends to suppress glucuronidation; this may explain why infants of nursing mothers show more prolonged jaundice than bottle-fed newborns.

Drug Elimination

The most important route of drug elimination is via the urinary tract.

Renal plasma flow is reduced in the neonate by approximately 30%, and kidney function, as assessed by urine volume, total osmolarity, urea clearance, and glomerular filtration rate, is limited during the first days of life, although glomerular development is completed in utero. The newborn is unable to excrete hydrogen ion through the renal tubules. Elimination of a water load or some antibiotics is greatly delayed (4). This limitation of renal function during the early postnatal period has been explained on the basis of glomerulo-tubular imbalance due, in part, to the decrease in glomerular filtration rate. There is also evidence that the supply of antidiuretic hormone is reduced and that the tubules do not respond maximally to the available ADH (1).

The decreased renal perfusion is possibly a result of low perfusion pressure, due to low arterial blood pressure (27). This is important for the anesthesiologist as renal blood flow may be further impaired by hypotension or vasoconstriction.

There are no specific data establishing a direct relationship between altered renal functions and sensitivity to anesthetic drugs in the human neonate, but the possibility should be kept in mind (20), particularly with the use of drugs such as tribromethanol and gallamine, which are primarily eliminated by the kidney (45).

Receptor Sensitivity

Drug receptor sensitivity is difficult to establish and has not been fully demonstrated with regard to drugs used in anesthesia. The assumption has been made that newborns may react differently to drugs because of modified receptor sensibility, but few quantitative studies are available. It has been shown that malnourished rodents are more susceptible to hexobarbital than well-fed animals, and this was explained on the basis of altered drug distribution as well as altered binding to brain receptors (47). Puppies and young rabbits are less sensitive than adult animals to the cardiac glycosides acetyl-strophantidin and ouabain, demonstrating immaturity of the cardiac receptors. Similarly, human neonates in heart failure may require larger doses of digoxin (17). In contrast, autonomic nervous system receptors appears to be fully developed in healthy term-infants. The neonatal response to adrenergic receptor stimulants and blocking agents resembles that of the adult (46). The reaction of the cardiovascular receptors of puppies to pressor agents is similar to that of older dogs (48). However, infants who were small for gestational age did not respond to the mydriatic property of tyramine suggesting that, in these disadvantaged newborns, the sympathetic system may not be fully developed (48).

The variation in neonatal response to different nondepolarizing muscle relaxants has been attributed to modified drug-receptor sensitivity. Neonates reacted to d-tubocurarine with a similar degree of muscle relaxation as adults when the drug was administered on a body-weight basis (7), but appeared to be more sensitive when the dosage was calculated on a body-surface basis (30). Newborns were also found to be resistant to the action of decamethonium. The response to pancuronium appeared enhanced, i.e., the potency, when compared with tubocurarine, was 6:1, from birth to 28 days. Sensitivity to nondepolarizing drugs was further increased in the presence of prematurity, acidosis, and hypothermia (3).

Conclusion

Increased drug sensitivity is a significant problem in the neonate. Rule-of-thumb dosage is convenient, but may be dangerous because of oversimplification. The complexity of the situation is exemplified by the neonatal response to depolarizing muscle relaxants. When succinylcholine was given to nine newborns on a body surface-dosage, the duration of neuromuscular blockade was close to that of adults in six of the infants and prolonged in three (43). The protracted effect in two neonates resulted from slow elimination of the drug, whereas in one, it was due, at least in part, to an unusual "dose-response" relationship (30). Another impressive example is the fate of meperidine in the newborn where practically all mechanisms described are involved. This accounts not only for the well-known respiratory depression, but also, as recently reported, for prolonged changes in the neurobehavioral status of the neonate (5, 9, 22, 44).

The systems involved in drug metabolism or excretion do not develop solely in proportion to the denominator, i.e., body weight or surface area. These processes also involve drug absorption, distribution, liver metabolism, and receptor reactivity, the age-dependent developments of which are expressed by a series of curves that are *not* identical (14). Therefore, as Fouts pointed out, the "recognition of the multiple causes and erratic nature of age-related changes in drug action and toxicity cannot be overemphasized."

References

1. Ames, R.G.: Urinary water excretion and neurohypophysial functions in full term and premature infants shortly after birth. Pediatrics **12**:272, 1953.
2. Bates, T.R., Gibaldi, M., Kanig, J.L.: Rate of dissolution of griseofulvin and hexoestrol in bile salt solutions. Nature **210**:1331, 1966.
3. Bennett, E.J., Ignacio, A., Patel, K., et al.: Tubocurarine and the neonate. Br. J. Anaesth. **48**:687, 1976.
4. Boe, R.W., Williams, C.P.S., Bennett, J.V., Oliver, T.K.: Serum levels of methicillin and ampicillin in newborn and premature infants in relation to postnatal age. Pediatrics **39**:194, 1967.
5. Brackbill, Y., Kane, J., Maniello, R.L., Abramson, D: Obstetric meperidine usage and assessment of neonatal status. Anesthesiology **40**:116, 1974.
6. Catz, C., Yaffe, S.J.: Strain and age variations in hexobarbital responses. J. Pharmacol. Exp. Ther. **155**:152, 1967.
7. Churchill-Davidson, H.C., Wise R.P.: Neuromuscular transmission in the newborn infant. Anesthesiology **24**:271, 1963.
8. Conney, A.H.: Pharmacological implications of microsomal enzyme induction. Pharmacol. Rev. **19**:317, 1967.
9. Corke, B.C.: Neurobehavioural responses of the newborn. The effect of different forms of maternal analgesia. Anesthesia **32**:539, 1977.
10. Crawford, J.S., Rudofsky, S.: The placental transmission of pethidine. Br. J. Anaesth. **37**:929, 1965.
11. Di Fazio, C.A., Brown, R.E.: Lidocaine metabolism in normal and phenobarbital pretreated dogs. Anesthesiology **36**:238, 1972.
12. Ehrnebo, M., Agurell, S., Jalling, B., Boréus, L.O.: Age differences in drug

binding by plasma proteins: Studies on human foetuses, neonates and adults. Eur. J. Clin. Pharmacol. **3**:189, 1971.
13. Eriksson, M., Yaffe, S.J.: Drug metabolism in the newborn. Annu. Rev. Med. **24**:29, 1973.
14. Fouts, R.J.: Microsomal mixed-function oxidases in the fetal and newborn rabbit, in Boréus, L.O. (ed.): Fetal Pharmacology. New York, Raven Press, 1973, p. 305.
15. Fouts, J.R., Adamson, R.H.: Drug metabolism in the newborn rabbit. Science **129**:897, 1959.
16. Fouts, J.R., Hart, L.G.: Hepatic metabolism during the perinatal period. Ann. N.Y. Acad. Sci. **123**:245, 1965.
17. Giacoia, G.P., Gorodisher, R.: Pharmacologic principles in neonatal drug therapy. Clin. Perinat. **2**:125, 1975.
18. Gillette, J.R., Stripp, B.: Pre- and postnatal enzyme capacity for drug metabolite production. Fed. Proc. **34**:172, 1975.
19. Gillette, J.R., Mitchell, J.R., Brodie, B.B.: Biochemical mechanisms of drug toxicity. Annu. Rev. Pharmacol. **14**:271, 1974.
20. Goldstein, A., Aronow, L., Kalman, S.M.: Principles of Drug Action: The Basis of Pharmacology, (2nd Ed.). New York, J. Wiley, 1974.
21. Halevy, S., Orkin, L.R.: Barbiturates in newborn animals: A drug response problem, in Marx, G.F. (ed.): Parturition and Perinatology. Philadelphia, F. A. Davis, 1973, p. 157.
22. Hodgkinson, R., Bhatt, M., Kim, S.S., Wang, C.N.: Double blind comparison of the neurobehavior of 920 neonates following the administration of different doses of meperidine to the mother. Abstracts of Scientific Papers, Annual Meeting of the American Society of Anesthesiologists, 1976, p. 255.
23. Hogben, C.A.M., Schanker, L.S., Tocco, D.J., Brodie, B.B.: Absorption of drugs from the stomach. II. The human. J. Pharmacol. Exp. Ther. **120**:540, 1957.
24. Jondorf, W.R., Maickel, R.P., Brodie, B.B.: Inability of newborn mice and guinea pigs to metabolize drugs. Biochem. Pharmacol. **1**:352, 1958.
25. Kalow, W.: Pharmacognetics. Heredity and Response to Drugs. Philadelphia, W. B. Saunders, 1962.
26. Katz, L., Hamilton, J.R.: Fat absorption in infants of birth weight less than 1,300 grams. J. Pediatr. **85**:608, 1974.
27. Kleinman, L.I.: Physiology of the perinatal kidney, in Stave, U. (ed.): Physiology of the Perinatal Period. New York, Appleton-Century-Crafts, 1970, p. 679.
28. Krasner, J., Giacoia, G.P., Yaffe, S.J.: Drug-protein binding in the newborn infant. Ann. N.Y. Acad. Sci. **226**:101, 1973.
29. La Du, B.N.: Pharmacogenetics: Defective enzymes in relation to reactions to drugs. Annu. Rev. Med. **23**:453, 1973.
30. Levy, G.: Pharmacokinetics of succinylcholine in newborns. Anesthesiology **32**:551, 1970.
31. Marx, G.F.: Altered drug response in obstetrics. Proceedings of the VI World Congress of Anaesthesiology, 1977, p. 532.

32. Morishima, H.O., Mueller-Heubach, E., Shnider, S.M.: Body temperature and disappearance of lidocaine in newborn puppies. Anesth. Analg. Curr. Res. **50**:938, 1971.
33. O'Donoghue, S.E.F.: Distribution of pethidine and chlorpromazine in maternal, foetal and neonatal biological fluids. Nature **229**:124, 1971.
34. Quinn, G.P., Axelrod, J., Brodie, B.B.: Species, strain and sex differences in metabolism of hexobarbitone, amidopyrine, antipyrine and aniline. Biochem. Pharmacol. **1**:152, 1958.
35. Ramboer, C., Thompson, R.P.H., Williams, R.: Controlled trials of phenobarbitone therapy in neonatal jaundice. Lancet **1**:966, 1969.
36. Rane, A., Lunde, P.K.M., Jalling, B., Yaffe, S.J., Sjöqvist, E.: Plasma protein binding of diphenylhydantoin in normal and hyperbilirubinemic infants. J. Pediat. **78**:877, 1971.
37. Schanker, L.S., Shore, P.A., Brodie, B.B., Hogben, C.A.M.: Absorption of drugs from the stomach. I. The rat. J. Pharmacol. Exp. Ther. **120**:528, 1957.
38. Schanker, L.S., Tocco, D.J., Brodie, B.B., Hogben, C.A.M.: Absorption of drugs from the rat small intestine. J. Pharmacol. Exp. Ther. **123**:81, 1958
39. Shore, P.A., Brodie, B.B., Hogben, C.A.M.: The gastric secretion of drugs: A pH partition hypothesis. J. Pharmacol. Exp. Ther. **119**:361, 1957.
40. Vesell, E.S.: Genetic and environmental factors affecting hexobarbital metabolism in mice. Ann. N.Y. Acad. Sci. **151**:900, 1968.
41. Vesell, E.S.: Factors altering the response of mice to hexobarbital. Pharmacology **1**:81, 1968.
42. Vesell, E.S.: Advances in pharmacogenetics, in Steinberg, A.G., and Bearn, A.G. (eds.): Progress in Medical Genetics, New York, Grune and Stratton, 1973, p. 291.
43. Walts, L.F., Dillon, J.B.: The response of newborns to succinylcholine and d-tubocurarine. Anesthesiology **31**:35, 1969.
44. Way, W.L., Costley, E.C., Way, E.L.: Respiratory sensitivity of the newborn infant to meperidine and morphine. Clin. Pharmacol. Ther. **6**:454, 1965.
45. Wylie, W.D., Churchill-Davidson, H.C.: A Practice of Anaesthesia, 3rd Ed. London, Lloyd-Luke, 1972.
46. Yaffe, S.J., Catz, C.S.: Pharmacology of the perinatal period. Clin. Obstet. Gynecol. **14**:722, 1971.
47. Yaffe, S.J., Juchau, M.R.: Perinatal pharmacology. Annu. Rev. Pharmacol. **14**:219, 1974.
48. Yaffe, S.J., Stern, L.: Clinical implications of perinatal pharmacology, in Mirkin, B.L. (ed.): Perinatal Pharmacology and Therapeutics. New York, Academic Press, 1976, p. 355.

9
Pulmonary Function in the Perinatal Period

Emile M. Scarpelli

To appreciate the formidable task that confronts the infant at the onset of breathing at birth, one must consider the state of the fetal lungs. The air spaces and terminal lung units are ·filled with liquid (the "liquid lung"), the volume of which is approximately the same as the functional residual capacity of the lung (67). When air breathing is generated at birth, the literally drowned lung must rapidly become a stable gas exchanger as the uteroplacental circulation is severed. Initially, air is dispersed in the prevailing liquid, producing gas entrapment in the lung primarily in the form of foam (the "foam lung") (66). During this short transitional state the vital cardiopulmonary adaptations of the newborn infant begin: alveolar-capillary gas exchange; increased pulmonary vascular perfusion; and functional elimination of right-to-left flow through the ductus arteriosus and foramen ovale. For the normal newborn infant, the foam lung disappears promptly, leaving behind a relatively liquid-free and stable air lung.

Measurement of function of the neonatal air lung has achieved rather remarkable sophistication. There are several recent reviews of the topic (4, 15, 21, 48). Several functions of the early neonatal and presumably foam lung have been recorded, and pulmonary function testing even prior to birth is now beginning to feel the "probes" of the clinician and clinical investigator.

The Prenatal Lung (Liquid Lung)

Fetal pulmonary development is marked as follows (36): The glandular stage persists through the 16th week of intrauterine life. It is characterized by what appears to be peripheral growth of the tracheobronchial system possessing terminal units of undifferentiated columnar epithelial cells. Biochemical immaturity and structural mass of the tissue would not permit normal function as an air lung. The canalicular stage extends to about the 29th week of gestation. Ultrastructurally, specific alveolar epithelial cell types appear; respiratory bronchioles emerge and develop. Again, structural and biochemical immaturity would not permit an air lung to function normally at this stage. The viable stage includes development and differentiation of the terminal lung units, the fetal alveoli. Potential viability as an air lung during this stage is determined by two basic factors. The first is structural maturation of the alveolar epithelial cells, whereby the two cell types become clearly differentiated. In the process, many of the cells become structurally attenuated and achieve the ultramicroscopic dimensions of mature cells; they become less resistant to expansion with air. Bulk tissue resistance due to structural immaturity could account for the "atelectasis of prematurity" originally described by Gruenwald (27) in the smallest premature infants. The second basic factor that determines potential viability of the neonatal lung is the maturation of appropriate enzyme systems that modulate the production and secretion of the pulmonary phospholipid surfactants.

Dipalmitoyl lecithin is the principal surfactant (60,64). It forms a surface film at the alveolar-air interface of the air lung and thereby reduces alveolar surface tension to very low values (near zero dynes/cm).* The observations that lecithin is secreted into fetal pulmonary fluid and that fetal pulmonary fluid may enter the amniotic fluid compartment (59) led to the development of the earliest tests of pulmonary function. It was shown that at about the 35th week of gestation the concentration of lecithin and the ratio of lecithin to sphingomyelin (L/S ratio) increases markedly (Fig. 9.1) (25), and that an $L/S > 2.0$ indicates biochemical pulmonary maturity and virtually no risk of alveolar collapse (respiratory distress syndrome) of the neonatal air lung. A similar test of surfactant concentration in amniotic fluid, in which the stability of foam produced from amniotic fluid is assayed (the "shake test") (14), also correlates well with apparent pulmonary maturity and stability of the neonatal air lung. These tests are of great value to the obstetrician, who must consider neonatal

---

* Surface tension produces a pressure which tends to collapse alveoli according to the LaPlace relationship,

$$P = \frac{2\gamma}{r}, \text{ where } P = \text{collapsing pressure}, \ \gamma = \text{surface tension}, \ r = \text{radius}.$$

The higher the surface tension, the greater the collapsing pressure. Once the fetus is able to synthesize sufficient quantities of surfactants to reduce γ to near zero, this potentially untoward force is eliminated and alveolar stability may be achieved.

viability when planning elective deliveries, and to the neonatologist, who can be made aware of the risk to respiratory distress syndrome before delivery and thus prepare appropriate immediate therapy. [Analogous tests, in which L/S is determined in tracheal aspirates (31), may also be of value for monitoring the course of respiratory distress syndrome in the newborn; it seems that the outcome of the infant can be predicted rather accurately by daily tests.]

The recent certification that the fetus normally makes breathing movements *in utero* (periods of breathing alternate with periods of apnea) (Fig. 9.2) has led to the suggestion that monitoring fetal breathing in human pregnancies by ultrasonography can provide a valuable direct measure of fetal activity, be a useful guide to fetal health during labor, and have predictive value both in the care of fetuses of hypertensive women and for identifying fetuses near term who may experience distress during labor (8).

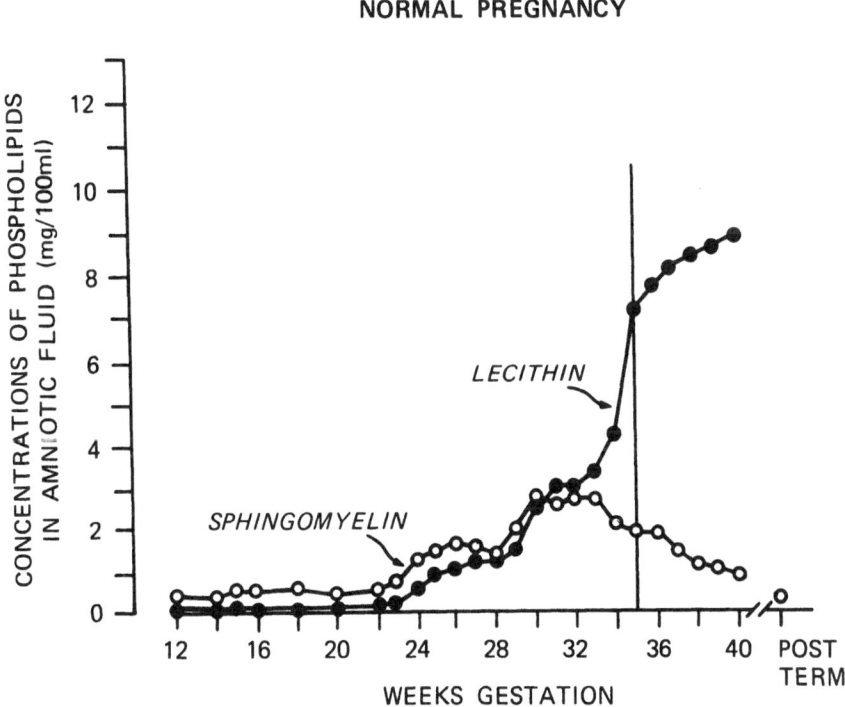

Fig. 9.1 Concentrations of acetone precipitable (surface active) lecithin and sphingomyelin in amniotic fluid are comparable until 30 to 32 weeks gestation. After 32 weeks gestation, concentration of lecithin increases sharply, while sphingomyelin decreases steadily until term. [From Gluck, L., Kulovich, M.V. (25).]

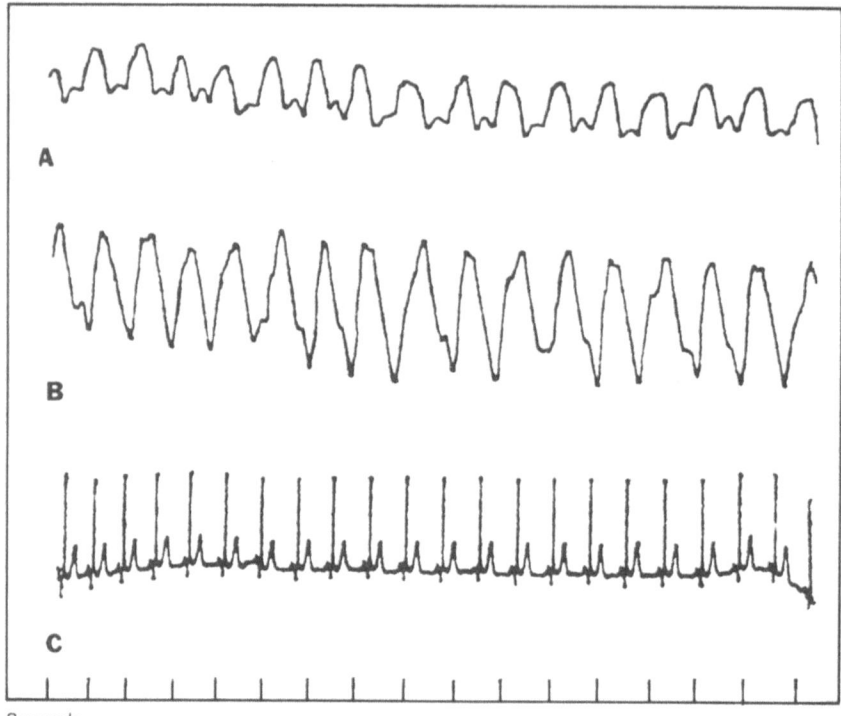

Seconds

Fig. 9.2 Human fetal breathing *in utero* transmitted through maternal abdominal wall. **A.** Maternal abdominal wall displacement at frequency of 60/minute. **B.** Fetal chest wall movements at frequency of 60/minute. **C.** Maternal pulse rate from ECG at frequency of 78/minute. (From Boddy, K., Mantell, C.D. Observations of fetal breathing movements transmitted through the maternal abdominal wall. Lancet **2**:1219, 1972.)

A most serious prognostic sign is the appearance of fetal gasping in association with diminution of normal breathing movements. Although these preliminary findings need to be confirmed, and it is apparent that ultrasonography for monitoring fetal breathing is not yet developed for routine clinical examinations, one may look forward to rapid advances of a practical nature in the recording of fetal pulmonary activity prior to birth. Of related interest are the recent demonstrations, in animal experiments, that fetal breathing *in utero* may be generated regularly by nonspecific somatic sensory stimulation and that both long- and short-acting barbiturates, in subclinical doses, can depress the respiratory center *in utero*, and thus presumably also after birth, for unexpectedly long periods of time (16).

The First Breaths (Foam Lung)

Transition from the fetal liquid lung to the stable neonatal air lung takes place rapidly once air breathing begins at birth and involves the removal of fetal pulmonary fluid and the establishment of alveolar-capillary gas exchange. Although direct measurement of pulmonary function is technically most difficult, enough direct and indirect measurements have been made—including measurements obtained in animal experiments—to permit a reasonable reconstruction of pulmonary function during this period.

Removal of Fetal Pulmonary Fluid

Compression of the infant's thoracic cage during passage through the birth canal has been recorded radiographically (10, 45, 46); in addition, intra-esophageal pressure, a reliable reflection of intrapleural pressure of the infant, has been measured directly during delivery (32, 33). Thoracic compression, with its accompanying increasingly positive intrapleural pressure, accounts for removal of a variable amount of fetal pulmonary fluid from the lung to the posterior pharynx, where it is presumably swallowed. Although as much as 20 ml of liquid has been measured from the infant's mouth during vaginal delivery (33), this volume would be only one-third the total estimated volume of liquid in the lung of a 3.0-kg infant (67). Thus, a considerable volume is left behind. In the case of an infant delivered by cesarean section, one may assume that the lung contains its full complement of liquid. Therefore, removal of liquid via peripheral pulmonary routes, i.e., directly into the pulmonary capillary circulation and into the interstices and lymphatics, is probably most important (63). Peripheral absorption of fetal pulmonary fluid is promoted by the osmotic pressure gradient between pulmonary fluid and blood, and also by opening of junctions between alveolar epithelial cells, thereby increasing permeability, as a consequence of the large transmural pressures produced at the onset of breathing (23). Despite these vigorous adaptive mechanisms, the newborn infant must manage to contend with large volumes of intrapulmonary liquid during the first breaths of extrauterine life.

Establishment of Alveolar-Capillary Gas Exchange

The first "inhalation" may begin before the first active inspiratory effort is made by the baby. As stated, thoracic compression during passage through the birth canal produces high intrapleural pressures. When the chest is delivered, the pressure is released and elastic recoil of the chest wall [which has low elasticity (high compliance), but is not completely plastic] may permit a considerable volume of air to enter the lung. This volume has been estimated at one-fourth to one-third functional residual capacity (32), a volume similar to the volume removed during the "vaginal squeeze." In addition, active laryngopharyngeal movements such as swallowing and "frog breathing" may augment both air distribution within the lung before the first breath and the inspiratory force of the diaphragmatic descent during the first breath (11).

Karlberg and his colleagues (32–35) have provided definitive studies of the forces produced and volumes exchanged during the first breaths. The following procedure was used: As soon as the infant's head was delivered, a water-filled, open-ended polyethylene catheter (1 mm internal diameter) was introduced into the nose and advanced to the upper to middle third of the esophagus for estimation of intrapleural pressure (20). A mask was placed tightly on the infant's face the moment it appeared at the introitus; the mask was connected by tubing to an inflexible 35-liter plastic container and the pressure changes produced in this closed system by breathing efforts were calibrated to give respiratory volume changes ("reversed plethysmography"). The first inspiration produced high intrapleural pressures, up to -70 cm H_2O, and the inspiratory volume (20 to 75 ml) was considerably higher than the resting tidal volume of the normal newborn infant. Most significantly, the volume of the first expiration, in which high positive intrapleural pressures were produced, was considerably less than that of the preceding inspiration, indicating that large quantities of

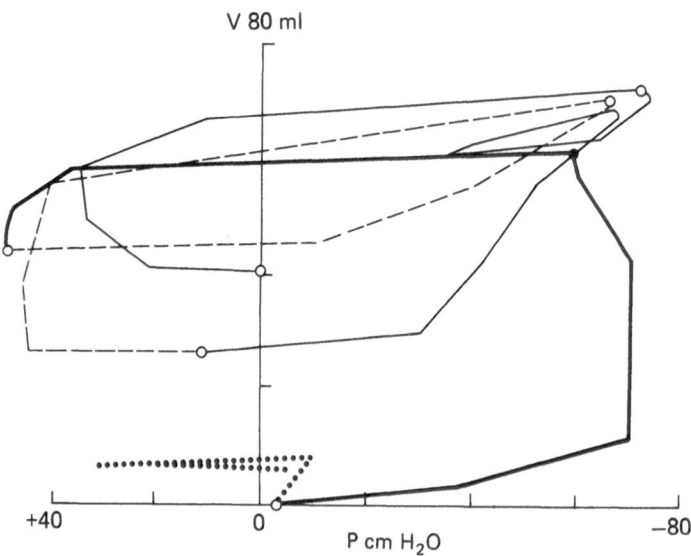

Fig. 9.3   Pressure-volume diagrams of 4.32-kg infant during first breath (heavy line), second breath (broken line), and third breath (thin line). [Adapted from Karlberg, P. et al. (35).]

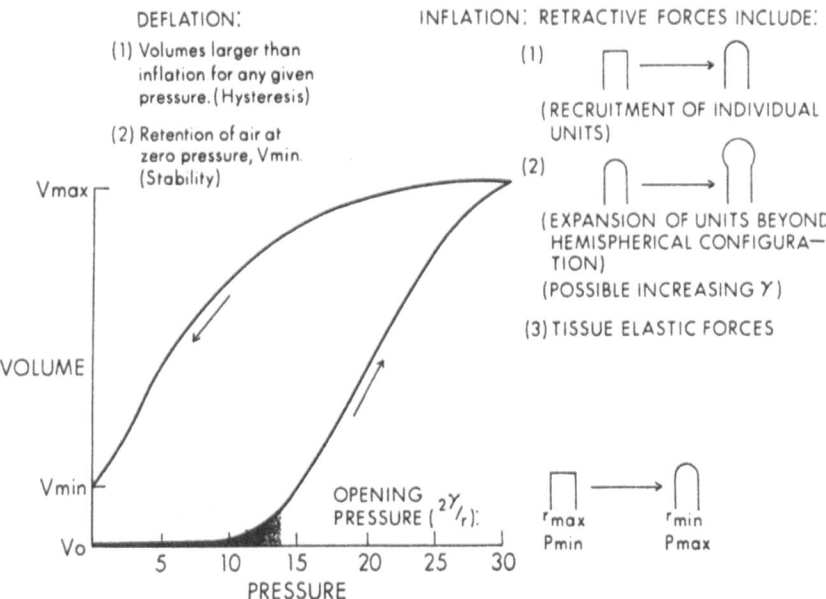

Fig. 9.4   Volume-pressure diagram, starting with degassed lung. Sketches represent terminal lung units, i.e., alveoli at end of conducting units. P_{min} and P_{max} are minimum and maximum pressures in individual terminal units; r_{max} and r_{min} are maximum and minimum radii of these units. [From Scarpelli, E.M. (60).]

air remained in the lung. Subsequent breaths had similar patterns, although peak pressures were generally smaller, so that the volume of air retained by the lung generally increased. Representative pressure-volume diagrams from the studies of Karlberg and co-workers are shown in Fig. 9.3. The hallmarks of the first breaths are rather extraordinarily high inspiratory and expiratory pressures and progressive increase of residual air volume in the lung.

The high pressures of the first breaths are required to overcome several resistive forces. Viscous resistance to the movement of fluid in the airways is maximal at the *beginning* of the first breath because the greatest displacement of liquid probably occurs in the trachea (2). Air inflation of terminal airways and alveoli requires considerable pressure, "opening pressure" (56), much as a soap solution requires high pressures before air may enter to form a bubble (Fig. 9.4). Beyond opening pressure, when lung volume increases rapidly with relatively small additional changes in pressure (Figs. 9.3 and 9.4), the pressure required is determined primarily by tissue elastic resistance, the reciprocal of compliance, and also by opening of additional peripheral lung units. Viscous resistance of the lung tissue itself is probably higher in the newborn lung than in the older air lung because of the relatively high content of liquid and tissue at birth (55). Total resistance to airflow is somewhat higher in the newborn infant than in the adult, no doubt because of the relatively high resistance to airflow through the nose of babies (43).

The progressive increase in the amount of air retained in the lung during the first breaths was thought to be due to peripheral displacement of liquid, formation of a surface-active film at the peripheral air-bulk liquid interface, and retention of air in the lung at end-expiration (7, 69). There are several objections to this concept,* which appear to have been resolved by the demonstration that the first air inflations of the excised liquid lung of the fetus produce considerable amounts of foam in airways and alveoli (Fig. 9.5) (66). The foam lung is consonant with the observed vital phenomena that mark cardiopulmonary adaptation at the onset of breathing.

* This concept does not take into account (1) the expectation that unabsorbed, bulk pulmonary fluid would effectively block alveolar gas transfer; (2) the observation that airways are *distended* at the end of the first expiration; (3) the observation that alveoli partially filled with liquid are unstable (68) and would either form bubbles or refill completely with liquid; and (4) the expectation that breathing movements should produce a dispersion of air in liquid, i.e., foam.

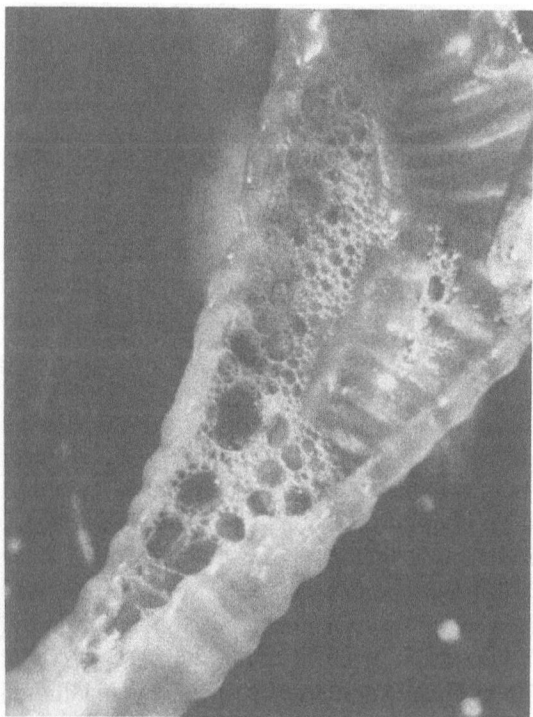

Fig. 9.5 Foam in cut trachea of normal newborn rabbit who had breathed less than 2 minutes before lungs were excised.

Much of the opening pressure (see above) is literally required for the formation of bubbles that constitute foam. Alveolar foam films would tend to be apposed to the epithelial surfaces and thus provide a rich supply of oxygen. This serves to reduce pulmonary arteriolar constriction (thereby increasing pulmonary blood flow) and to oxygenate the blood rapidly so that pulmonary venous blood has virtually normal oxygen pressure. The foam films, which are rich in phospholipid surfactants, would provide a highly surface-active film for the alveolar epithelial surfaces when the bubbles collapse as liquid is resorbed and the air lung is formed. The "entrapped" foam would sustain dilated airways at the onset of breathing (28) and would account for some of the "trapped gas" that characterizes the neonatal lung (see below). As the rate of liquid absorption increases after the onset of breathing, the rate of foam production decreases and the rate of bubble collapse increases until the normal, stable air lung is established (66).

The Neonatal Lung (Air Lung)

Most parameters of pulmonary function are measureable in the newborn infant, generally by techniques that were developed and standardized originally for adults. Thus, methods for determining parenchymal pulmonary stability, airway function, and alveolar-capillary gas exchange are available to the clinical investigator and have revealed much of the functional characteristics of the neonatal lung. However, these often ingenious methods are difficult to administer and sometimes confound interpretation, primarily because of the natural intransigence of the subject. Unlike the adult, the infant will not be regimented, and most of the pulmonary function tests must be carried out while he is either asleep or awake and inactive. The spontaneous agitation of the sick infant adds to the problem of making reliable determinations of pulmonary function in this group, but in spite of this, the pulmonary neonatologist's dedication, creativity, and dogged persistence have prevailed.

Gas Pressures and pH

Of all pulmonary function tests, the most valuable, reliable, and easiest to conduct repeatedly is determination of gas pressures and pH of peripheral blood. Arterial samples are preferred; determination of oxygen pressure of systemic venous blood (P_vO_2) is a completely useless task. In extremis, systemic venous blood may be used to estimate arterial Pco_2 and pH, since the arteriovenous differences are relatively small and generally do not introduce a substantial error in the estimation. Nonetheless, systemic arterial blood should be used. The relative ease with which it may be sampled in

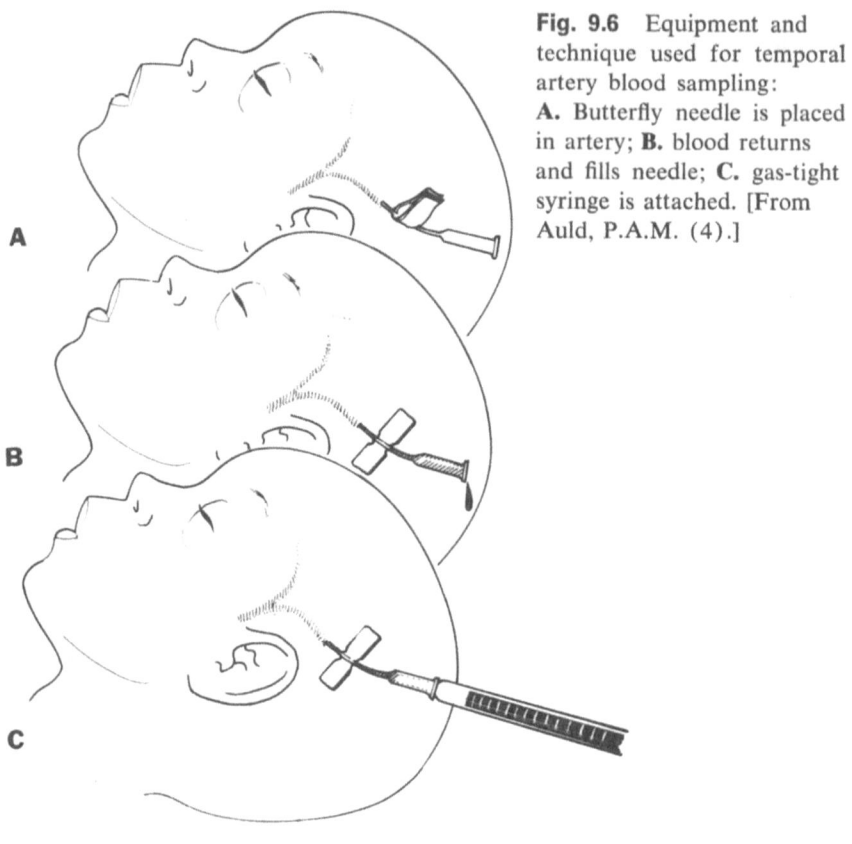

Fig. 9.6 Equipment and technique used for temporal artery blood sampling: **A.** Butterfly needle is placed in artery; **B.** blood returns and fills needle; **C.** gas-tight syringe is attached. [From Auld, P.A.M. (4).]

infants and the small volumes required to determine Pao_2, $Paco_2$, and pH, make this the "routine" pulmonary function test in any setting that cares for the newborn. Arterial blood is obtained easily by direct puncture of the temporal, radial, or brachial artery (Fig. 9.6). When repeated blood samples are required, consideration must be given to the placement of an indwelling arterial needle or to placement of an umbilical arterial catheter, with awareness of the possible complications of catheterization. In the presence of right-to-left shunt through the ductus arteriosus, it must be recalled that blood samples from below the level of the ductus will probably contain lower Po_2 than those from above. The recently developed "transcutaneous technique" permits continuous estimation of Pao_2 from a noninvasive electrode placed on the skin (Fig. 9.7) (29, 58). This technique, in which problems of strict quantification of Pao_2 and calibration *in vivo* persist, holds great promise as a potential standard method for infant monitoring.

Fetal Pao_2 is low *in utero* and may fall further during labor, especially if labor is associated with marked or sustained reduction of uteroplacental blood flow. Thus, umbilical arterial Po_2 is low during the first minutes of air breathing, whereas pulmonary venous Po_2 may be substantially higher (Fig. 9.8). The relatively low Pao_2 during the first hours of life of the normal infant is a result of persistent shunting from right to left through the foramen ovale, ductus arteriosus, and the lungs. The relative contribution of intrapulmonary shunts versus ductal and foramen shunts is reflected in the pulmonary venous and umbilical arterial Po_2 respectively. However, when there is respiratory distress syndrome of the newborn, the intrapulmonary shunt may become the primary pathophysiologic derangement, accounting for the severe systemic hypoxemia of these infants (61).

Because the hemoglobin-oxygen dissociation curve of the fetus is shifted to the left in comparison with the adult curve and because transition of the dissociation curve to the adult configuration takes place gradually over a period of months after birth (Fig. 9.9), neonatal blood is well saturated with oxygen shortly after breathing begins at birth. For example, using the data of Fig. 9.8, an umbilical arterial Po_2 of 56.3 mm Hg at 15 minutes of life would produce a hemoglobin-oxygen saturation of about 95%. In addition, although the hemoglobin concentration of cord blood may vary considerably (54), it is apparent that the normal full-term neonate generally has substantial amounts of hemoglobin (mean values ranging from about 15 to 17 g/100 ml) and that the oxygen content of arterial blood is at "adult" levels even with "low" Pao_2. However, because of the shape

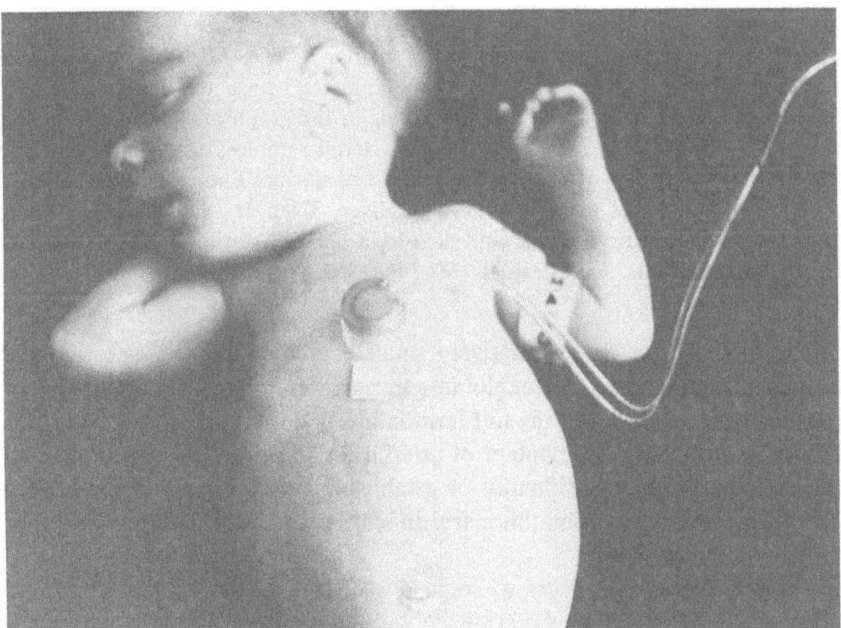

Fig. 9.7   Transcutaneous oxygen electrode in place. [From Rooth, G. (58).]

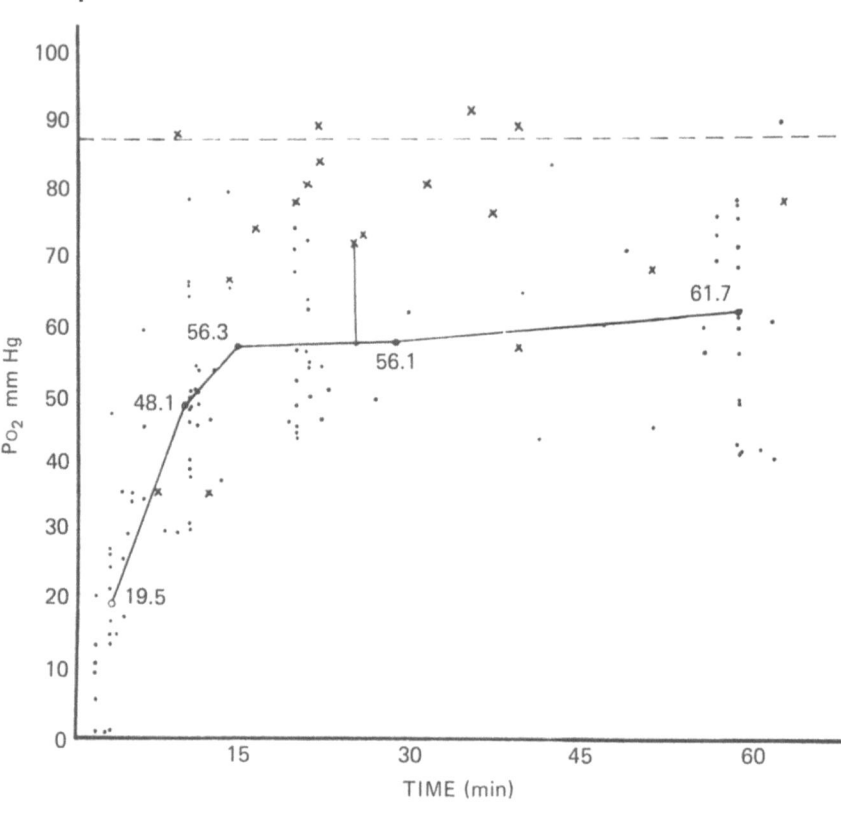

Fig. 9.8 Pao_2 versus time during the first hour of life. All subjects were mature neonates by weight except for three subjects whose weights were 2.495, 2.407, and 2.280 kg, respectively. Numerals in the graph are the means of the five time periods. Dots indicate umbilical arterial samples; crosses indicate left atrial samples. Dashed line is the lower limit of normal Pao_2 for older children and adults (i.e., ~88 mm Hg). (From Oliver, T.K., Jr., Demis, J.A., Bates, G.D. Serial blood-gas tensions and acid-base balance during the first hour of life in human infants. Acta Paediatr. **50**:346, 1961.)

of the dissociation curve, relatively small decreases of Pao_2 substantially reduce oxygen content. Hemoglobin concentration of the premature infant may be lower than that of the full-term infant (54) and, if so, would reduce the oxygen capacity and content of arterial blood at birth. This, along with the apparently greater difficulty of establishing an air lung at birth, may add to the risk of cardiopulmonary difficulties in the premature infant at the onset of breathing.

Fetal hypercapnia occurs to some degree during the course of normal labor and delivery (30) as uteroplacental flow is compromised during contractions. $Paco_2$ tends to be higher at delivery than it is in the fetus before the onset of labor and in the newborn infant after air breathing is established (42). With the onset of respiration $Paco_2$ falls rapidly; at one hour of life it is slightly below 40 mm Hg in the normal infant (Fig. 9.10). $Paco_2$ remains at this level during the neonatal period. Its elevation during the course of both central and peripheral respiratory disease is an ominous sign of respiratory insufficiency or failure (65).

Lung Volumes and Capacities

The establishment of alveolar-capillary gas exchange is the end point toward which neonatal cardiopulmonary adaptation is directed. For the lung, this requires removal of fetal pulmonary fluid from the airways and alveoli and establishment and maintenance of a stable gas volume, the functional residual capacity (FRC), in the lung. The transitional stage from fetal liquid lung to neonatal air lung was discussed in the preceding section.

Functional residual capacity is the volume of gas in the lung at the end of normal expiration; its volume is about 30 ml/kg body weight in both the mature infant and adult (Table 9.1) and in most mammalian species. Its physiologic importance rests on several points:

[1] It provides a significant "buffer volume" which minimizes the changes of Pao_2 and $Paco_2$ that might occur if each breath ("tidal volume") were

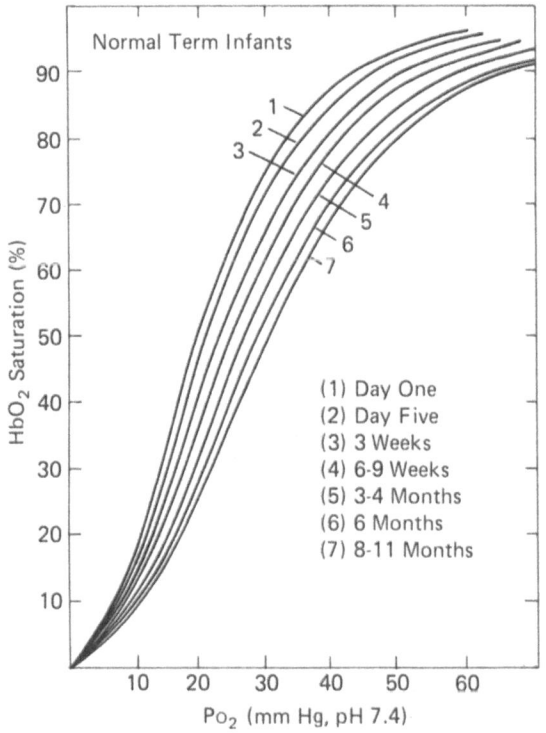

(1) Day One
(2) Day Five
(3) 3 Weeks
(4) 6-9 Weeks
(5) 3-4 Months
(6) 6 Months
(7) 8-11 Months

Fig. 9.9 Comparison of curves from blood of infants at different postnatal ages. (From Delivoria-Papadopoulos, M. et al. Postnatal changes in oxygen transport of term, premature and sick infants: the role of red cell 2,3-diphosphoglycerate and adult hemoglobin. Pediatr. Res. **5**:235, 1971.)

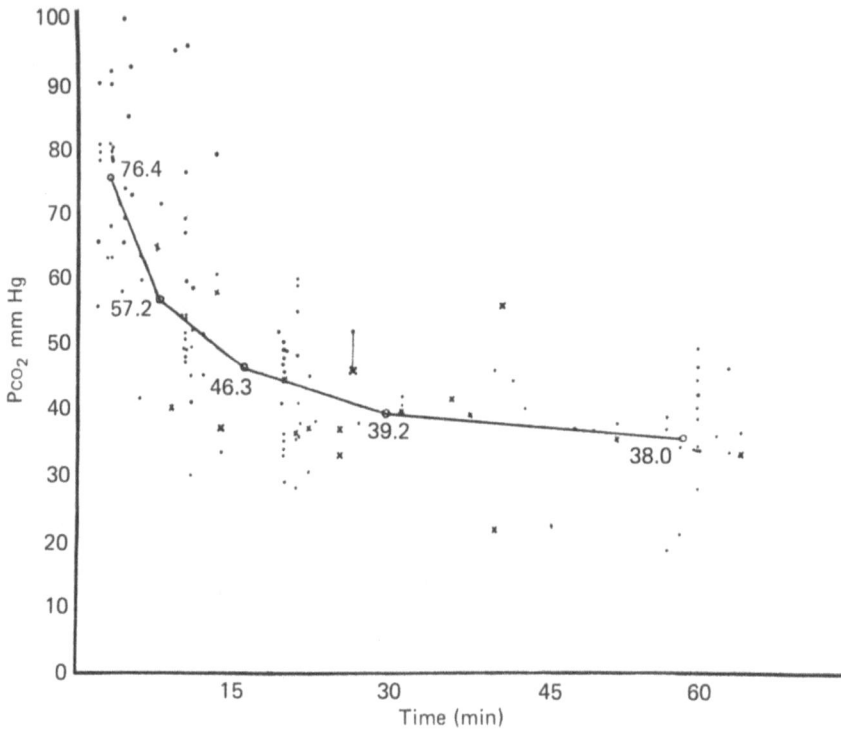

Fig. 9.10 Paco$_2$ versus time during the first hour of life. Subjects and symbols are the same as in Fig. 8. (From Oliver, T.K., Jr., Demis, J.A., Bates, G.D. Serial blood-gas tensions and acid-base balance during the first hour of life in human subjects. Acta Paediatr. **50**:346, 1961.)

taken into a virtually airless lung. In the latter case, $P_{A}O_2$ would be highest at end-inspiration, then fall to low values at end-expiration. Analogously, $P_{A}CO_2$ would be highest at end-expiration and fall to very low values at end-inspiration. Thus, blood gas pressures would fluctuate widely with each breath. These potentially extreme shifts are minimized by the FRC, since tidal volume is only about 20% FRC (Table 9.1).

[2] Functional residual capacity normally is established by expanded, stable alveoli; thus, the pressure required for each inhalation is needed only for minimal expansion of lung tissue and airflow into the lung. Conversely, the virtually airless lung or the lung at low FRC, which contain collapsed alveoli, require significantly higher pressures ("opening pressures") for ventilation (Fig. 9.4).

[3] It is the resting volume of the lung in thorax at which the retractile forces of lung tissue and chest wall are counterbalanced so that active work is not required to sustain the aerated lung.

Since the chest wall is highly compliant at birth, the more so in the premature infant, it may seem surprising to find that the resting volume, or FRC, of the infant is equal to that of the adult when expressed as volume per unit body weight, i.e., about 30 ml/kg (Table 9.1), and somewhat larger than that of the adult when expressed as a percentage of total lung capacity. In fact, the two observations are probably not incompatible because the total lung capacity of the infant is measured as the crying response to noxious stimulation and therefore may yield an underestimation when compared with the volume moved during a maximum voluntary breathing effort as required of the adult. Also, the highly compliant chest wall of the infant may not be able to produce maximum lung expansion. In addition, the *excised* neonatal lung is just as expandable as the lung of the adult. Thus, neonatal FRC may not be higher than that of the adult when related to true total lung capacity.

Functional residual capacity of infants has been measured by the standard methods of either helium dilution (24) or nitrogen washout (50, 70). The method of "helium rebreathing" (40) is rapid, apparently accurate, and particularly well suited to the infant. With the helium dilution or rebreathing methods the subject breathes from a source containing a known concentration of helium in respiratory gas. Breathing is effected in a closed circuit until helium concentration is equilibrated between lung and source and FRC is calculated as follows:

$$(V_s)(F_I He) = (V_s + FRC)(F_F He)$$

where V_s is the total volume of the source, $F_I He$ is the initial helium concentration in the source, and $F_F He$ is the final helium concentration at

Table 9.1   Lung Volumes, Capacities, and Ratios of Infants and Adults*

	Infant (ml/kg)	Adult (ml/kg)
Total lung capacity (TLC)	63	82
Inspiratory capacity (IC)	33	52
Thoracic gas volume (TGV)	30–36	30
Functional residual capacity (FRC)	30	30
Vital capacity (VC)	40	66
Closing capacity (CC)	35	23
Tidal volume (V_T)	6	7
Expiratory reserve volume (ERV)	7	14
Closing volume (CV)	12	7
Residual volume (RV)	23	16
ERV/FRC	0.23	0.47
RV/TLC	0.37	0.20
FRC/TLC	0.48	0.37
V_T/FRC	0.20	0.23

* From reference 48.

equilibration. With the nitrogen washout method, expired gas is collected breath by breath, in a nonrebreathing system, as the subject breathes 100% oxygen. Measurement of N_2 concentration at the mouth provides an accurate index of the point at which the nitrogen has been washed out of the lung. FRC is calculated as follows:

$$FRC = \frac{(V_s)(F_sN_2)}{F_LN_2},$$

where V_s is the volume collected, F_sN_2 is the concentration of N_2 in the collected gas, and F_LN_2 is the concentration of N_2 in the lung before washout (about 0.8). In performing these tests care must be taken to maintain an effective seal between the oronasal mask and the infant's skin, and to begin the test at the end of normal expiration, when the lung is at FRC.

Thoracic gas volume (TGV) is the total amount of gas in the thorax that is both in communication with the airways and trapped within the lung or pleura. Thus TGV is FRC plus trapped gas. Normally TGV equals FRC, since gas trapping is negligible in the air lung, but in the early newborn infant the former is considerably larger than the latter. Whereas FRC is relatively constant during the first few days of life, TGV is high at first, and then falls during the subsequent postnatal days (40, 50, 72). In fullterm infants TGV becomes equal to FRC at about the third to fourth days, whereas the inequality may persist for 10 days or more in the premature infant. Thus "gas trapping" is a normal phenomenon in the newborn and it is obvious that the trapped gas is intrapulmonary. The mechanism by which gas trapping occurs has not been defined, but possibilities include trapping beyond films of unabsorbed fetal pulmonary fluid and trapping behind collapsed airways. Discovery of the normal neonatal foam lung (66) seems to provide the best explanation for "gas trapping" in the newborn infant. In contrast to trapping associated with airway collapse, gas trapped as foam could play an important physiologic role in the cardiopulmonary adaptations at birth (see preceding section and reference 2).

Measurement of TGV in the infant has been accomplished by the standard plethysmographic method adapted to the neonate (5, 24, 40, 50). The baby is placed entirely within a plethysmograph and breathes through an oronasal mask that can be occluded. Airway pressure and pressure within the plethysmograph are measured directly. At the desired point in the respiratory cycle (at the end of normal expiration), the breathing piece is occluded and the subject continues to make breathing movements against the obstruction. Pressures are recorded before and at the end of inspiration and substituted in Boyle's law ($PV = P'V'$) to solve for TGV:

$$(P)(TGV) = (P')(TGV + \Delta V)$$

where P is airway pressure (atmospheric) before inspiration; P' is airway pressure at end inspiration; and ΔV is the increase in volume at end inspiration.

Vital capacity is the total volume of gas that may be expired by maximal expiration after maximal inspiration. It has been approximated in infants by measurement of respired volumes during crying (19), but the method has been criticized on the basis that artificially induced crying is not strong or sustained enough for the test to be valid. Closing volume is the volume remaining in the lung during a vital capacity maneuver when there is the first evidence that airflow out of alveoli (usually the dependent alveoli) stops as intrapleural pressure increases. As the vital capacity maneuver continues, airflow ceases in a progressively larger number of alveoli until expiratory flow stops completely at residual volume. (Closing capacity is the sum of closing volume and residual volume.) The closing volume phenomenon is attributed to collapse of airways as intrapleural pressure increases. The high closing volumes of young subjects suggest that some airways may close even during normal quiet breathing, perhaps because of the high compliance of young airways. Closing volumes have not been measured extensively in the neonate. Since the procedure requires patient cooperation, extrapolations from determinations on young children (3, 47) provide the best approximation at this time.

Pulmonary Mechanics (Static)

Pulmonary compliance is an expression of the force required to produce a given volume change in the lung, i.e., $\Delta V/\Delta P$ (where ΔP is transpulmonary pressure), and specific pulmonary compliance is compliance related to lung volume (usually FRC) at the time the determination was made. Both measurements have been made in the newborn infant by a number of investigators (13, 18, 24, 41) (Table 9.2). The compliance of the lung (C_L) is a static mechanical property determined primarily by the elastic recoil of the tissue and, especially in certain pathologic conditions where

Table 9.2   Compliance of Newborn Infants*

Source and Reference	Age	Birth Weight	Compliance (ml/cm H_2O)	Specific Compliance (ml/cm H_2O/ml)
Geubelle et al. (24)	<2 hours	Full term	—	0.036
	24 hours	Full term	—	0.049
Chu et al. (13)	<3 hours	Full term	4.75	0.0406
	>24 hours	Full term	6.24	0.0548
Cook et al. (18)	2 hours–7 days	Full term	4.9	—
Krauss et al. (41)	1–52 days	Nondistressed premature 0.8–2.0 kg	0.41–3.4	0.012–0.052

* From reference 4.

alveolar surface tension is high, by surface forces at the alveolar-air interface of the lung (60). Chest wall compliance (C_w), i.e., $\Delta V/\Delta P$ (where
ΔP is transthoracic pressure) is a function of the elastic recoil of the chest
cage. The total compliance of the respiratory system (C_T) is determined
as follows:

$$1/C_T = 1/C_L + 1/C_W$$

In the few studies in which C_L and C_W have been determined for the same
infants (57, 73), it was found that chest wall and lung compliance equal
the compliance of the lung alone (the chest wall of the infant is very compliant). Thus it has been estimated that of the total static mechanical ("elastic") resistance to volume change in the respiratory system, the chest wall
accounts for 15% in the newborn infant. Comparatively, C_w accounts for
37% of C_T in children 5 to 16 years of age and 50% in adults (48). The
high compliance of the chest wall and relatively low compliance of the
lung of the newborn infant make him particularly dependent on intrinsic
factors that modulate pulmonary tissue stability, such as low to near-zero
surface tension and, perhaps, production of foam at birth. When surface
tension is abnormally high, as in respiratory distress syndrome, the lung
becomes highly unstable, and alveoli collapse (61).

Specific pulmonary compliance (C_L/FRC) has been reported to increase
during the first eight hours of age (13) and C_L increases in the full-term
infant from birth to one to seven days of life (22). In premature infants,
C_L/FRC may be low for days and weeks after birth even though the infant
shows no signs of respiratory distress (41). The compliance of the lung
probably decreases during growth of the individual; studies of pressure-
volume diagrams (1) with relation to age suggest that the decrease of
C_L continues up to about the age of 16 to 20 years. Chest wall compliance
probably increases rapidly after birth (1); whether this is due to "stiffening"
of the chest cage or to change in the position of the diaphragm, or both,
has not been determined (1, 6, 48). Nonetheless, as the chest wall grows
and ossifies, C_w does fall with age.

Measurement of C_L of the newborn infant is a complex task generally
reserved for the clinical investigative laboratory (Fig. 9.11). For the newborn infant, C_L is measured while he is breathing spontaneously ("dynamic" compliance). The infant is placed in a plethysmograph with his head
exposed to the outside and sealed as shown in Fig. 9.11. Volume change
is recorded from the plethysmograph and intrapleural pressure from an intraesophageal tube or balloon. At points of zero airflow—at end-inspiration
and end-expiration—ΔV and ΔP are determined and C_L is calculated.

Alveolar Ventilation

Factors that determine alveolar ventilation $(\dot{V}_A)$ are listed in Table 9.3.
Since the volume of gas reaching the alveoli with each breath equals tidal

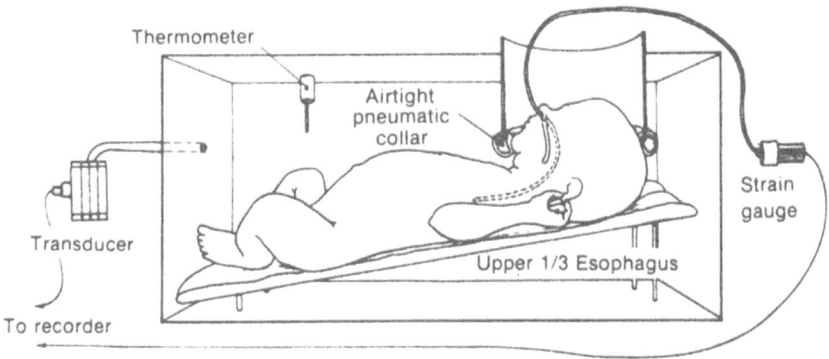

Fig. 9.11   Body plethysmograph with infant's face exposed to outside but sealed by pneumatic collar. Intraesophageal balloon is in upper third of esophagus and connected to strain gauge. Transducer detects chamber pressure which is calibrated in terms of volume and thus permits recording of V_T. (From Griffin, A.J. et al. Pulmonary compliance. Amer. J. Dis. Child. **123**:89, 1972.)

volume (V_T) minus dead space (V_D), the product $(V_T - V_D)$ (f) is the volume of gas ventilating the alveoli per minute $(\dot{V}_A)$, when f is the number of breaths per minute. Normally, V_D is anatomic dead space (the volume of gas that ventilates conducting airways in which no gas exchange with pulmonary capillaries takes place). In certain circumstances unperfused alveoli may be ventilated, in which case there is an added dead space, the "alveolar dead space." Alveolar dead space plus anatomic dead space equals total wasted ventilation, or the paradoxically named physiologic dead space. The following points of interest are apparent from the data presented in Table 9.3: (1) V_T, V_A and V_D per breath are similar in infants

Table 9.3   Pulmonary Ventilation*

	Infant	Adult	
Respiratory frequency (f)	34–45	13	BPM
Tidal volume (V_T)	6–8	7	ml/kg
Alveolar volume (V_A)	3.8–5.8	4.8	ml/kg
Dead space volume (V_D)	2–2.2	2.2	ml/kg
Minute ventilation $(\dot{V}_E)$	200–260	90	ml/kg/min
Alveolar ventilation $(\dot{V}_A)$	100–150	60	ml/kg/min
	2.3	2.4	L/m²/min
Wasted (dead space) ventilation $(\dot{V}_D)$	77–99	30	ml/kg/min
Dead space/tidal volume (V_D/V_T)	.27–.37	.3	
Oxygen consumption $(\dot{V}_{O_2})$	6–8	3.2	ml/kg/min

* Adapted from Nelson, N.M. Respiration and circulation before birth, in Smith, C.A., Nelson, N.M. (eds.): The Physiology of the Newborn Infant, 4th ed. Springfield, Charles C Thomas, 1976, p. 209.

and adults when expressed as ml/kg. Thus, V_T and V_D can be predicted from the same simple formulae used for adults. (2) Whereas $\dot{V}_A$ is much higher in the infant than in the adult when related to body weight (ml/kg/minute), $\dot{V}_A$ is the same for each when related to body surface area (2.3–2.4 liters/m²/minute). Therefore, alveolar ventilation per unit surface area remains unchanged with age. Since oxygen consumption is also rather constant in relation to surface area, it is apparent that $\dot{V}_A$ is modulated to meet the oxygen needs of the infant and the adult in much the same way.

Tidal volume is best measured in infants by collecting expired gas in a Neoprene bag over a fixed period of time during which f is determined. Special nonrebreathing valves for insertion into the infant's nostrils can be made locally (26). A number of pneumographs can be used to monitor f and relative V_T (15). Some of these (e.g., electromagnetic coils) appear to be more accurately quantifiable than others (e.g., mercury strain gauges), but they all lack precision.

Anatomic dead space of premature and full-term infants has been determined by a number of investigators (17,49). The usual method is to record respired gas concentrations and respired volume simultaneously and to use the Fowler method (Fig. 9.12) for calculating V_{Danat}. The difficulties and possible errors in this method have been reviewed (49); they center on the reliability and reproducibility of recording end-tidal gas concentrations in an infant who is breathing rapidly and moving small volumes of gas with each breath. Estimation of physiologic dead space can be made by determination of the difference between alveolar and arterial P_{CO_2} (4). This again requires the sampling of end-tidal gas. The standard Bohr equations may be used to calculate both V_{Danat} and $V_{Dphysiol}$:

$$V_{Danat} = \frac{(F_{ACO2} - F_{ECO2})}{F_{ACO2}} V_E$$

The volume expired per breath (V_E) and the CO_2 concentration in V_E (F_{ECO_2}) can be obtained easily by collecting expired gas from the nonrebreathing nasal valve mentioned previously. However, determination of alveolar CO_2 concentration (F_{ACO2}) is made from end-tidal gas.

$$V_{Dphysiol} = \frac{(P_{aCO_2} - P_{ECO_2})}{P_{aCO_2}} V_E$$

is more easily determined since end-tidal sampling is not required

The ratio V_D/V_T is a useful determination: When $V_{Dphysiol}$ is used, any increase above the normal V_D/V_T (0.27 to 0.37) indicates that excessive ventilation is being wasted, that alveolar and thus physiologic dead space has increased.

The distribution of ventilated gas within the lungs of the newborn infant has been studied by a number of investigators (9, 12, 50, 70), who find that distribution is generally uniform throughout the lung. This is in con-

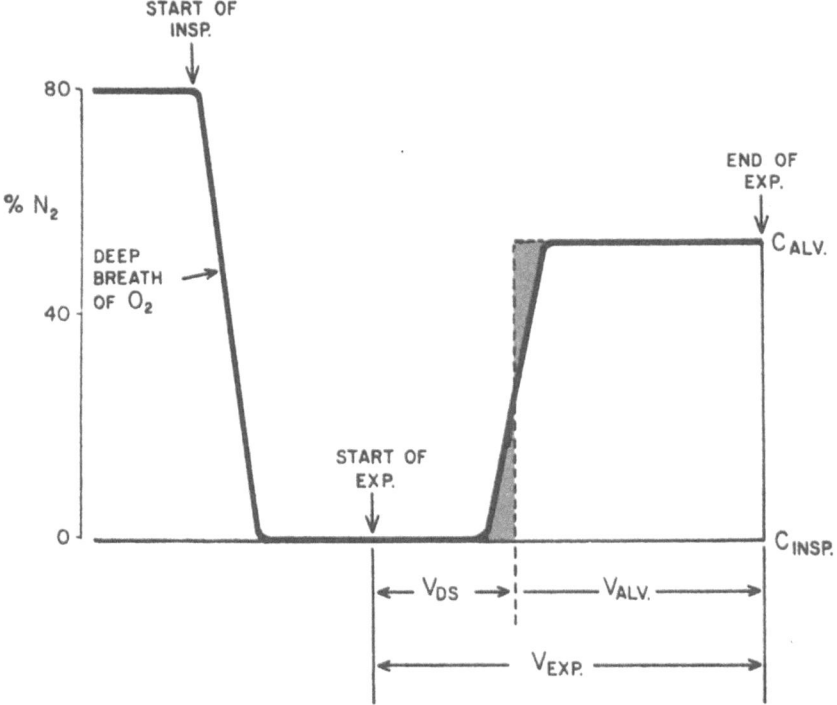

Fig. 9.12   Fowler method for calculating anatomic dead space. [From Clutario, B.C. (15). Modified from Bates, D.V., Macklem, P.T., Christie, R.V.: Respiratory Function In Disease, 2nd ed. Philadelphia, W.B. Saunders Co., 1971.]

trast to the adult, who normally shows fast- and slow-ventilated spaces. The standard method of monitoring nitrogen clearance (15) while the subject is breathing oxygen is used most frequently.

Alveolar Ventilation and Pulmonary Vascular Perfusion ($\dot{V}A/\dot{Q}$)

Along with establishment of $\dot{V}_A$ at birth, there is an "opening up" of the pulmonary circulation in which pulmonary vascular resistance falls and pulmonary blood flow increases. (At the same time the ductus arteriosus narrows and flow from right to left atrium falls as the foramen ovale begins to close functionally.) The increased pulmonary blood flow serves the needs of alveolar-capillary gas exchange best when $\dot{V}_A$ and $\dot{Q}$ are matched. Conventionally, $\dot{V}_A$ is determined as total alveolar ventilation and $\dot{Q}$ as total pulmonary blood flow, and normally the ratio $\dot{V}_A/\dot{Q}$ is 0.8 to 0.9. In fact, it is known that $\dot{V}_A$ and $\dot{Q}$ vary in different zones of the lung (e.g., $\dot{V}_A/\dot{Q}$ is about 3.3 near the apex and 0.63 near the base of the lung of the adult in the erect position) and that this variation is related to gravity effects on pleural and vascular pressures (74). Nonetheless, the lung as a whole functions at a mean $\dot{V}_A/\dot{Q}$ of 0.8 to 0.9. Under these conditions the mean difference between alveolar and arterial Po_2 ($AaDo_2$) is 4 mm Hg; the $aADco_2$ is 1 mm Hg; and the $aADN_2$ is 3 mm Hg. When $\dot{V}_A/\dot{Q}$ increases (e.g., when alveolar capillary perfusion is reduced), the $aADco_2$ will rise, since alveoli of hypoperfused capillaries remove little CO_2 from the blood and thus contribute little CO_2 to expired gas. When $\dot{V}_A/\dot{Q}$ decreases (e.g., underventilated alveoli with relatively normally perfused capillaries), the $aADN_2$ will rise, since the PN_2 of these alveoli and their capillaries increases, and the $AaDo_2$ will rise, as Pao_2 falls to a greater extent than Po_2 of end-tidal gas. An elevated $AaDo_2$ will develop also in the presence of right-to-left shunts—intrapulmonary as well as extrapulmonary shunts—whereas elevations of $aADco_2$ and $aADN_2$ do not develop to the same extent (Table 9.4).

aA and Aa gradients have been monitored in the newborn infant to determine the nature and time course of $\dot{V}_A/\dot{Q}$ adjustments in the early neonatal period (37, 39, 51–53, 71). These studies indicated that the well-known reduced Pao_2 of normal premature infants is caused primarily by right-to-left shunts, since the abnormal $AaDo_2$ persists during oxygen breathing. The shunting was attributed to either nonventilated or poorly ventilated but perfused alveolar units. The studies also showed that normal full-term infants maintain an elevated $AaDo_2$ on air and on oxygen for the first several days of life. This was consonant with observations that significant shunts may be measured up to seven days of life. In addition, these studies showed that $aADN_2$ is high at birth but falls to normal values in hours. Therefore, uniformity of gas distribution is achieved shortly after birth. These findings have not been corroborated in one study (44), a dis-

Table 9.4 Some Distinguishing Characteristics of Respiratory Pathophysiologic Processes*

Pathophysiologic Condition	Distinguishing Characteristics	
Hyperventilation	Low P_Aco_2, $Paco_2$	High, P_Ao_2, Pao_2
Hypoventilation	High P_Aco_2, $Paco_2$	Low P_Ao_2, Pao_2
Right-to-left shunt	$AaDo_2$ breathing O_2 shunt on 100% O_2	Low Pao_2
Diffusion defect	$AaDo_2$ especially with exercise low diffusing capacity	Low Pao_2
$\dot{V}_A/\dot{Q}$ abnormality		
Weighted high	$AaDo_2$, $aADco_2$ breathing air wasted $\dot{V}$; $V_{Dphysiol}$-effect	Low, normal, high Pao_2
Weighted low	$AaDo_2$, $aADN_2$ breathing air wasted $\dot{Q}$; shunt-effect	Low Pao_2

* From Scarpelli, E.M. Concepts in respiratory pathophysiology, in Scarpelli et al. (eds.): Pulmonary Disease of the Fetus, Newborn and Child. Philadelphia, Lea and Febiger, 1978.

crepancy which has not been explained. An additional point was that significant $\mathrm{aADco_2}$ exists in both normal full-term and premature infants during the first two days of life; the more immature the infant the longer the gradient persists. These studies indicate that there are areas of high $\dot{V}_A/\dot{Q}$ normally in the lungs of healthy full-term and premature infants during the early neonatal period.

Thus, evidence is presented for intrapulmonary shunting and "wasted" ventilation as normal features of the neonatal lung. This is not surprising in view of the fact that the period is marked by transition of the liquid lung through the foam lung to the air lung. The neonatal lung is a polyphasic system of bulk liquid, foam, and bulk gas, with the relative proportions of each determining overall $\dot{V}_A/\dot{Q}$ at any given moment. For example, areas of bulk liquid would be areas of shunts; areas of foam, if also ventilated, could be areas of "wasted" ventilation; and areas of bulk gas would be areas of normal $\dot{V}_A/\dot{Q}$, the end point to which the other areas must advance.

References

1. Agostoni, E., Mead, J.: Statics of the respiratory system, in Fenn, W.O. and Rahn, H. (eds.): Handbook of Physiology, Section 3, Respiration. Washington, D.C., American Physiological Society, 1965.
2. Agostoni, E., Taglietti, A., Agostoni, F., Setnikar, I.: Mechanical aspects of the first breath. J. Appl. Physiol. 13:344, 1958.
3. Anthonisen, N.R., Danson, J., Robertson, P.C., Ross, W.R.D.: Airway closure as a function of age. Respir. Physiol. 8:58, 1969.
4. Auld, P.A.M.: Pulmonary physiology of the newborn infant, in Scarpelli, E.M. and Auld, P.A.M. (eds.): Pulmonary Physiology of the Fetus, Newborn, and Child. Philadelphia, Lea and Febiger, 1975, p. 140.
5. Auld, P.A.M., Nelson, N.M., Cherry, R.B., et al.: Measurement of thoracic gas volume in the newborn infant. J. Clin. Invest. 42:476, 1963.
6. Avery, M.E., Cook, C.D.. Volume-pressure relationships of lungs and thorax in fetal, newborn, and adult goats. J. Appl. Physiol. 16:1034, 1961.
7. Avery, M.E., Fletcher, B.D.: The Lung and its Disorders in the Newborn Infant. Philadelphia, W. B. Saunders Company, 1974.
8. Boddy, K., Dawes, G.S., Robinson, J.S.: A 24-hour rhythm in the foetus, in Barcroft Symposium of Foetal and Neonatal Physiology. Cambridge, Cambridge University Press, 1973.
9. Bolton, D.P.G., Cross, K.W.: Lung volume and mixing efficiency in the new-born infant. J. Physiol. (London) 208:25P, 1970.
10. Borell, U., Fernstrom, I.: The shape of the foetal chest during its passage through the birth canal. Acta Obstet. Gynec. Scand. 41:213, 1962.
11. Bosma, J.F., Lind, J.: Roentgenologic observations of motions of the upper airway associated with establishment of respiration in the newborn infant. Acta Paediatr. Scand. (Suppl. 123) 49:18, 1960.

12. Chu, J., Clements, J.A., Cotton, E.K., et al.: Neonatal pulmonary ischemia. Pediatrics **40**:709, 1967.
13. Chu, J., Dawson, P., Klaus, M., Sweet, A.Y.: Lung compliance and lung volume measured concurrently in normal full-term and premature infants. Pediatrics **34**:525, 1964.
14. Clements, J.A., Platzker, A.C.G., Tierney, D.F., et al.: Assessment of the risk of the respiratory distress syndrome by a rapid test for surfactant in amniotic fluid. N. Engl. J. Med. **286**:1077, 1972.
15. Clutario, B.C.: Clinical pulmonary function, in Scarpelli, E.M. and Auld. P.A.M. (eds.): Pulmonary Physiology of the Fetus, Newborn, and Child. Philadelphia, Lea and Febiger, 1975, p. 299.
16. Condorelli, S., Scarpelli, E.M.: Fetal breathing: Induction in utero and effects of vagotomy and barbiturates. J. Pediatr. **88**:94, 1976.
17. Cook, C.D., Cherry, R.B., O'Brian, D., et al.: Studies in respiratory physiology in the newborn infant. I. Observations on normal fullterm and premature infants. J. Clin. Invest. **34**:975, 1955.
18. Cook, C.D., Sutherland, J.M., Segal, S., et al.: Studies of respiratory physiology in the newborn infant. III. Measurements of the mechanics of respiration. J. Clin. Invest. **36**:440, 1957.
19. Deming, J., Hanner, J.P.: Respiration in infancy. Study of rate, volume and character of respiration in healthy infants during neonatal period. Am. J. Dis. Child. **51**:823, 1936.
20. Dinwiddie, R., Russell, G.: Relationship of intraesophageal pressure to intrapleural pressure in the newborn. J. Appl. Physiol. **33**:415, 1972.
21. Doershuk, C.F., Fisher, B.J., Matthews, L.W.: Pulmonary physiology of the young child, in Scarpelli, E.M. and Auld, P.A.M. (eds.): Pulmonary Physiology of the Fetus, Newborn, and Child. Philadelphia, Lea and Febiger, 1975, p. 166.
22. Drorbaugh, J.E., Segal, S., Sutherland, J.M., et al.: Compliance of lung during first week of life. Am. J. Dis. Child. **105**:63, 1963.
23. Egan, E.A., Olver, R.E., Strang, L.B.: Changes in non-electrolyte permeability of alveoli and the absorption of lung liquid at the start of breathing in the lamb. J. Physiol. (London) **244**:161, 1975.
24. Geubelle, F., Karlberg, P., Koch, G., et al.: L'aeration du poumon chez le nouveau-né. Biol. Neonat **1**:169, 1959.
25. Gluck, L., Kulovich, M.V.: Lecithin/sphingomyelin ratios in amniotic fluid in normal and abnormal pregnancy. Am. J. Obstet. Gynec. **115**:539, 1973.
26. Golinko, R.J., Rudolph, A.M.: A valve for respiratory studies on infants. Pediatrics **27**:645, 1961.
27. Gruenwald, P.: Normal and abnormal expansion of the lungs of newborn infants obtained at autopsy. III. The pattern of aeration as affected by gestational and postnatal age. Anat. Rec. **146**:337, 1963.
28. Hirvonen, R., Peltonen, R., Peltonen, T.: Disappearance of tracheobronchial fluid at birth in the lamb. Ann. Chir. Gynaecol. **64**:170, 1975.
29. Huch, R. Lübbers, D.W., Huch, A.: Reliability of transcutaneous monitoring of arterial PO_2 in newborn infants. Arch. Dis. Child. **49**:213, 1974.

30. James, L.S., Weisbrot, I.M., Prince, C.E., et al.: The acid-base status of human infants in relation to birth asphyxia and the onset of respiration. J. Pediatr. **52**:379, 1958.
31. Kanto, W.P., Jr., Borer, R.C., Jr., Barr, M., Jr., Roloff, D.W.:Trachael aspirate lecithin/sphingomyelin ratios as predictors of recovery from respiratory distress syndrome. J. Pediatr. **89**:612, 1976.
32. Karlberg, P.: The adaptive changes in the immediate postnatal period with particular reference to respiration. J. Pediatr. **56**:585, 1960.
33. Karlberg, P., Adams, F.H., Geubelle, F., Wallgren, G.: Alternations of the infant's thorax during vaginal delivery. Acta Obstet. Gynecol. Scand. 41: 223, 1962.
34. Karlberg, P., Cherry, R.B., Escardo, F.E., Koch, G.: Respiratory studies in newborn infants. I. Apparatus and methods for studies of pulmonary ventilation and the mechanics of breathing. Acta Pediatr. Scand. **49**:345, 1960.
35. Karlberg, P., Cherry, R.B., Escardo, F.E., Koch, G.: Respiratory studies in newborn infants. II. Pulmonary ventilation and mechanics of breathing in the first minutes of life, including the onset of respiration. Acta Paed. Scand. **51**:121, 1962.
36. Kikkawa, Y.: Morphology and morphologic development of the lung, in Scarpelli, E.M., and Auld, P.A.M. (eds.): Pulmonary Physiology of the Fetus, Newborn, and Child. Philadelphia, Lea and Febiger, 1975, p. 37.
37. Koch, G.: Alveolar ventilation, diffusing capacity and the A-a Po_2 difference in the newborn infant. Respir. Physiol. **4**:168, 1968.
38. Klaus, M.H., Tooley, W.H., Weaver, K.H., Clements, J.A.: Lung volume in the newborn infant. Pediatrics **30**:111, 1962.
39. Krauss, A.N., Auld, P.A.M.: Ventilation-perfusion abnormalities in the premature infant. Triple gradient. Pediatr. Res. **3**:255, 1969.
40. Krauss, A.N., Auld, P.A.M.: Pulmonary gas trapping in premature infants. Pediat. Res. **5**:10, 1971.
41. Kraus, A.N., Klain, D.B., Dahms, B., Auld, P.A.M.: Vital capacity in premature infants. Am. Rev. Respir. Dis. **108**:1361, 1973.
42. Kubli, F.W., Berg, D.: The early disagnosis of foetal distress. J. Obstet. Gynec. Brit. Comm. **72**:507, 1965.
43. Lacourt, G., Polgar, G.: Interaction between nasal and pulmonary resistance in newborn infants. J. Appl. Physiol. **30**:870, 1971.
44. Ledbetter, M.K., Homma, T., Farhi, L.E.: Readjustment in distribution of alveolar ventilation and lung perfusion in the newborn. Pediatrics **40**:940, 1967.
45. Lind, J., Tahti, E.: Roentgenologic studies of the human fetal lungs at midterm. Ann. Paed. Fenn. **12**:25, 1966.
46. Lind, J., Tahti, E., Hirvensalo, M.: Roentgenologic studies of the size of the lungs of the newborn baby before and after aeration. Ann. Paed. Fenn. **12**:20, 1966.
47. Mansell, A., Bryan, C., Levison, H.: Airway closure in children. J. Appl. Physiol. **33**:711, 1972.
48. Nelson, N.M. Respiration and circulation after birth, in Smith, C.A. and

Nelson, N.M. (eds.): The Physiology of the Newborn. Springfield, Charles C Thomas, 1976, p. 117.

49. Nelson, N.M., Prod'hom, L.S., Cherry, R.B., et al.: Pulmonary function in the newborn infant. I. Methods: Ventilation and gaseous metabolism. Pediatrics **30**:963, 1962.

50. Nelson, N.M., Prod'hom, L.S., Cherry, R.B., et al: Pulmonary function in the newborn infant. V. Trapped gas in the normal infant's lung. J. Clin. Invest. **42**:1850, 1963.

51. Nelson, N.M., Prod'hom, L.S., Cherry, R.B., et al.: Pulmonary function in the newborn infant, the alveolar-arterial oxygen gradient. J. Appl. Physiol. **18**:534, 1963.

52. Nelson, N.M., Prod'hom, L.S., Cherry, R.B., et al.: Pulmonary function in the newborn infant. II. Perfusion-estimation by analysis of the arterial-alveolar carbon dioxide difference. Pediatrics **30**:975, 1962.

53. Nourse, C.H., Nelson, N.M.: Uniformity of ventilation in the newborn infant: Direct assessment of the arterial-alveolar N_2 difference. Pediatrics **43**:226, 1969.

54. Pearson, H.A. The blood, in Smith, C.A. and Nelson, N.M. (eds.):The Physiology of the Newborn Infant. Springfield, Charles C Thomas, 1976, p. 263.

55. Polgar, G., String, S.T.: The viscous resistance of the lung tissues in newborn infants. J. Pediatr. **69**:787, 1966.

56. Radford, E. P., Jr.: Static mechanical properties of mammalian lungs, in Fenn, W.O. and Rahn, H. (eds.): Handbook of Physiology, Section 3, Respiration. Washington, D.C.: American Physiological Society, 1964.

57. Richards, C.C., Bachman, L.: Lung and chest wall compliance of apneic paralyzed infants. J. Clin. Invest. **40**:273, 1961.

58. Rooth, G.: Transcutaneous technique for continuous oxygen tension measurements. Rev. Perinatal Med. **1**:179, 1976.

59. Scarpelli, E.M.: The lung, trachael fluid and lipid metabolism of the fetus. Pediatrics **40**:941, 1967.

60. Scarpelli, E.M.: The Surfactant System Of The Lung. Philadelphia, Lea and Febiger, 1968.

61. Scarpelli, E.M.: Lung surfactant: dynamic properties, metabolic pathways, and possible significance in the pathogenesis of the respiratory distress syndrome. Bull. N.Y. Acad. Med. **44**:431, 1968.

62. Scarpelli, E.M., Perinatal respiration, in Scarpelli, E.M. and Auld, P.A.M. (eds.):Pulmonary Physiology of the Fetus, Newborn and Child. Philadelphia, Lea and Febiger, 1975, p. 116.

63. Scarpelli, E. M.: Fetal pulmonary fluid. Rev. Perinatal Med. **1**:49, 1976.

64. Scarpelli, E.M.: The surfactant system of the lung. Int. Anesthesiol. Clin. **15** (4):19, 1977.

65. Scarpelli, E.M.: Concepts in respiratory pathophysiology, in Scarpelli, E.M., Auld, P.A.M., and Goldman, H.S. (eds.): Pulmonary Disease of The Fetus, Newborn and Child. Philadelphia, Lea and Febiger, 1978.

66. Scarpelli, E.M.: Intrapulmonary foam at birth: An adaptational phenomenon. Pediatr. Res. **12**:1070, 1978.

67. Scarpelli, E.M., Condorelli, S., Cosmi, E.V.: Lamb fetal pulmonary fluid. I. Validation and significance of method for determination of volume and volume change. Pediatr. Res. 9:190, 1975.
68. Staub, N.C., Nagano, H. Pearce, M.L.: Pulmonary edema in dogs, especially the sequence of fluid accumulation in lungs. J. Appl. Physiol. 22:227, 1967.
69. Strang, L.B.: Uptake of liquid from the lungs at the start of breathing, in De Reuck, A.V.S. and Porter, R. (eds.): Development Of The Lung. Boston, Little, Brown and Company, 1967.
70. Strang, L.B., McGrath, M.W.: Alveolar ventilation in normal newborn infants studied by air wash-in after oxygen breathing. Clin. Sci. 23:129, 1962.
71. Thibeault, D.W., Poblete, E., Auld, P.A.M.: Alveolar-arterial O_2 and CO_2 differences and their relation to lung volume in the newborn. Pediatrics 41:574, 1968.
72. Thibeault, D.W., Wong, M.M., Auld, P.A.M.: Thoracic gas volume changes in premature infants. Pediatrics 40:403, 1967.
73. Tooley, W. H.: In Normal and Abnormal Respiration of Children, 37th Ross Conference on Pediatric Research, 1960. Published by Ross Laboratories.
74. West, J.B.: Regional differences in gas exchange in the lung of erect man. J. Appl. Physiol. 17:893, 1962.

10
The Meconium Aspiration Syndrome

Jean F. Hobbs and Arthur I. Eidelman

Aspiration of meconium-stained amniotic fluid during the birth process is a common event that can have catastrophic results. In fact, meconium aspiration syndrome has emerged as a leading cause of death in the neonatal period, with a mortality rate in the term infant as high as 20 times that of all other causes combined (22). Moreover, the impact on infant and family of the prolonged hospitalization, complications, and sequelae of the neonatal disease can be enormous and devastating.

In the past decade, intrapartum aspiration and the subsequent respiratory distress have received considerable attention from clinicians and investigators as other causes of neonatal mortality and morbidity have yielded to the techniques of newborn intensive care. Although the pathophysiology of meconium aspiration syndrome is not clearly defined, it has become apparent that the course and prognosis are mostly determined in the delivery room, perhaps even before the first breath is taken. The direction of current management is therefore toward anticipation and prevention of the syndrome; once pulmonary disease is established, there is little to offer but supportive therapy. The challenge for the physician is first to identify the infant at risk for aspiration and then to choose appropriate measures to prevent or at least minimize the developing symptoms.

Incidence

In general, the incidence of meconium aspiration parallels that of meconium passage *in utero*, although the physiologic mechanisms for the two processes may be quite different. Even with optimal obstetric management, 8.8% (14) to 29% (18) of vertex deliveries occur through meconium.

Of course, breech presentation is associated with far higher rates of meconium passage during delivery, but this is of no clinical significance if the rush of amniotic fluid following the aftercoming head is clear. Until recently, as many as 20% (14) to 35% (4) of infants born through meconium have been reported to develop respiratory symptoms ranging from mild to most severe, making this a leading cause of extended hospital stay in the term or postterm infant. In our experience, as many as 20% of the admissions to our newborn intensive care unit have been for treatment of meconium aspiration.

Pathophysiology (Fig. 10.1)

Meconium passage *in utero* can occur as a natural phenomenon in the maturation of a fetus and is, in fact, most common when gestational age is greater than 42 weeks. However, the incidence of meconium-stained amniotic fluid also increases with signs of fetal distress, specifically low-scalp pH or heart-rate abnormalities. Hyperperistalsis and relaxation of the anal sphincter have been associated with umbilical cord compression and the resultant fetal bradycardia (18).

Although Dawes and others have clearly demonstrated fetal breathing and gasping under normal and stressed conditions, it is not clear whether movement of amniotic fluid into the fetal lung occurs in sufficient quantity

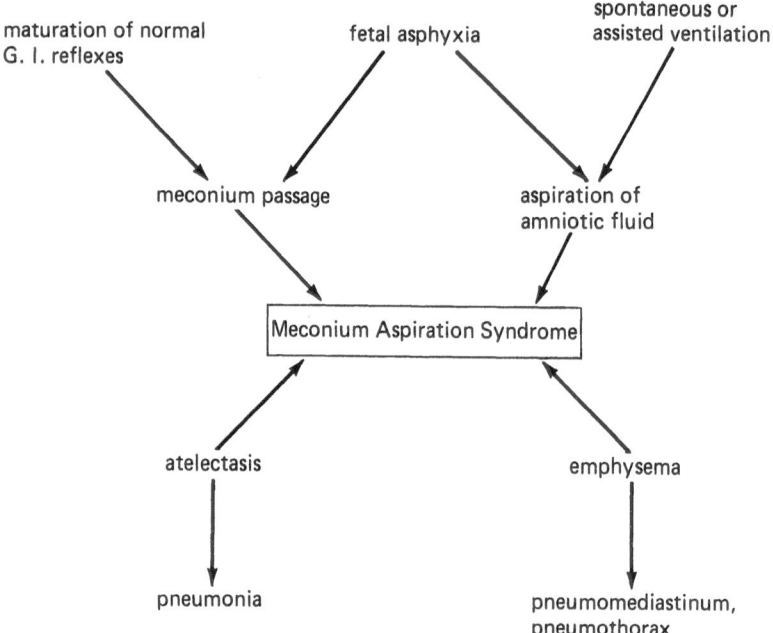

Fig. 10.1 Pathophysiology of meconium aspiration syndrome.

to cause massive *in utero* aspiration. During labor and delivery, however, material taken into the mouth and trachea moves into the smaller airways and alveoli as air breathing is initiated. Particulate or very thick meconium can cause airway obstruction so severe that ventilation is impossible. Smaller plugs distributed throughout the tracheobronchial tree create some areas of atelectasis and others of compensatory emphysema. Rupture of alveoli can cause interstitial emphysema and pneumothorax, while dissection of air along vessel walls can lead to pneumomediastinum. These complications may be secondary to positive pressure ventilation with bag or respirator, but can also occur spontaneously, especially in a vigorous term infant capable of generating intrathoracic pressures as high as 70 cm of water with initial breaths (21).

Gooding et al. (11) have shown in an animal model that migration of tantalum-labelled meconium from the tracheobronchial tree to the periphery of the lung takes place within one hour. In our clinical experience, efforts to retrieve aspirated meconium by endotracheal suction are futile if initiated more than 30 to 60 minutes after delivery. Chest x-rays taken at this time often document parenchymal disease.

Meconium consists of bile, bile acids, and swallowed amniotic fluid contents containing lanugo, vernix caseosa, and epithelial cells. It also contains varying concentrations of intestinal and pancreatic secretions theoretically capable of causing a chemical pneumonitis. Goodlin (13) was not able to demonstrate this effect in newborn rabbits, but pathologic changes in puppies (12) and human neonates (21) are suggestive of an inflammatory reaction. Material aspirated *in utero* is sterile unless, of course, prolonged rupture of membranes has led to chorioamnionitis. However, organisms aspirated from the birth canal or introduced during endotracheal manipulation may superimpose a bacterial pneumonia on the already compromised lung.

In a small proportion of infants, the degree of hypoxemia is more profound than can be accounted for by the airway or parenchymal manifestations of aspiration. This may be the result of marked right-to-left shunting of blood in three locations: within the pulmonary vascular bed, through the foramen ovale, and across a patent ductus arteriosus. Clinical conditions associated with increased shunting include acidosis, hypothermia, hypotension, and hypoglycemia. These infants require prompt and maximal intervention. Even with intensive therapy, however, deep hypoxemia and intractable metabolic acidosis often lead to fatal intracerebral or pulmonary hemorrhages.

Clinical Presentation

The meconium aspiration syndrome occurs almost exclusively in term or postterm infants, whether normally-grown, small, or large for gestational age. The incidence is greatest over 40 weeks estimated gestational age; Gregory et al. reported an average length of gestation of 290 days (range 268 to 322) (14). Several authors have found no affected infants born at less than 37 weeks (14, 18, 23). Ting and Brady (22) reported that, of 125 infants delivered through meconium, none was less than 32 weeks and only six were preterm. In fact, of these six only the three infants who were over 34 weeks estimated gestational age displayed symptoms of aspiration.

A definite diagnosis of meconium aspiration syndrome requires evidence of meconium in the oropharynx or trachea, clinical respiratory distress, and radiographic changes consistent with aspiration pneumonia. Initial clinical findings vary considerably. At one end of a spectrum are the vigorous, well-developed term infants with good Apgar scores who appear completely normal in the delivery room despite passage through meconium-stained amniotic fluid. The great majority of such babies remain well, but a few within the first four hours of life will develop tachypnea and flaring as evidence of mild pulmonary involvement and vomiting or poor feeding secondary to meconium gastritis.

At the other extreme are the term or postterm dysmature infants with respiratory symptoms in the immediate postpartum period. These infants can be recognized by their dry and scaling skin, lack of vernix caseosa, wrinkled skin folds over knees and elbows, and generally wasted appearance. If they have been exposed to meconium *in utero* for several hours they will have deeply stained skin, nails, and umbilical cord. If the meconium is thick, such a neonate may be choking and gasping, unable to clear his major airways or to establish adequate ventilation. If sufficient time has elapsed for the meconium to move into the smaller airways, the infant may have many signs of respiratory distress including tachypnea, nasal flaring, grunting, retractions, central cyanosis, and hyperexpanded chest. Auscultation of the chest reveals diffuse rales and rhonchi, with alveolar breath sounds at times entirely replaced by tubular noises. If significant intrapartum asphyxia has caused the aspiration, the need for immediate resuscitation may be evident by low Apgar scores, hypotonia, absent or irregular ventilatory effort, and deep cyanosis. Sudden deterioration with asymmetry of breath sounds may occur secondary to pneumomediastinum or pneumothorax. Seizures may develop within the first 24 hours of life as a result either of the precipitating asphyxic insult or of failure subsequently to establish and maintain adequate oxygenation and acid-base balance.

It is important to emphasize that since meconium aspiration is a condition of obstructed ventilation, it cannot in itself be the cause of significant neonatal depression in the first moments of life before pulmonary air exchange is required. Specifically, the infant born with a heart rate less than 100 or with an Apgar score at one minute of less than 7 is suffering from an insult that may be either primary or incidental to the aspiration. Identification and correction of this underlying condition must take priority in initial management of the infant even at the risk of worsening the potential aspiration pneumonia.

Radiographic Features

The classic x-ray changes of meconium aspiration syndrome were described in 1955 by Peterson and Pendleton (19). They noted bilateral, patchy, asymmetric infiltrates and uneven aeration with both atelectatic and emphysematous areas (Fig. 10.2). The pattern is clearly different from the fine, granular appearance of hyaline membrane disease. However, the infiltrates are impossible to distinguish from those of congenital pneumonia or pulmonary hemorrhage and both of these conditions may occur secondarily, thus complicating the serial x-ray findings.

In general, the prominence of the x-ray changes correlates with the

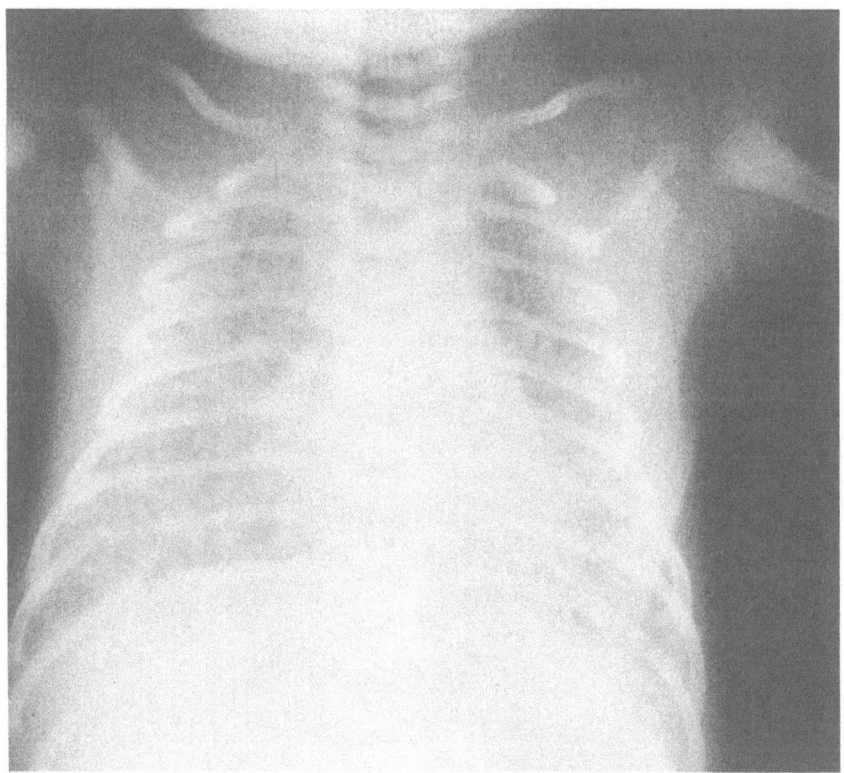

Fig. 10.2 A-P chest film showing bilateral infiltrates secondary to severe meconium aspiration.

severity of the clinical symptoms, although respiratory distress may precede the appearance of infiltrates. In some infants, however, the deteriorating clinical condition marked by poor oxygenation may be in part secondary to intra- and extra-pulmonary right-to-left shunting that is not reflected radiographically.

Gooding and Gregory (11) studied chest x-rays in a sample of 75 infants delivered through meconium, almost all of whom had received endotracheal suction in the delivery room. Forty-five of these neonates were clinically well and had clear lungs within the first hour of life, except for fluid in the minor fissure or costophrenic sulci. The remainder had pulmonary consolidation classified as slight, moderate, or severe. Serial x-rays documented clearing of infiltrates within 24 to 72 hours in all but one infant; however, resolution in cases of severe or massive aspiration can be considerably prolonged.

Other findings of Gooding and Gregory (11) included pneumomediastinum or pneumothorax in seven infants, only two of whom had associated severe pulmonary consolidation. Tension pneumothorax may be a cause of rapid deterioration and, if unrecognized and untreated, of death (Fig. 10.3). It is important to remember that in the supine neonate the lung tends to collapse behind the anterior air collection. In such an infant,

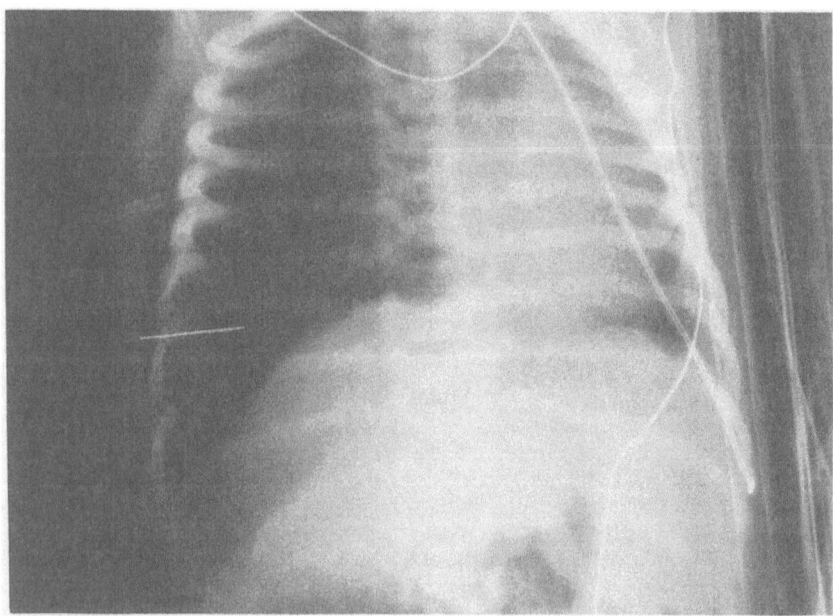

Fig. 10.3 A-P chest film of right tension pneumothorax with mediastinum shifted to left.

lung markings may still be visible to the periphery and the only sign of pneumothorax or anteroposterior chest film may be increased lucency on the affected side. A cross-table lateral view can aid in diagnosis.

Management Considerations

Risk Profile

It is evident that in the great majority of cases, aspiration of meconium occurs during rather than prior to delivery. It is also clear that the syndrome is a result of a sequence of events starting with airway obstruction and progressing to alveolar disease within as short a time as one hour. Since we have no specific therapy for the parenchymal disease, attempts must be made to interrupt the sequence proximal to the alveoli, either by oropharyngeal or endotracheal suction. Recommendations for initial management are actively debated in the obstetric, anesthesia, and pediatric literature, while practices at individual hospitals often are based on the exigencies of delivery room equipment and staffing.

Many physicians feel that the presence of meconium in the trachea of the normal, healthy infant is of no clinical significance, and that, in such a neonate, airway suction under direct visualization is both unnecessary and potentially hazardous. Moreover, a majority of infants born through meconium do not develop meconium aspiration syndrome. It is important to know, therefore, whether a particular constellation of fetal and maternal factors can clearly define the population of infants who will become symptomatic without suction of the pharynx or trachea. In the past five years, several authors have examined correlations between various risk factors and outcome. They differ considerably in the specific questions asked, prospective or retrospective nature of the studies, selection of the patient samples, delivery room management during the study intervals, results, and conclusions. Nevertheless, a review of the data can be used to develop a profile of the infant at greatest risk, which can then serve as a base for management guidelines.

Maternal Factors

Maternal age and parity do not appear to be related to either passage (18) or aspiration (17, 22) of meconium by the fetus. Concurrent diseases with the possible exception of toxemia (4, 15, 18, 22) are also unrelated. In our experience, infants of narcotic-addicted mothers do not appear at increased risk for meconium aspiration (16). However, meconium passage and aspiration can occur even *prior* to delivery if the fetus of a narcotic-addicted mother undergoes in utero withdrawal (20).

Intrapartum Conditions

Gregory, the only author to address this issue, found that prolonged labor increased the risk of meconium aspiration syndrome (14). However, duration of meconium staining, time of rupture of membranes, and type and duration of anesthesia are not related (14, 22). The higher incidence of aspiration with delivery by mid-forceps (17), vacuum extraction (14), or Cesarean section (14) probably reflects as much the fetal indication as the mode of intervention. Specific complications such as abruptio placentae (14) or cord abnormalities (22) do not occur more frequently in symptomatic than in asymptomatic infants.

The thickness or viscosity of the meconium in the amniotic fluid is an interesting variable. Miller (18) reported that thick, in contrast to thin, meconium was associated with lower mean one and five-minute Apgar scores, and Hobel (15) found in a series of 76 patients that a subgroup defined by thick meconium had the highest morbidity (i.e., respiratory distress) and mortality. Gregory did not find a statistical correlation between consistency of meconium in the trachea and incidence of meconium aspiration syndrome; nevertheless he recommends that the thick, particulate, or "pea soup" nature of the meconium should be a key factor in prompting endotracheal suction (14).

Fetal Variables

Meconium passage and aspiration occur in the term or postterm infant. In Gregory's series of 88 infants born through meconium, the average gestational age was 41½ weeks (range 38 to 46 weeks) and the average birth weight was 2911 g with only two infants under 2500 g (14). As cited above, in the large group of meconium-stained infants studied by Ting and Brady there were only six prematures, and of these only the three over 34 weeks' gestation were symptomatic of aspiration (22). Ting's data also suggests that the proportion of infants who are symptomatic increases with postmaturity.

Since continuous monitoring of fetal heart rate (FHR) and fetal scalp blood sampling are now available for most high-risk pregnancies, the obstetrician may have criteria other than historic ones for evaluating the fetus in the presence of meconium-stained amniotic fluid. FHR abnormalities fall into four main categories: accelerations (tachycardia over 160/minute) and decelerations, which are early, late, or variable with regard to uterine contractions. Tachycardia or early decelerations are not associated with either meconium passage or symptomatic aspiration (18, 14), although the former may carry a high neonatal mortality from other causes (15). Infants born through meconium appear to have no greater incidence of moderate-to-severe decelerations than matched controls (18). However, the presence of both features is ominous. Gregory has reported a significant increase in "sick" versus "well" infants when fetal heart rates are below 120/minute (14), and Miller has correlated meconium passage and late decelerations occurring with greater than 10% of contractions with low 5-minute Apgar scores (18).

The other essential element in the fetal profile is the scalp pH. Hobel (15) measured blood pH serially during labor, and correlated aberrations with the presence of meconium, FHR abnormalities, umbilical cord pH values, Apgar scores, morbidity, and mortality. He found that meconium staining of the amniotic fluid, whether light or heavy, with or without FHR abnormality, was associated with pH values below normal throughout labor and subsequently in the umbilical artery and vein. In early labor (2 to 4 cm cervical dilatation), heavy meconium and moderate-to-severe FHR decelerations were found in conjunction with the lowest scalp pH values and the highest base deficits; although scalp pH tended to rise during labor, umbilical artery acidosis was marked (7.19 ± 0.10) and the UA/UV pH differential was large.

Where there has been no *in utero* monitoring, the one-minute Apgar score may be used to estimate the degree of intrapartum asphyxia and therefore the likelihood of aspiration. However, a good initial score does not rule out the possibility of aspiration, and moreover, if the physician waits one or certainly five minutes before intervening, he may miss a critical opportunity to abort the disease.

Delivery Room Intervention

The factors that place the infant at highest risk for meconium aspiration syndrome are postmaturity, maternal toxemia, prolonged labor, thick or "pea-soup" meconium, moderate to severe FHR decelerations, and low scalp pH (Table 10.1). If even one of the risk factors is present, we recommend that the obstetrician suction the mouth and nose with the bulb

Table 10.1   High Risk Factors in Meconium Aspiration Syndrome

Location	Risk
Maternal	Toxemia
Intrapartum	Prolonged labor
	Thick meconium
Fetal	Postmaturity
	Moderate to severe FHR decelerations
	Low scalp pH

syringe and that the infant then be promptly given to the most skilled attendant for endotracheal intubation and suction. The mother, and father if present, should be informed of this possibility prior to delivery, since the otherwise desirable practice of resting the infant on the mother's abdomen or in her arms will have to be delayed, and the manipulation of the neonate can be distressing to an unprepared family.

It is important to use a sufficiently large endotracheal tube to permit passage of a #8 French suction catheter. This is rarely a problem, since term or postterm infants almost always accept a 3.5- or 4.0-mm endotracheal tube. If the meconium is very viscous, it may be necessary to reintubate with a fresh tube; however, we do not recommend routine reintubation because of the risk of trauma to the larynx or trachea.

The trachea must be suctioned until the return is free of meconium. The procedure should be frequently interrupted to allow the infant to breathe. Increased F_{IO_2} or positive pressure ventilation can be given as needed, but should be delayed until after the initial suctioning when possible.

A therapeutic issue raised by Burke-Strickland (4) is that of tracheal lavage. If a sufficient amount of instilled saline is not promptly removed, ventilation may be impaired. Carson (5) has stated that lavage in the absence of meconium may lead to iatrogenic "wet lung disease" requiring oxygen therapy. Burke-Strickland, however, cited that in the nine cases in which x-rays were taken before and after lavage, there was no evidence of increased pulmonary fluid. If the meconium is very thick, a commercial preparation of N-acetylcysteine, "Mucomyst," may be diluted to 2% in alkaline solution and used a few times for tracheal lavage. However, in higher concentrations, or with prolonged use, this preparation can cause irritation of mucous membranes, paralysis of cilia, and bronchospasm.

The benefits of prompt and aggressive intervention have been documented. Ting and Brady (22) reported that a retrospective analysis of morbidity and mortality rates of 125 infants delivered through meconium-stained amniotic fluid showed a markedly improved outcome after tracheal suction in the delivery room became common practice at their hospital. Gregory et al. (14) also commented that although there were no deaths in their current series, they did find that, prior to initiation of a policy of delivery room endotracheal intubation and suction, three infants with meconium aspiration syndrome had died from widespread bronchopneumonia.

It is also evident that suctioning meconium from the mouth after the onset of air breathing is not sufficient because infants with clear oropharynx may already have drawn material into the trachea. Burke-Strickland reported in 1973 the results of a two-year prospective study attempting to determine which infants require aggressive therapy in the delivery room (4). By study design, infants born through meconium, but with clear oropharynx, were not intubated. Of this group of infants, all had Apgar scores of five or more at one and five minutes, and eight of 17 had changes on x-ray consistent with aspiration syndrome as described by Peterson and Pendleton. These patients were all term or postterm and required an average hospital stay of 10 days, and two of the 8 had pneumothoraces. A study by Gregory et al. (14) in 1974 confirmed that an infant with clear mouth and larynx may have meconium in the trachea, but neither of these authors attempted to relate the presence of risk factors to aspiration in such cases.

In skilled hands, intubation has a very low complication rate. Nevertheless, it can never be entirely benign and, at best, has not been shown to completely prevent meconium aspiration syndrome. Recently Carson et al. (5) cited experience with De Lee suction of the nasopharynx as soon as the head of the neonate appeared on the perineum before the first breath was taken, and suggested this procedure as an alternative to routine intubation. This technique was stimulated by the work of Gooding et al. (12), which showed that in fetal pups aspiration and migration of meconium into the lung parenchyma did not occur until the onset of air breathing. Carson reported that this method of suctioning by the obstetrician significantly reduced the incidence of meconium aspiration syndrome without creating hazardous effects such as reflex bradycardia. However, this complication has been well documented by others (6), and Carson did not state whether she monitored the fetal heart during delivery. Carson has recommended that when meconium is present at the level of the vocal cords after the onset of respiration, intubation and suction should proceed at once. This would necessitate routine laryngoscopic examination of the cords whenever meconium-stained amniotic fluid is present. Since this procedure can also cause reflex bradycardia, we recommend it only when intubation is to be performed. Examination of the vocal cords *per se* has not been shown to add to the previous assessment of the infant.

Currently, our recommendations for management of the vigorous term infant, born through meconium but without additional risk factor for aspiration, do not include deep nasopharyngeal suction, laryngoscopy, or endotracheal intubation. We feel that such an infant routinely requires no more than careful suctioning of the nose and mouth with a bulb syringe upon delivery of the head. A cord pH should be obtained because the infant may have suffered a silent *in utero* asphyxic insult which has caused metabolic acidosis of some severity. This presumably healthy infant should also be observed in an incubator for the first six to eight hours of life to detect any signs of respiratory distress. If none develop, he may subsequently be returned to routine well-baby care.

An additional procedure to be done in the delivery room is the removal of swallowed meconium from the stomach to prevent secondary aspiration during stabilization or transport.

Subsequent Nursery Care

If meconium has been suctioned from the trachea, the infant should remain intubated for subsequent pulmonary toilet and should be transferred to a special care nursery for chest x-ray and arterial blood gas sampling. Once meconium aspiration syndrome is established, treatment consists of support of ventilation and oxygenation, minimizing the development of further atelectasis, and prophylaxis against infection. Critical factors in respiratory management are high humidity, preferably via heated nebulizer, skilled percussion of the chest, and postural drainage. Equipment for management of pneumothorax should be kept at the bedside. When hypoxemia is severe, mechanical ventilation may be required, and Fox et al. (7) have shown continuous distending pressure (CDP) to be of some benefit. We were at first reluctant to use CDP because of the risk of pneumothorax. However, we have found that in cases of moderate to severe disease, levels of CDP to 7 or 8 cm H_2O may improve oxygenation whether by decreasing pulmonary fluid retention or by opening collapsed alveoli. In addition, we agree with Fox that this level of CDP has not increased the incidence of pneumothorax or pneumomediastinum.

However, in cases of significant right-to-left intra- and extrapulmonary shunting, high levels of CDP may worsen the hypoxemia by increasing intrathoracic pressures. In this situation, it may be necessary to modify the use of CDP and to consider the use of a pulmonary vasodilator such as tolazoline, which has been employed with some success in a few very severe cases (8) (10). In extreme situations, one group has even employed extracorporeal membrane oxygenation with venoarterial bypass (2).

Although meconium is sterile at birth, antibiotic coverage, i.e., a penicillin and an aminoglycoside, is generally used for several reasons. As mentioned above, the lung findings cannot be differentiated from those of congenital pneumonia. Also, the presence of a high carbohydrate substance in a wet lung provides an excellent culture media for organisms introduced by tracheal manipulation. Bryan (3) has demonstrated in rats that the addition of meconium to aspirated amniotic fluid significantly increases susceptibility to bacterial pneumonia.

It has been suggested that steroids might be of use in the treatment of meconium pneumonitis (1). However, a controlled study of glucocorticoid therapy in rabbits (9) indicated that, despite less severe pulmonary histologic changes after administration of steroids, there was no clinical improvement; in fact, survival rates in the treated sample were less than in controls. Recently, a double-blind study in human neonates failed to document any improvement in the steroid-treated sample. To the contrary, these infants had greater morbidity as indicated by duration of respiratory symptoms and requirement for increased oxygen (24).

Although the primary concern is the pulmonary disease, the infant may have other problems as well. In particular, if a significant amount of meconium has been swallowed, it may be necessary to lavage the stomach with saline to minimize gastritis. Even when this has been done, many infants may have difficulty with the initiation of formula feedings and so should be watched for gastric distention or vomiting.

Our recommendations for management are briefly summarized in Table 10.2.

Prognosis

Although anticipation and aggressive therapy in the delivery room have significantly decreased the incidence of severe meconium aspiration syndrome, it remains a leading cause of death in the term or postterm infant. As recently as 1973, for example, the mortality rate for classic meconium aspiration syndrome at Cook County Hospital was 28% (21). There is now some indication that prompt intervention, whether by clearing the

Table 10.2 Management of the Infant Born Through Meconium when an Additional Risk Factor is Present

In the delivery room
1. Obtain cord pH.
2. Clear oropharynx and nose with bulb syringe or De Lee prior to first breath.
3. Intubate with large ET tube if possible.
4. Aspirate by mouth.
5. Remove ET tube if obstructed; reintubate and leave in place.
6. Avoid positive pressure; if required for resuscitation, give only after initial aspiration of ET tube.
7. Instill 0.5-cc sterile saline and suction until clear. If meconium is very thick, instill 1 cc of 2% Mucomyst* solution and suction.

1 cc 20% Mucomyst*
1.5 cc M NaHCO$_3$
7.5 cc DW
_____
10.0 cc

8. Empty stomach.
9. Transfer to special care nursery.

In the nursery
1. Attach cardiorespiratory monitor.
2. Draw arterial blood gas.
3. Obtain chest x-ray.
4. Continue intermittent ET lavage wtih sterile saline.
5. Begin postural drainage and percussion.
6. Administer warm, high humidity.
7. Cover with broad-spectrum antibiotics.
8. Keep NPO; lavage stomach if necessary.

nasopharynx before the first breath (5) or by suctioning via an endotracheal tube (14), may all but eliminate the mortality of this syndrome. With optimal management, the majority of milder cases resolve in two to four days without sequelae. A few infants remain tachypneic for weeks, even after resolution of x-ray findings. Chronic lung disease is not a sequela of meconium aspiration syndrome except in severe cases where changes secondary to increased FI_{O_2} and respirator therapy are superimposed.

There is an incidence of central nervous system abnormalities, especially following prolonged periods of hypoxemia or acidosis. Some of these problems, however, may have existed prior to birth and contributed to the etiology of the aspiration syndrome. Since neurologic examinations in the neonatal period have unreliable prognostic value, infants with severe disease, seizures, or a history of marked blood gas or acid-base abnormalities should be followed until school age to watch for sequelae.

References

1. Avery, M.E., Fletcher, B.D.: The Lung and Its Disorders in the Newborn infant, 3rd Ed. Philadelphia: W. B. Saunders Co., 1974.
2. Bartlett, R.H., Gazzaniga, A.B., Jeffries, M.R., et al.: Extracorporeal membrane oxygenation (ECMO); cardio-pulmonary support in infancy. Trans. Am. Soc. Artif. Intern, Organs 22:80, 1976.
3. Bryan, C.S.: Enhancement of bacterial infection by meconium. John Hopkins Med. J. 121:9, 1967.
4. Burke-Strickland, M., Edwards, N.B.: Meconium aspiration in the newborn. Minn. Med. 56:1031, 1973.
5. Carson, B.S., Losey, R.W., Bowes, W.A., Simmons, M.A.: Combined obstetric and pediatric approach to prevent meconium aspiration syndrome. Am. J. Obstet. Gynecol. 126:712, 1976.
6. Cordero, L., Hon, E.: Neonatal bradycardia following nasopharyngeal stimulation. J. Pediatr. 78:441, 1971.
7. Fox, W.W., Berman, L.S., Downes, J.J., Peckham, G.J.: The therapeutic application of end-expiratory pressure in the meconium aspiration syndrome. Pediatrics 56:214, 1975.
8. Fox, W.W., Gewitz, M.H., Dinwiddie, R., et al.: Pulmonary hypertension in the perinatal aspiration syndromes. Pediatrics 59:205, 1977.
9. Frantz, I.D., Wang, N.S., Thach, B.T.: Experimental meconium aspiration: Effects of glucocorticord treatment. J. Pediatr. 86:438, 1975.
10. Goetzman, B.W., Sunshine, P., Johnson, J.D., et al.: Neonatal hypoxia and pulmonary vasopasm: Response to tolazoline. J. Pediatr. 89:617, 1976.
11. Gooding, C.A., Gregorp, G.A.: Roentgenographic analysis of meconium aspiration of the newborn. Radiology 100:131, 1971.
12. Gooding, C.A., Gregory, G.A., Taber, P., Wright, R.R.: An Experimental

model for the study of meconium aspiration of the newborn. Radiology **100**:137, 1971.

13. Goodlin, R.C.: Meconium aspiration. Obstet. Gynecol. **32**:94, 1968.
14. Gregory, G.A., Gooding, C.A., Phibbs, R.H., Tooley, W.H.: Meconium aspiration in infants—a prospective study. J. Pediatr. **85**:848, 1974.
15. Hobel, C.J.: Intrapartum clinical assessment of fetal distress. Am. J. Obstet. Gynecol. **110**:336, 1971.
16. Kandall, S.B., Albin, S., Gartner, L.M., et al.:The narcotic dependent mother: fetal and neonatal consequences. Early Human Development, 1/2: 159, 1977.
17. Leake, R.D., Gunther, R., Sunshine, P.: Perinatal aspiration syndrome: its association with intrapartum events and anesthesia. Am. J. Obstet. Gynecol. **118**:271, 1974.
18. Miller, F.C., Sacks, D.A., Yeh, S., et al.: Significance of meconium during labor. Am. J. Obstet. Gynecol. **122**:573, 1975.
19. Peterson, H.G., Pendleton, M.E.: Contrasting roentgenographic pulmonary patterns of the hyaline membrane and fetal aspiration syndromes. Am. J. Roentgen. Radium Ther. Nucl. Med. **74**:800, 1955.
20. Rememteria, J.L., Nunag, N.N.: Narcotic withdrawal in pregnancy: Stillbirth incidence with a case report. Am. J. Obstet. Gynecol. **116**:1152, 1973.
21. Schaffer, A.J., Avery, M.E.: Diseases of the newborn, 3rd Ed. Philadelphia, W.B. Saunders Co., 1971.
22. Ting, P., Brady, J.P.: Tracheal suction in the meconium aspiration. Am. J. Obstet. Gynecol. **122**:767, 1975.
23. Vidyasagar, D., Yeh, T.F., Harris, V., Pildes, R.S.: Assisted ventilation in infants with meconium aspiration syndrome. Pediatrics **56**:208, 1975.
24. Yeh, T.F., Srinivasan, G., Harris, V., Pildes, R.S.: Hydrocortisone therapy in meconium aspiration syndrome: a controlled study. J. Pediatr. **90**:140, 1977.

11
Treatment of Neonatal Metabolic Acidosis

Arthur I. Eidelman and Jean F. Hobbs

The maintenance of a normal acid-base state in the newborn infant is a challenge both to the neonate's inherent regulatory mechanisms and to the clinician's skill in compensating for the biochemical and physiologic consequences when these mechanisms fail. The birth process and the immediate neonatal period are frequently associated with clinical conditions that lead to an acidotic state. This chapter will address itself to a discussion of perinatal acidosis, with special emphasis on the etiology and management of metabolic acidosis in the newborn period.

Acid Base Regulatory Mechanisms

Acidosis results from the production of both volatile and nonvolatile acids in excess of the capacity of the organism to buffer and excrete these acids. The elimination of the volatile acids is dependent on a normally functioning ventilatory system, while an adequate renal excretory mechanism is required for the elimination of the nonvolatile acids. Both types of acids are buffered by a combination of bicarbonate and nonbicarbonate buffers. The interrelationship of the excretory mechanism and the buffering system is illustrated by the fact that the end product of bicarbonate buffering is carbon dioxide, which must be eliminated by the lungs. In addition, much of the bicarbonate and nonbicarbonate buffering systems is dependent on mature renal function.

Daily metabolic processes produce hydrogen ions that consume equal amounts of buffer. The kidney is the only organ that can restore the buffer

Table 11.1   Buffer System

		Percent	
Bicarbonate	Plasma	35⎫	53
	RBC	18⎭	
Nonbicarbonate	Hemoglobin	35⎫	
	Plasma proteins	7⎬	47
	Phosphates	5⎭	

Adapted from Winters, R. W., Dell, R. B. Regulation of acid-base equilibrium, in Yamamoto, W. S. and Brobeck, J. R. (eds.): Physiological Controls and Regulations. Philadelphia, W. B. Saunders, 1965.

at rates equal to the daily rate of consumption. The normal renal tubule reabsorbs a large load of filtered bicarbonate. The renal threshhold for bicarbonate reabsorption sets the plasma bicarbonate level and thus determines the availability of the bicarbonate buffer. In addition, the nephron actively secretes hydrogen ion and in the process generates new bicarbonate. This acidification of the urine is dependent on the buffering of secreted hydrogen ion with phosphate and other buffers, and the conversion of ammonia synthesized in the renal tubules to ammonium.

Table 11.1 summarizes the components of the buffering system and quantifies the contribution of each element.

Elevation of the plasma carbon dioxide tension above normal as a primary disturbance leads to respiratory acidosis. Metabolic acidosis results from accumulation of excess nonvolatile acids, either from increased production or from loss of buffering capacity. Production may increase in hypoxemic states, e.g., when lactic acid accumulates. Loss of buffering capacity may occur when organic anions are excreted in large amounts in diarrheal stools, or when a low renal threshhold for bicarbonate reabsorption exists, as in the premature infant.

Neonatal Limitations

The newborn infant is particularly handicapped on all levels in his attempt to maintain a normal acid-base state. His relatively immature renal function limits his capacity to excrete excess hydrogen ion. McCance (75) documented that infants during the first days of life may not excrete a strongly acid urine. Fomon (48) noted that breast-fed infants excrete little phosphate in their urine and thus cannot excrete large loads of titratable acid. Similarly Hatem (58) and Kildberg (67) reported that infants excrete less ammonia than older subjects when challenged with ammonium chloride loads.

Of major significance is the lower renal bicarbonate threshhold that leads directly to a lower buffering capacity. Edelmann and co-workers (42) demonstrated that newborn infants have a bicarbonate threshhold of 21.5 to 22.5 mmoles per liter compared with 26 to 28 mmoles in adults. Sulyok (123) noted that in premature infants the level was as low as 12 mmoles per liter.

Buffering capacity via plasma proteins and oxygenated hemoglobin is also reduced in the premature infant. Albumin levels are particularly low (108) and disturbances in ventilation leading to the desaturation of hemoglobin are frequent (13).

Ventilatory insufficiency eventually leads to retention of carbon dioxide and respiratory acidosis. In addition, the newborn infant, especially the premature, cannot significantly hyperventilate in an attempt to compensate for a developing metabolic acidosis (100). The adult can hyperventilate to the point of lowering his $Paco_2$ below 20 torr. The lack of a compensatory ventilatory response for the elimination of CO_2 in face of a metabolic acidosis is of particular significance when buffers such as bicarbonate are infused into a patient. To be effective these buffers require the elimination of CO_2 (91). Clinical states that simulate a closed system therefore result in a paradoxical failure of buffering. Figure 11.1 graphically demonstrates the difference between open and closed systems when hydrogen ions are added. Figure 11.2 compares the change in pH as increments of $NaHCO_3$ are added to open and closed flasks. In the closed system the CO_2 is retained and limits the buffering capacity of the additional HCO_3. Opening the system allows for the elimination of CO_2 and a rise in pH.

In summary, the newborn infant, especially if preterm, is limited on a developmental basis in his capacity to excrete hydrogen ion, acidify the urine, and maintain an adequate plasma bicarbonate buffering level. In addition, the neonate is frequently afflicted with pulmonary disease that interferes with his ability to excrete the volatile acids produced both by normal metabolism and by the buffering process.

Clinical Conditions

Physicians involved with the care of the fetus and the newborn are frequently faced with clinical situations in which acidosis develops. This section will review the most common conditions that the anesthesiologist must recognize and evaluate.

Normal Labor and Delivery

Angiographic and manometric studies performed on both humans and monkeys (17, 98, 99) have demonstrated conclusively that during normal

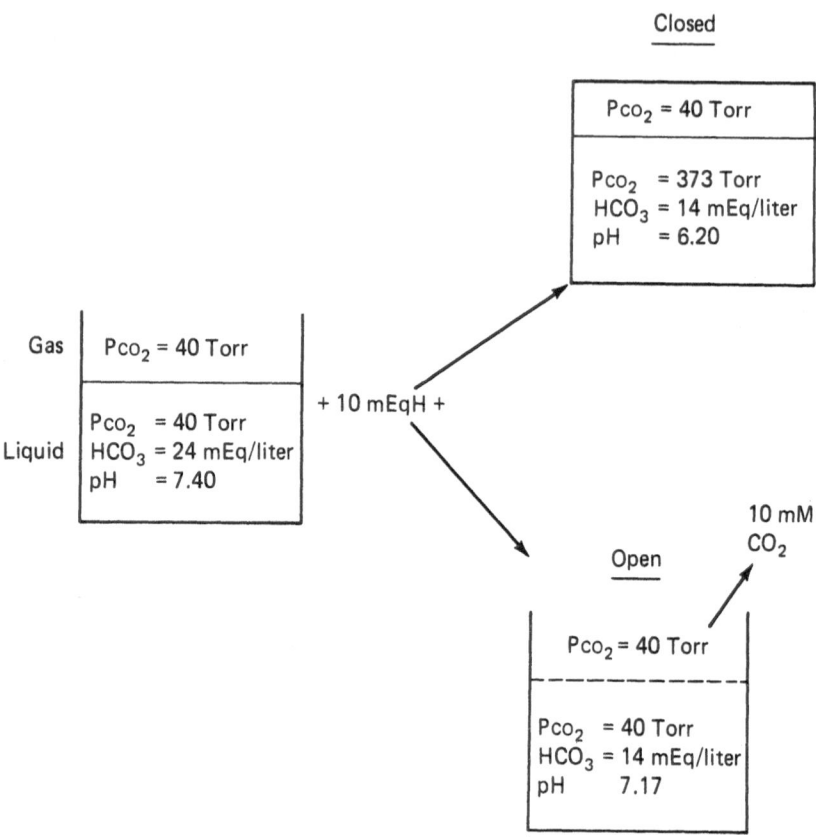

Fig. 11.1 Effect of H+ on an open and closed system. (Adapted from Dell, R.B. Normal acid base regulation, in Winters, R.W.: The Body Fluids in Pediatrics. Boston: Little, Brown and Company, 1973.)

labor there is progressive impairment of blood flow from the uterine arteries to the intervillous space. During the early part of the first stage of labor the intervillous space pressure varies from 10 to 50 torr during a uterine contraction (124). As mean uterine artery pressure is normally above 30 torr and the interruption of blood flow is only of brief duration (104), intervillous oxygen tension does not change. Fetal oxygenation is also dependent on the total amount of oxygen in the intervillous space. The volume of the intervillous space in a normal term placenta has been estimated to be from 150 ml to 300 ml (133). Given a normal maternal hemoglobin level of 12 g/dl and a saturation of 100%, the oxygen content of this volume of blood would be approximately 50 ml. As the total term fetal and placental oxygen requirements are in the range of 20 to 25 ml per minute, the oxygen reserve would be exhausted only after complete cessation of blood flow for two to two and a half minutes (127). Thus, during the first stage of labor there is little if any effect on fetal acid-base status. Dawes' studies of mature monkey fetuses documented a decreased arterial Po_2 but no change in pH during contractions (34), and other investigators (109, 134) have noted no change at all in either fetal Po_2 or pH.

As the cervix becomes fully dilated and the second stage of labor begins, intraamniotic pressure may increase to 120 torr, causing complete interruption of uterine blood flow to the intervillous space (93, 98). Repeated and prolonged interruptions during labor will begin to exhaust the intervillous space reserve capacity and changes in fetal acid base status inevitably occur. The length of the second stage of labor has been correlated with increased fetal acidosis (135, 136), with the most pronounced fall in pH when the head is crowning (Fig. 11.3). During the second stage the in-

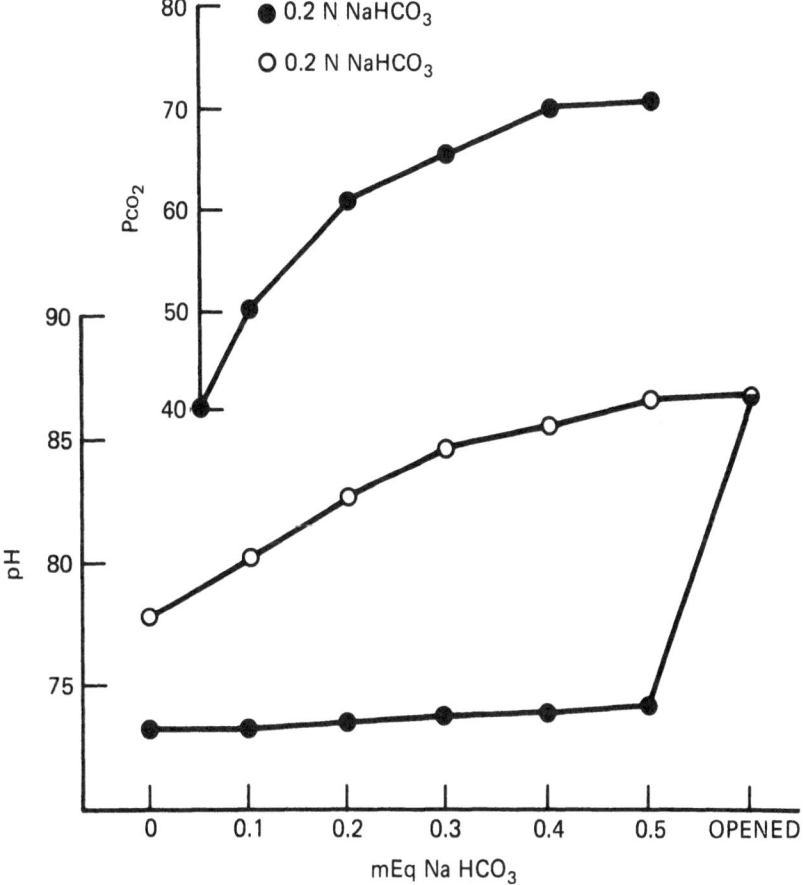

Fig. 11.2   Effect of $NaHCO_3$ on blood pH in a closed and open system. Serial addition of $NaHCO_3$ to blood in the sealed system (closed circles) was associated with progressive elevations of Pco_2 without a significant rise in pH. [Adapted from the Journal of Pediatrics (91).]

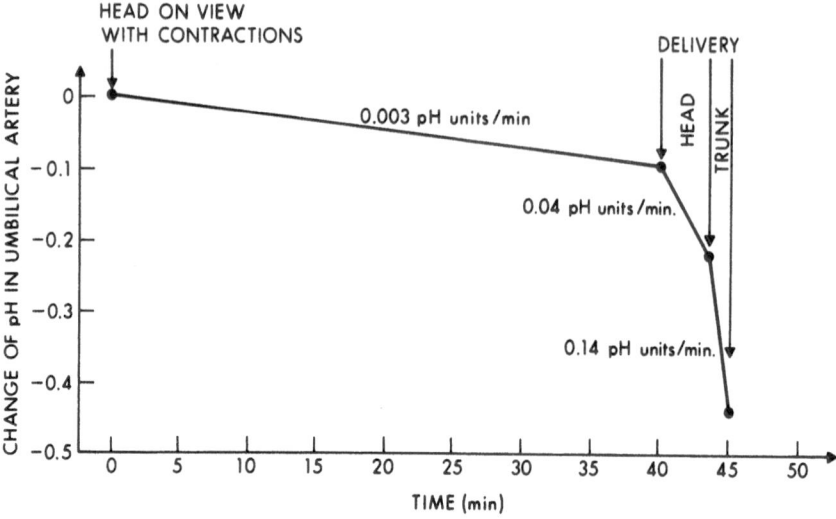

Fig. 11.3 Effect of delivery on umbilical artery pH. (Adapted from Wood, C., Ng, K.H., Hounslow, D., et al.: J. Obstet. Gynaecol. Br. Comm. **80**:295, 1973.)

creased duration, frequency, and intensity of uterine contractions can cause both umbilical cord and head compression, which may further contribute to the developing fetal acidosis.

The normal process of labor should thus be viewed as an asphyxial stress resulting in an inevitable mild degree of fetal acidosis (65). Table 11.2 summarizes the biochemical changes during the course of labor and the immediate neonatal period. The fall of pH is a result of both CO_2 retention and increased lactic acid production. Lactic acid accumulation primarily reflects the degree and duration of anaerobic metabolism (30). Since fetal

Table 11.2 Biochemical Changes Secondary to Labor and Delivery

	Stage	pH	PO₂ torr	PCO₂ torr	Base excess mEq/liter	Lactate mM/liter
Fetus	Prior to labor	7.37	25	40	−2	1.5
	End of labor	7.25	0 to 20	55	−5	2.8
Newborn	10 min. of age	7.20	50	48	−10	4.0
	1 hour of age	7.35	70	35	−5	2.0

Adapted from Brady, J. B.: Homeostatic adjustment of the fetus and neonate, in Aladjem, S. and Brown, A. K. (eds.): Clinical Perinatology. St. Louis, C. V. Mosby Co., 1974.

P_{O_2} normally drops below 20 torr during the second stage of labor, an inevitable degree of anaerobic glycolysis occurs during each delivery. Kubli (70) and Beard (9) confirmed that the fall in pH reflects the stage of dilatation of the cervix. Mean fetal pH values varied from 7.29 to 7.36 early in the first stage of labor, from 7.28 to 7.31 in the latter part of the first stage and early in the second stage, and from 7.19 to 7.28 at the end of the second stage.

Maternal pH at the onset of labor is in the range of 7.40 to 7.45 secondary to hypocapnea (28, 30). As labor progresses, especially when there are prolonged and vigorous contractions, a maternal metabolic acidosis develops with pH dropping to 7.35, the base deficit rising to 5 mEq/liter, and the maternal lactic acid accumulating to 2 mmoles/liter (30). This maternal lactic acidosis contributes to some degree to the fetal acidosis documented in cord blood at the time of delivery.

Postnatally, there is a further decrease in pH in the first 5 to 10 minutes of life (18, 44). As the infant begins to breathe there is a lag in establishing adequate gas exchange, with further elevation of P_{CO_2} and persistence of the hypoxemic state. By the third or fourth minute of life the infant is usually in positive respiratory balance, i.e., he eliminates carbon dioxide at a rate greater than its production. However, as tissue perfusion improves, the lactic acid previously generated is mobilized and contributes to a further fall in pH (30). Within an hour the normal infant adjusts his pH to a mean of 7.35.

Perinatal Asphyxia

While normal labor is a mild asphyxiating process, clinical conditions such as prolapse of the umbilical cord, abruptio placenta, and delivery of the aftercoming head in a breech presentation (20) may be associated with severe and complete interruption of maternal-fetal gas exchange. Unexpected severe asphyxia may occur even with normal labor when there are predisposing maternal conditions associated with pathologic alterations of the placenta, e.g., hypertension, toxemia of pregnancy, diabetes, and postmaturity (72).

Excessive use of oxytocin can lead to increased uterine basal tone and activity leading to decreased uterine blood flow and lower fetal pH (71). A supine maternal position during labor may lead to uterine compression of the inferior vena cava and the lower aorta, causing maternal hypotension, decreased uterine blood flow, and fetal asphyxia.[10]

Intrapartum asphyxia of a degree evident by an Apgar score of less than 3 at one minute is accompanied by a marked degree of acidosis. Dawes and co-workers (32, 34, 35, 37), in a series of classical studies of experimental asphyxia in newborn lambs and rhesus monkeys, have elucidated the time course of the consequences of severe asphyxia. Figure 11.4 outlines the relationships of the physiologic and biochemical changes during the various phases of complete asphyxia.

The initial clinical response, which lasts one minute, is hyperpnea with an associated tachycardia and elevation of blood pressure. Retention of carbon dioxide and fall in arterial oxygen tension occur, but pH remains reasonably stable since the full-term newborn has sufficient plasma buffers to titrate the accumulation of both volatile and nonvolatile acids.

The second period, the primary apneic phase with a duration of one to two minutes, is marked physiologically by a bradycardia and biochemically by a mixed acidosis. The third period is heralded by reflex gasping and is characterized by persistent bradycardia and falling blood pressure as the pH drops below the 7.0 level. Both CO_2 retention and elevation in lactic acid secondary to anaerobic glycolysis account for this profound acidosis. The gasping phase may last as long as five minutes. As the pH falls at a rate of 0.04 to 0.06 pH units per minute of complete asphyxia, a total of eight minutes is frequently associated with pH values as low as 6.8 and a base excess over 20 mEq/liter. The pH at the onset of asphyxia is correlated with the physiologic response. For example, if the arterial pH at the time of delivery is 7.0, then no hyperpneic response occurs; if it is 6.8, there will not be a gasping phase.

The fourth and final period is that of secondary apnea. Its duration may

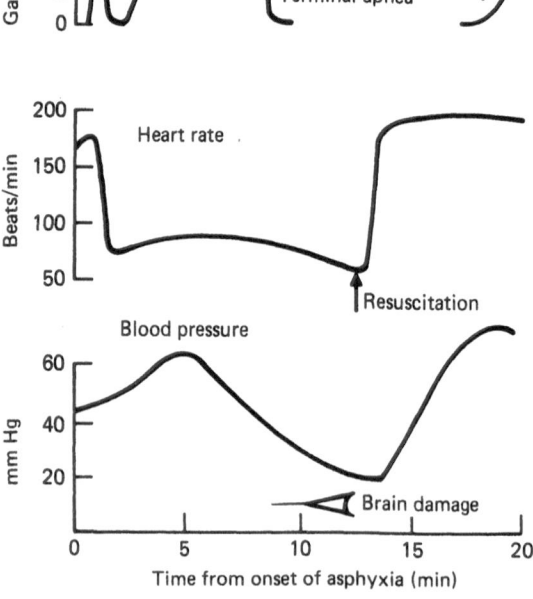

Fig. 11.4   Schematic diagram of changes in rhesus monkeys during asphyxia and on resuscitation by positive pressure ventilation. Brain damage was assessed by histological examination some weeks or months later. (Adapted from Dawes, G.S.: Birth asphyxia, resuscitation and brain damage, in Dawes, G.S.: Foetal and Neonatal Physiology. Chicago. Yearbook Medical Publishers, 1968.

be as long as ten minutes although histologic evidence of brain damage occurs within one to two minutes of the onset of this terminal phase (33). Both the time to the last gasp and the duration of secondary apnea are proportional to the initial cardiac carbohydrate concentration (36). Irreversibility of asphyxia is defined in the animal model as the inability to resuscitate to the point of independent respiration and heart rate. The terminal event is associated with depletion of cardiac muscle glycogen. Depletion of cardiac glycogen stores by repeated intrauterine stresses or paralysis of glycolysis by experimental use of fluoride or iodacetate will shorten survival time (60).

The human correlates of the experimental model are fortunately relatively rare, representing less than 2% of all deliveries (5). Far more frequently partial asphyxia occurs and progressive acidosis develops (19). In clinical situations such as intrauterine growth retardation, post-maturity, and maternal diabetes, fetal hypoglycemia may develop (57). The hypoglycemia in association with acidosis may lead to fetal cardiac decompensation at a much earlier phase of asphyxia than anticipated (82).

Respiratory Distress Syndrome

Respiratory distress syndrome is a disease of developmental immaturity of the pulmonary surfactant system (52, 53). The physiologic consequence of this biochemical disorder is diminished alveolar stability leading to reduced lung volume (6) and a marked ventilation-perfusion imbalance (97). The increased work of breathing, nearly seven-fold compared to that of the asymptomatic infant, leads to an accumulation of lactic acid even before critical levels of hypoxemia are reached (29). As the disease progresses, ventilatory failure with retention of carbon dioxide develops (130). The acidosis itself further decreases the ability of the infant to maintain normal oxygenation by increasing pulmonary vascular tone and intrapulmonary and intracardiac right-to-left shunting (26, 81, 117). In addition, ongoing surfactant synthesis may also be inhibited by acidemia, leading to further deterioration of the ventilatory capacity (53, 77).

Blood Transfusions

Exchange transfusion or massive blood replacement with donor blood prepared with either of the two standard anticoagulants, acid-citrate-dextrose (ACD) or citrate-phosphate-dextrose (CPD), presents the newborn infant with a large amount of metabolic acid (Table 11.3). The citric acid load alone in ACD blood is 18 mEq/liter, and blood that is more than 48 hours old contains over 20 mEq of acid per liter due to the production of non-

Table 11.3   Anticoagulant Solutions

	ACD (75 ml)	CPD (63 ml)
Citric acid	600 mg	206 mg
Sodium citrate	1.65 g	1.66 g
Dextrose	1.84 g	1.61 g
Sodium biphosphate	—	140 mg
pH	6.9	7.1
Titratable acid	20 mEq/liter	8 mEq/liter

volatile acids and carbon dioxide by the continued metabolism of red blood cells (21, 73). CPD blood has less than half the acid load (51) of ACD blood. In addition, the increased phosphate in CPD blood maintains red blood cell viability for a longer period, minimizing the large load of acid that accumulates when red cells lyse. The pH range of donor blood at the time of drawing is 6.8 to 7.0 for ACD (96) blood and 7.0 to 7.10 for CPD blood (51). Within 48 hours the pH of ACD blood drops to a range of 6.4 to 6.8 (92) while the pH in CPD blood drops to levels of 6.9 to 7.0 (51).

The normal full-term infant can handle this infusion. The citrate administered either as citric acid or as sodium citrate will be metabolized by the liver to bicarbonate and ultimately to carbon dioxide and water.

As an exchange transfusion proceeds there is an initial fall of the infant's pH from 7.35 to the range of 7.25 to 7.30. By the end of the exchange the pH is stabilized as the hepatic metabolism of the citrate handles the acid infused. In addition, the initial acidosis stimulates ventilation leading to increased elimination of CO_2. Post transfusion, as the respiratory drive and the metabolism of citrate continue, a significant alkalosis may develop (16, 92, 96).

The premature infant with hepatic immaturity and the newborn with respiratory insufficiency will not tolerate these large acid loads. The delay in hepatic metabolism of the citric acid will lead to progressive acidemia, often with pH values of less than 7.20 (92). In addition, the inability of the infant to increase ventilation to eliminate the CO_2 load from the donor blood (Pco_2 in donor blood $>$ 100 torr) and that generated by the metabolism of citrate leads to a persistent respiratory acidosis.

Hypothermia

Full-term newborn infants subjected to hypothermic stress markedly increase their metabolic rate in an attempt to maintain normal core temperature (120). Oxygen consumption increases three-fold (86) and plasma levels of glycerol, lactate, and free fatty acids rise (4, 76, 110). As a consequence a variable degree of metabolic acidosis develops (49). Initially, glucose levels increase, but as glycogen stores are depleted and as nonesterified fatty acid levels rise, hypoglycemia ensues (25, 57). In addition, the fall in pH itself may interfere with glycolysis and prevent full utilization of the available glycogen stores.

The newborn primarily responds to a cold stress by an increase in chemical thermogenesis. Dawkins (39) has suggested that the thermogenesis occurs predominantly in the brown fat by the lipolysis of triglycerides and the oxidation of the nonesterified fatty acids. This reaction is mediated by norepinephrine (110, 121). The increased catecholamine response to cold stress also has a marked effect on vascular tone, and so there is an increase in pulmonary vascular resistance and thus right-to-left shunting of blood (119). Constriction of peripheral vessels leads to poor perfusion of tissue and a further increase in metabolic acidosis (4).

Infants who are preterm or small for gestational age have even less capacity to withstand hypothermia (120). Their greater surface-area-to-mass ratio facilitates heat loss and they have diminished glycogen reserves, inadequately developed brown fat, and little ability to conserve heat by constriction of surface vessels. Therefore, severe hypothermia, hypoxemia, hypoglycemia, and metabolic acidosis can occur when such infants are kept in an inadequate thermal environment. Moreover, during the rewarming phase lactic acid may be mobilized from previously poorly perfused tissues, leading to a persistent acidosis.

Consequences of Acidosis

The biochemical and physiologic consequences of acidosis have varied and profound clinical implications for the sick newborn infant. A fall in pH limits critical intracellular reactions, affects organ systems as a whole, interferes with plasma transport and binding of toxic agents, and may ultimately be a factor in the demise of the patient.

Acidemia, regardless of etiology, causes changes in intracellular pH and intracellular biochemical processes. There is a quantitative difference, however, when there is retention of a volatile versus a nonvolatile acid. Adler (3) has demonstrated that intracellular pH drops when the plasma pH reaches 7.1 secondary to CO_2 retention, while no change is noted intracellularly in a metabolic acidemia until the plasma pH drops to 6.9. This occurs because carbon dioxide diffuses across cell membranes and equilibrates with the intracellular medium more rapidly than does bicarbonate.

A comparable phenomenon occurs in the relationship of cerebrospinal fluid (CSF) pH to acidemia. Acute metabolic acidemia stimulates carotid body chemoreceptors causing hyperventilation and subsequent hypocapnia in both the plasma and CSF. Since CSF bicarbonate levels remain stable, a mild alkaline pH develops (79). Similarly, during a rapid intravascular infusion of bicarbonate the rise in plasma pH is accompanied by a paradoxical CSF acidosis. This results from the immediate accumulation of CO_2 in the CSF, both from the decreased ventilation secondary to the rise in plasma pH and from the buffered bicarbonate (15).

The selective permeability of the blood-brain barrier protects both the CSF pH and central nervous system function against most changes in blood acid base status (78). However, overtreatment with bicarbonate or inadequate ventilatory support can overcome this protective mechanism and lead to secondary central nervous system dysfunction (94, 95).

Chronic systemic acidosis of any type limits the delivery of oxygen to the tissues. Acidosis causes a decrease in the amount of 2,3-disphosphoglycerate (2,3-DPG) by inhibiting 2,3-DPG mutase and phosphatase (90). As a result, the oxygen dissociation curve shifts to the left, reflecting the decreased ability of hemoglobin to release oxygen at any given oxygen tension (89). Tissue hypoxia will cause a metabolic acidosis which in turn will further limit the synthesis of 2,3-DPG and perpetuate the vicious cycle (41).

Acidosis inhibits specific biochemical processes including glycolysis (38). Lactate production reflects the rate of glycolysis and is reduced as pH drops (1). The effect of pH is independent of oxygenation. Acidosis diminishes the myocardial response to catecholamine: as pH falls, the direct inotropic effect of epinephrine on myocardial contractility is abolished (87).

Acidemia and hypoxemia together have a synergistic and deleterious effect on cardiac function. Isolated heart perfusion studies demonstrate gross deterioration in left ventricular function if the pH falls below 7.1 (88). In vivo animal studies, however, have shown that function continues as long as pH remains above 6.9. Goodyear (55) similarly noted little effect on cardiac function in intact dogs which were infused with hydrochloric acid as long as normal Po_2 was maintained. Downing (40) reported that in lambs a Po_2 of 25 torr and a normal pH, or a pH of 6.9 with normal Po_2, had little effect on ventricular function; however, when hypoxemia and acidosis occurred together a marked change in myocardial contractility ensued.

The effect of acidosis on cardiac function has been related primarily to its inhibition of glycolysis (87). Below critical levels of oxygen tension, cardiac muscle is totally dependent on anaerobic metabolism of glucose. Therefore, infusion of base during asphyxia will help to sustain glycolysis and maintain cardiac function (1, 35).

Studies of all mammalian species have documented that the newborn can survive longer periods of anoxia than the adult. This is due in large part to the greater glycogen stores in the infant heart (88). This difference in survival between the newborn and adult animal can be abolished experimentally by the chemical inhibition of glycolysis, thus emphasizing the need to maintain pH during prolonged hypoxemia (60).

A deleterious effect of combined hypoxemia and acidemia has also been demonstrated in studies of oxygen consumption by fetal sheep brains (68). With fixed cerebral blood flow and oxygen saturation below 40%, a fall in pH from 7.39 to 7.02 reduced oxygen consumption of the brain 80%.

The effects of pH on the vascular tone in general and the pulmonary vessels in particular have been well studied. Rudolph (105) has clearly demonstrated that in calves pulmonary vascular resistance is unchanged even at Po₂ as low as 30 torr, as long as the pH is maintained above 7.35. However, at a pH of 7.1, changes in resistance begin at Po₂ of 50 to 75 torr, and even at Po₂ over 100 torr a fall in the pH from 7.30 to 7.1 will increase resistance 300% (Fig. 11.5). Similar studies by Cassin (24) and Campbell (22, 23) confirm the effect of pH on pulmonary vasculature tone. Under conditions of perinatal stress the human infant is frequently subjected to hypoxemia and acidosis to a degree which could lead to a similar profound decrease in pulmonary perfusion.

The synthesis of surface active phospholipids by the alveolar lining is critical to the infant's pulmonary function. The preterm infant has marginal amounts of surfactant and is dependent on its ongoing production to maintain alveolar stability. Gluck (53) and co-workers have demonstrated that acidosis interferes with the production of lecithin, the critical phospholipid, especially that fraction derived from the methylating pathway. Merrit (77) confirmed the decrease in pulmonary lecithin synthesis in

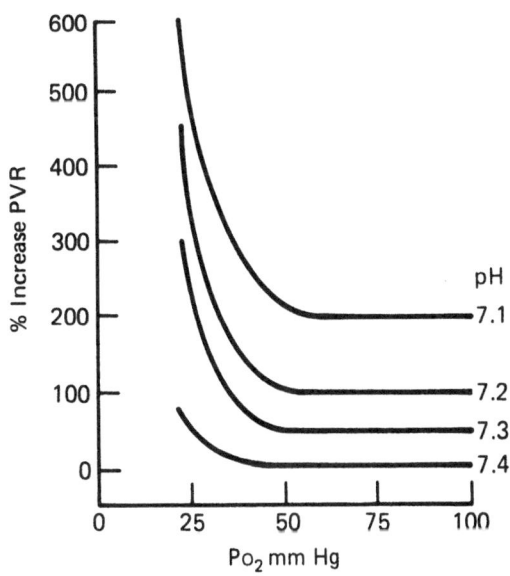

Fig. 11.5 Changes in pulmonary vascular resistance (PVR) at various Po₂ and pH. (Adapted from Rudolph, A.M., Yuan, S.: J. Clin. Invest. 45:399, 1966.)

acidosis, although his data indicated that the reduction was secondary to diminished choline incorporation.

Treatment of Acidosis

A major therapeutic goal in the treatment of metabolic acidosis is the correction of pH by restoring the buffering capacity of the blood. The most commonly used therapy is the infusion of an alkalinizing agent such as sodium bicarbonate or THAM.

Sodium Bicarbonate

The efficacy of sodium bicarbonate rests primarily on the fact that the acid form of the buffer, H_2CO_3, dissociates into water and a volatile gas, CO_2:

$$Na^+ + HCO_3^- + HA \rightarrow Na^+ A^- + H_2CO_3 \tag{1}$$

$$H_2CO_3 \rightarrow H_2O + CO_2 \tag{2}$$

The maximum capacity of a buffer to directly affect pH occurs when the ratio of the acid and its dissociated anion is 1:1. For the bicarbonate system, this occurs at the pK value of 6.1 which does not fall within physiologic range. The ability of normal patients to rapidly eliminate CO_2 from the lungs, however, shifts the equation to the right and affects the pH even when the ratio of HCO_3 : P_{CO_2} is 20:1. Were it not for this continual elimination of CO_2, bicarbonate would be a very poor buffer for the human organism. This has been demonstrated by a series of *in vitro* experiments by Ostrea and Odell (91). When bicarbonate was added to a closed system, P_{CO_2} rose without a significant rise in pH (Fig. 11.2). When similar quantities of bicarbonate were added to an open system, pH dramatically increased. Steichen (118) confirmed this in a study of acidotic dogs that were mechanically ventilated at a fixed rate of CO_2 elimination. Rapid infusion of hypertonic bicarbonate caused little rise in pH and, in fact, caused the pH to fall when the acidosis was accompanied by hypoxia. In addition, the direct effect of hypercapnia generated from infused bicarbonate caused an acute decrease in P_{O_2} (Fig. 11.6), presumably secondary to pulmonary vasoconstriction and increased right-to-left shunting.

An isotonic (0.15 M) infusion of 3 mEq of $NaHCO_3$ per kilogram of body weight to an infant with a pH of 7.1 will generate approximately 0.43 mmoles of CO_2 per kilogram. The endogenous production of CO_2 in such an infant is approximately 0.3 mmoles per kilogram per minute. Thus, a typical infusion of isotonic $NaHCO_3$ generates an amount of CO_2 equal to that produced endogenously in about one and a half minutes. In a closed system this would acutely raise the P_{CO_2} 15 torr.

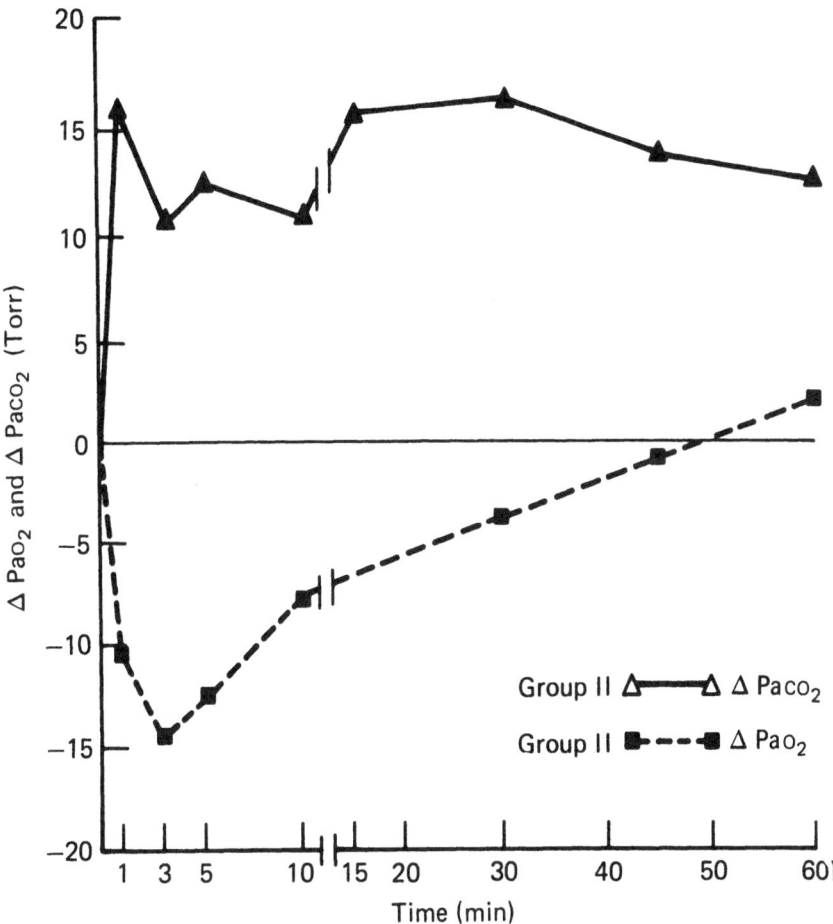

Fig. 11.6   Change in $Paco_2$ (Δ $Paco_2$) and concomitant change in Pao_2 (Δ Pao_2) during rapid infusion of HCO_3. (Adapted from Steichen, J.J., Kleinman, L.I.: J. Pediatr. **91**:287, 1977.)

Moreover, sodium bicarbonate is frequently infused in hypertonic concentrations. The dose schedule is either an empiric infusion of 2 to 3 mEq per kilogram per dose, or based on the following equation:

$$\frac{\text{birth weight}}{3} \times \frac{\text{base deficit}}{2} = \text{mEq } HCO_3$$

Molar bicarbonate (1 mEq/ml) is 1800 mOsm per liter, over six times the normal tonicity of blood. Hypertonic solutions have a direct affect on acid base balance and in a paradoxical way minimize the potential benefit of any infused bicarbonate (91, 116). The addition of relatively nonpermeable solute causes a shift of water from the intracellular compartment. Within the erythrocyte, hemoglobin and potassium became more concentrated. The increased ionic strength of the intracellular medium causes hemoglobin to dissociate more readily. The protons released from the hemoglobin in turn titrate both intracellular and extracellular bicarbonate. As a result, hypertonic bicarbonate infused into a closed system causes a greater elevation in Pco_2 than occurs when equal amounts of bicarbonate are injected in an isotonic concentration (Fig. 11.7) (91).

Hyperosmolarity secondary to sodium bicarbonate infusion has been associated, in retrospective studies by some authors, with an increased incidence of intracranial hemorrhage (114). Experimental studies with kittens and rabbits confirm that hypertonic infusion of saline or bicarbonate can lead to intracranial hemorrhage (69, 129). In a prospective study by Thomas (126) of human infants of less than 33 weeks' gestation, intraventricular hemorrhage was noted to correlate with a serum osmolality over 320 mOsm per kilogram of water. Hypernatremia itself, without concomitant hyperosmolality over this level, was not associated with intraventricular hemorrhage. Baum and Robertson (8) have demonstrated that infusions of 5 to 10 mililiters of molar bicarbonate in preterm infants with respiratory distress syndrome lead to a mean increase in osmolality of 25 mOsm. Among those infants with changes over 25 mOsm was one infant with a peak increase of 64 mOsm. Finberg (46) has previously suggested an increase of 25 mOsm as a maximal safe rise. This would correlate with the absolute levels of 320 mOsm specified by Thomas (126). Osmolar changes above this level presumably lead to major fluid shifts into the

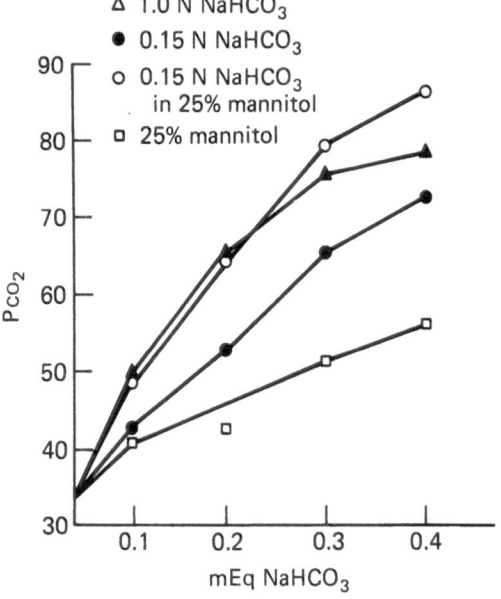

Fig. 11.7   Effect of hypertonic solutions on CO_2 tension in a closed *in vitro* system. (Adapted from Ostrea, E.M., Jr., Odell, G.B.: J. Pediatr. **80**:672, 1972.)

vascular compartment, distention of intracranial capillaries, elevation of venous pressure, and thus intracranial hemorrhage.

Rapid infusions of hypertonic sodium bicarbonate solutions have been associated with other complications. Tissue necrosis and thrombosis have been reported as results of the direct corrosive effect of the highly alkaline fluid. Hypernatremia has caused renal damage in experimental animals and in infants with salt poisoning (47, 106).

THAM

An alternative to the use of sodium bicarbonate as an alkalinizing agent is trishydroxy methyl amino methane (THAM) (122), an amino alcohol with a molecular weight of 121. It is a weak base, 70% ionized at pH 7.4 (pK 7.84) and nearly 90% in the more acid intracellular environment. It is not protein bound and therefore does not compete with bilirubin for albumin binding sites.

THAM buffers as follows:

$$R - NH_2 \text{ (THAM)} + HA \rightarrow R\text{-}NH^+_3 + A^- \tag{1}$$

In addition THAM reacts with dissolved CO_2 to form bicarbonate:

$$CO_2 \text{ (dissolved)} + H_2O \rightarrow H_2CO_3 \tag{2}$$

$$H_2CO_3 \rightarrow H^+ + HCO^-_3 \tag{3}$$

$$R - NH_2 \text{ (THAM)} + H^+ + HCO^-_3 \rightarrow R\text{-}NH^+_3 + HCO^-_3 \tag{4}$$

THAM reportedly buffers the intracellular milieu at rates faster than bicarbonate. Although it penetrates the CSF slowly, the change of pH in the CSF is in the same direction as in plasma, in contrast to the paradoxical fall in CSF pH when HCO_3 is administered (62). This simultaneous lowering of the Pco_2 in both plasma and CSF with increase in CSF pH and correlated EEG improvement explains the efficacy of THAM in treatment of CO_2 narcosis.

THAM is not metabolized and is excreted primarily by glomerular filtration. It may be administered orally, intravenously, or intraperitoneally. Commercial solutions of THAM (THAM-E Abbot) are prepared by dissolving 36 g of lyophilized powder in 1000 cc of water resulting in a 0.3 M (36 mg per milliliter) solution with an electrolyte concentration of 30 mEq per liter sodium, 5 mEq per liter potassium, and 35 mEq per liter of chloride. The pH of this solution is very highly alkaline (10.6) and is damaging to vessels. The 0.3 M solution is only slightly hypertonic, i.e., 367 mOsm/liter.

THAM infusion can have several side effects. Hypoglycemia develops only after rapid administration of doses greater than 500 mg/kg (14 ml/kg of 0.3 M solution) and may be avoided by reconstituting THAM in 5% dextrose (11). However, this raises the osmolality to approximately 650 mOsm/liter. The respiratory depression that is manifested initially by a decrease in tidal volume and subsequently by frank apnea is a factor of the rapid change of pH (103) and not an effect of the THAM molecule itself (83). The risk of respiratory depression may be minimized by a slow infusion, but ventilatory support should be available. Additional side effects have included hyperkalemia and vessel and tissue necrosis secondary to the irritating effect of the alkaline solution (54). Therefore, infusion of THAM either should be limited to administration through large vessels or should be given at a very slow rate. In patients with decreased renal function the use of THAM is limited.

The dosage schedule of THAM has yet to be clearly defined. Physicians should use either the following equation:

$$\text{ml THAM (0.3 M)} = \text{Wt (kg)} \times \frac{\text{Base deficit}}{2}$$

or an empiric dosage of 3 to 5 cc per dose.

Total daily dose should not exceed 20 mM per kilogram per day (60 cc/kg of the 0.3 M solution). Cardiovascular collapse has been described above this level (102). THAM is stable in liquid form but because of its alkalinity it erodes conventional glass containers and should be discarded within 24 hours of reconstitution.

Asphyxia Neonatorum

The experimental models described by Dawes and co-workers (32, 34, 35, 37) have provided an opportunity to test the value of infusing alkalinizing agents during progressive asphyxia and resuscitation.

Combined infusion of glucose and a potent base (such as sodium carbonate) during the entire course of asphyxia in both immature and mature fetal lambs and monkeys prolongs the duration of gasping and accelerates the response to artificial ventilation (35, 37, 38). Infusion of either sodium carbonate or THAM beginning 6.5 minutes after onset of asphyxia restores the pH and increases heart rate and blood pressure. The gasping period is prolonged and the monkeys respond to subsequent resuscitation measures more rapidly. When THAM and glucose are infused as part of the resuscitation procedure the time required to establish spontaneous breathing is reduced by 33% (1).

The ability to restore cardiovascular function by an infusion of base irrespective of oxygenation derives from the fact that glycolysis is a pH dependent process. Inhibition of glycolysis by acidosis limits the energy available to the myocardium and the brain. In those animals infused with base, lactic acid continues to accumulate during asphyxia as anaerobic metabolism continues (1). This maintenance of glycolysis during asphyxia and resuscitation is reflected in the prolongation and improvement of cardiovascular function and in the reduced incidence and extent of brain damage. Dawes (33) studied monkeys which were asphyxiated for a total of 12.5 minutes and which were infused with saline, THAM, sodium carbonate, or sodium bicarbonate beginning at 6.5 minutes after onset of asphyxia. All of those monkeys which did not receive any base had extensive bilateral brain damage. The treated monkeys, regardless of the type of base infused, showed significantly less damage.

The choice of which base to use during resuscitation has been much discussed. Since all experimental models have utilized infusion of hypertonic solutions, it has been argued that the cardiovascular effect is solely a result of the expansion of the circulating volume and the subsequent restoration of blood pressure and tissue perfusion. This argument is supported by Johnson (66), who demonstrated that equal volumes of hypertonic (930 mOsm/liter) sodium bicarbonate, sodium chloride, or dextrose led to similar increases in pulmonary blood flow and decreases in pulmonary vascular resistance. Dawes (35), however, demonstrated that there was no increase in survival time or response to resuscitation in lambs infused with a hypertonic glucose-saline solution, but that an alkali-glucose solution clearly prolonged gasping and cardiovascular function.

Adamson (2) compared the efficacy of infusing different bases in asphyxiated monkeys. Sodium carbonate proved to be too caustic and caused necrosis of the liver from direct umbilical vein infusions. THAM was suggested as the base of choice; compared with sodium bicarbonate, less volume was required to maintain pH. Haworth (59) compared THAM and bicarbonate in the resuscitation of piglets and concluded that bicarbonate was as effective as THAM and possibly safer. Berg (12) and co-workers studied asphyxiated adult rabbits who were infused with either 0.5 to 1 mmole per kilogram of THAM or 1 to 2 mmole per kilogram of sodium bicarbonate. They concluded that THAM only provided an advantage before artificial ventilation was established and that bicarbonate should be used subsequent to restoration of ventilation.

Comparable human experiments testing various therapeutic regimens during resuscitation have not been done. Evans (45) and co-workers, in an interesting controlled study, tested the efficacy of bicarbonate administered intragastrically or intravenously to asphyxiated acidotic human neonates. The infants were studied in the period following the resuscitation. Those infants who had received alkali in the delivery room were excluded. The infants were breathing spontaneously at the time of the study and had a mean pH of 7.20 and Pco_2 of 34. Administration of bicarbonate by either route did not change pH significantly compared to controls treated only with dextrose. CO_2 retention offset the change in base deficit with no net gain in pH. Hypercapnia occurred despite the fact the infants maintained a clinically normal respiratory pattern. The absence of a normal hyperventilation response to hypercarbia was a result of the loss of central drive secondary to the previous cerebral anoxia.

The clinician who is faced with the therapeutic decision to infuse alkali or not during resuscitation of an asphyxiated newborn must consider both the clear evidence of the efficacy of base in maintaining and restoring cardiovascular function and the risk of infusing hypertonic solutions. An appropriate compromise rests in limiting the infusion only to those infants who fail to respond to ventilation alone, as evidenced by persistent brady-cardia below 80 with concomitant hypotension. In such cases, base should be infused in a 1:5 dilution of molar bicarbonate (360 mOsm/liter). Since hypotension is part of the asphyxia syndrome (56), infusion of a relatively large volume (10 to 15 cc per kilogram) is warranted both to restore pH and to maintain blood pressure. In cases where the institution of ventilation is delayed or inadequate, 3 to 5 cc per kilogram of 0.3M THAM (367 mOsm/liter) is an appropriate alternative. Both of these infusions will avoid the effects of hypertonicity on the volume and pH of body fluid and should correct approximately half the base deficit associated with severe asphyxia.

Respiratory Distress Syndrome

Infusion of alkali has been recommended for nearly 20 years for the treat-ment of the acidosis that accompanies the respiratory distress syndrome of infancy (130). The rationale for this therapy has rested on the studies documenting the deleterious effects of acidosis on pulmonary vascular tone (105) and on surfactant synthesis (53, 77). Correction of acidosis, it is postulated, improves pulmonary perfusion and gas exchange while alveolar stability is enhanced secondary to increased availability of surface-active lecithin.

Since Usher's (131) initial report there have been various recommenda-tions as to choice of alkali and rate of infusion. Usher, Hutchinson (63), and Russel (107) have advocated the use of sodium bicarbonate. Troelstra (128) has recommended THAM. Usher has recommended a slow con-tinuous infusion while Russel, Hutchinson, Davies (31) and others have suggested that rapid "pushes" of hypertonic bicarbonate are most effi-cacious. In a controlled study, Usher demonstrated that bicarbonate low-ered the mortality rate in infants over 1500 g suffering from RDS. Sinclair (115), Teck (118), and Bland (14), however, were not able to demon-strate any therapeutic advantage from bicarbonate infusions. Hoebel (61) noted no difference if bicarbonate was infused within the first hour of life or after a few hours. Vliet and Gupta (132), while demonstrating that THAM had a slight statistical advantage over bicarbonate, did not compare either treated group with a control population.

The lack of any firm evidence as to the therapeutic benefit of alkali therapy in the treatment of the respiratory distress syndrome is of concern, especially in view of the retrospective clinical reports of increased intracranial hemorrhage associated with bicarbonate therapy. While the association of bicarbonate therapy with intracranial hemorrhage is much debated (see above), both Siegel (113) and Rhodes (101) have noted changes in osmolality secondary to administration of bicarbonate to preterm infants with RDS. Infusion of molar bicarbonate in both studies in doses of approximately 3 mEq/kg and at rates of 1 to 2 ml per minute caused an increase in osmolality of 10 mOsm/liter. Baum (8), in a prospective study, compared the immediate effects of rapid infusions of 0.58M THAM and 1.0 M bicarbonate in the treatment of severe RDS. While P_{CO_2} fell after THAM infusion and rose after bicarbonate therapy, the pH rose in all infants. Changes in P_{O_2} were variable and were not significantly different in the two study groups. The most pronounced changes in osmolality were noted when molar bicarbonate was infused over a 30-second period, with an average of nearly 20 mOsm change. In one patient a rise of 60 mOsm was documented. The smallest change in osmolality resulted from a bicarbonate infusion over five minutes (less than 10 mOsm per kg of water).

A prospective study of infants with RDS comparing infusions of sodium bicarbonate, glucose, salt-poor albumin, and a combination of albumin and bicarbonate was reported by Bland and co-workers (14). The infusions were given over a 5 to 10 minute period. No therapeutic benefit from alkali infusion with or without albumin was noted. Glucose alone did as well (Table 11.4). Of particular interest was the fact that intracranial hemorrhage occurred only in those infants infused with hypertonic bicarbonate.

Thus to date the usefulness of rapid infusions of alkali in the treatment of RDS has not been proven and genuine concern regarding the deleterious effects of the traditional use of hypertonic solution has emerged. A therapeutic approach is recommended on the basis of the following principles (43).

1. Alkali infusions are not a substitute for adequate ventilation. Retention of CO_2 should be treated with ventilatory assistance. The normal infant's response to a metabolic acidosis is to hyperventilate and to lower its P_{CO_2} to a level of 20 to 30 torr, and ventilatory assistance should aim for that level.
2. When, despite ventilatory compensation, the pH is still below 7.20, alkali infusion should be used.
3. Alkali should be infused in a nearly isotonic concentration (0.3M

Table 11.4   Comparison of Nonalkali and Alkali Infusions* Given to Infants with RDS

Infants	Nonalkali		Alkali	
	Glucose	Albumin	NaHCO₃	Albumin and NaHCO₃
Number	13	14	13	13
RDS	5	6	8	5
Died	1	4	6	5
Intracranial hemorrhage	0	0	3	1

Adapted from Bland, R.D., Clarke, T.L., Harden, L.B.: Rapid infusion of sodium bicarbonate and albumin into high risk premature infants soon after birth: A controlled prospective trial. Am. J. Obstet. Gynecol. **124**:263, 1976.
* Infusions given over a 5 to 10 minute period.

THAM, 0.15 M sodium bicarbonate) to minimize any osmotic effect on the body fluids.

4. When bicarbonate is infused it should be administered slowly, over a period of not less than 5 minutes and preferably over at least 10. This rate minimizes the contribution of the CO_2 generated by the buffering of bicarbonate to that produced endogenously and allows sufficient time for elimination by the lungs.

5. THAM should be restricted in the treatment of RDS to situations where hypernatremia or hypercarbia are major problems and where ventilatory support has already been instituted. THAM should be infused over a minimum of at least 5 minutes and at single doses of less than 500 mg per kg per dose.

Blood Transfusions

Exchange transfusion for Rh hemolytic disease or massive transfusion during major surgery is a serious metabolic stress to a small sick infant (86, 92, 96, 112, 120). Buffering of blood with alkali has been recommended to reduce this stress (7, 27, 50, 92, 111).

Experimentally it has been shown that transfusion of THAM-buffered blood reduces the mortality in hypovolemic dogs when compared to transfusion with nonbuffered blood. Similarly, low weight infants exchanged with THAM-buffered blood had less change in electrolytes and a pH closer to normal than infants exchanged with nonbuffered blood (85, 92).

Sodium bicarbonate is a poor choice for the titration of donor blood which is hypernatremic, hypercarbic, and hyperosmolar. Bicarbonate buffer will only generate more CO_2 in the closed system of the donor blood bag. If one uses hypertonic bicarbonate, a greater degree of hypernatremia and hyperosmolality will ensue. If one dilutes the bicarbonate to an isotonic concentration, the amount needed to buffer the donor blood will dilute the red cell mass by over 20%. THAM has been found to be highly effective in buffering blood without causing any deleterious side effects (85, 92). The addition of 25 cc of 0.3 M THAM will raise the pH to 7.1 or 7.2, thus lowering the acid load to a safe level for most infants. However, in more unstable or immature neonates there is greater need to accurately measure the pH of the donor blood and to titrate it with serial infusions of THAM. Frequent measurements of the infant's pH during transfusion are mandatory.

Conclusion

Acidosis has profound effects on the newborn infant. Some of these effects are obvious clinically; others are detectable only at a cellular level. The primary goal of the physician is to anticipate those situations in which intervention may prevent serious acid-base derangements. When this has failed, the challenge is to correct abnormality without introducing new complications. It is toward this end that we have directed the discussion of therapeutic issues: the selection of bicarbonate or THAM as buffer, the mode of administration, and the special considerations of specific clinical conditions. It is painfully obvious that many questions remain. As in most of perinatal medicine, ideal prophylaxis and therapy are still far from reality.

References

1. Adamsons, K., Jr., Behrman, R., Dawes, G.S., et al.: The treatment of acidosis with alkali and glucose during asphyxia in foetal Rhesus monkeys. London, J. Physiol. **169**:679, 1963.
2. Adamsons, K., Jr., Behrman, R., Dames, G.S., et al.: Resuscitation by positive pressure ventilation and trishydroxymethylaminomethane of rhesus monkeys asphyxiated at birth. J. Pediatr. **65**:807, 1963.
3. Adler, S., Roy, A., Relman, A.S.: Intracellular acid base regulation I. The response of muscle cells to changes in CO_2 tension or extracellular bicarbonate concentration. J. Clin. Invest. **44**:8, 1965.
4. Alexander, G., Bell, A.W., Hales, J.R.S.: The effect of cold exposure on the plasma levels of glucose, lactate, free fatty acids, and glycerol, and on the blood gas and acid base status in young lambs. Biol. Neonate **20**:9, 1972.
5. Apgar, V.: The newborn (Apgar) scoring system. Reflections and advice. Pediatr. Clin. N. Am. **13**:645, 1966.
6. Auld, P.A.M., Nelson, N.M., Cherry, R.B., et al.: Measurement of thoracic gas volume in the newborn infant. J. Clin. Invest. **42**:476, 1963.
7. Barrie, H.: Acid base control during exchange transfusions. Lancet **2**:712, 1965.

8. Baum, J.D., Robertson, N.R.C.: Immediate effects of alkaline infusion in infants with respiratory distress syndrome. J. Pediatr. **87**:255, 1975.

9. Beard, R.W., Morris, E.D., Clayton, S.G.: pH of fetal capillary blood as an indicator of the condition of the fetus. J. Obstet. Gynaecol. Br. Common. **74**:812, 1967.

10. Beard, R.W., Roberts, G.M.: Supine hypotension syndrome. Br. Med. J. **2**:297, 1970.

11. Bennett, T.E., Tavail, R.: The hypoglycemic activity of 2-amino-2-hydroxy-methyl-1,3 propanediol. Ann. N.Y. Acad. Sci. **92**:651, 1961.

12. Berg, D., Mulling, M., Saling, E.: Use of THAM and sodium bicarbonate in correcting acidosis in asphyxiated newborns. Arch. Dis. Child. **44**:318, 1959.

13. Bland, R.D.: Cord blood total protein levels as a screening aid for the idiopathic respiratory distress syndrome. N. Engl. J. Med. **287**:9, 1972.

14. Bland, R.D., Clarke, T.L., Harden, L.B.: Rapid infusion of sodium bicarbonate and albumin into high risk premature infants soon after birth: A controlled prospective trial. Am. J. Obstet. Gynecol. **124**:263, 1976.

15. Bleich, H.L., Berkman, D.M., Schwartz, W.B.: The response of cerebrospinal fluid composition to sustained hypercapnea. J. Clin. Invest. **43**:11, 1964.

16. Boda, D., Toth, G.Y., Muranyi, L., Eck, E.: Acid base and electrolyte changes during exchange transfusion. Acta Paediatr. Scand. **56**:217, 1966.

17. Borell, V., Fernstrom, I., Ohlson, L. Wiquist, N.: Influence of uterine contractions on the uteroplacental blood flow at term. Am. J. Obstet. Gynecol. **93**:44, 1965.

18. Brady, J.: Homeostatic adjustments of the fetus and neonate, in Aladjem, S., and Brown, A.K. (eds.): Clinical Perinatology. St. Louis, C.V. Mosby Co., 1974.

19. Brann, A.W., Jr., Dykes, F.D.: The effect of intrauterine asphyxia on the full term neonate. Clin. Perinatol. **4**:149, 1977.

20. Brenner, W.E., Bruce, R.D., Hendricks, C.H.: The characteristics and perils of breech presentation. Am. J. Obstet. Gynecol. **118**:700, 1974.

21. Calladine, M., Gairdner, D., Naidoo, B.L., Orrell, D.H.: Acid base changes following exchange transfusion with citrated blood. Arch. Dis. Child. **40**:626, 1965.

22. Campbell, A.G.M., Cockburn, F., Dawes, G.S., Milligan, J.E.: Pulmonary vasoconstriction in asphyxia during cross circulation between twin foetal lambs. London, J. Physiol. **192**:111, 1967.

23. Campbell, A.G.M., Dawes, G.S., Fishman, A.P., Hyman, A.T.: Pulmonary vasoconstriction and changes in heart rate during asphyxia in immature fetal lambs. London, J. Physiol. **192**:93, 1967.

24. Cassin, S., Dawes, G.S., Ross, B.B.: Pulmonary blood flow and vascular resistance in immature fetal lambs. London, J. Physiol. **171**:80, 1964.

25. Char, V.C., Creasy, R.K.: Glucose and oxygen metabolism in normally oxygenated and spontaneously hypoxemic fetal lambs. Am. J. Obstet. Gynecol. **127**:499, 1977.

26. Chu, Clements, J.A., Cotton, E.K., et al.: Neonatal pulmonary ischemia. Pediatrics (suppl) **40**:709, 1967.

27. Clark, L.C., Jr.: The use of amine buffers in cardiovascular surgery. Ann. N.Y. Acad. Sci. **133**:134, 1966.
28. Cohen, A., Schulman, H., Romney, S.: Maternal acid base metabolism in normal human partuition. Am. J. Obstet. Gynecol. **107**:933, 1970.
29. Cook, C.D.: Respiration and metabolism of newborn infants. Exhibition at VII International Congress of Pediatrics Copenhagen, 1956, in Avery, M.E. (ed.): The Lung and Its Development in the Newborn Infant. Philadelphia, W.B. Saunders Co., 1964.
30. Daniel, S.S., Adamsons, K., Jr., James, L.S.: Lactate and pyruvate as an index of prenatal oxygen deprivation. Pediatrics **37**:942, 1966.
31. Davies, P.A., Robinson, R.J., Scopes, J.W., et al.: Medical care of Newborn Babies. Philadelphia, J.B. Lippincott, 1972.
32. Dawes, G.S.: Birth asphyxia, resusitation, and brain damage, in Dawes, G.S.: Foetal and Neonatal Physiology. Chicago, Yearbook Medical Publishers, 1968.
33. Dawes, G.S., Hibbard, E., Windle, W.F.: The effect of alkali and glucose infusions on permanent brain damage in rhesus monkeys asphyxiated at birth. London, J. Pediatr. **65**:801, 1964.
34. Dawes, G.S., Jacobson, H.N., Mott, J.C., Shelley, H.J.: Some observations in foetal and newborn rhesus monkeys. London, J. Physiol. **152**:271, 1960.
35. Dawes, G.S., Jacobson, H.N., Mott, J.C.: The treatment of asphyxiated mature foetal lambs and rhesus monkeys with intravenous glucose and sodium carbonate. London, J. Physiol. **168**:43, 1963.
36. Dawes, G.S., Mott, J.C., Shelley, H.J.: The importance of cardiac glycogen for the maintenance of life in foetal lambs and newborn animals during anoxia. London, J. Physiol. **146**:516, 1959.
37. Dawes, G.A., Mott, J.C., Shelley, H.S., Stafford, A.: The prolongation of survival time in asphyxiated immature foetal lambs. London, J. Physiol. **168**:43, 1963.
38. Dawes, G.S., Mott, J.C., Stafford, A.: Prolongation of survival in the anoxic foetal lamb. London, J. Physiol. **153**:16, 1960.
39. Dawkins, M.R.J., Hull, D.: Brown adipose tissue and the response of newborn rabbits to cold. London, J. Physiol. **172**:216, 1964.
40. Downing, S.E., Talner, N.S., Gardner, T.H.: Influence of arterial oxygen tension and pH on cardiac function in the newborn lamb. Am. J. Physiol. **211**:1203, 1966.
41. Duc, G.V., Engel, K.: Hemoglobin oxygen affinity and erythrocyte 2, 3 diphosphoglycerate (DPG) content in hyaline membrane disease and cardiac malformations. Proc. Soc. Pedr. Res. 1970, p. 79.
42. Edelmann, C.M., Jr., Rodriquez-Soriano, J., Boichis, H,. et al.: Renal bicarbonate reabsorption and hydrogen ion excretion in infants. J. Clin. Invest. **46**:1309, 1967.
43. Eidelman, A.I., Nash, M.A., Edelmann, C.M., Jr.: Sodium bicarbonate therapy for respiratory distress syndrome. J. Pediatr. **82**:172, 1973.
44. Engstrom, L., Karlberg, P., Rooth, G., Turnell, R.: The onset of respiration—a study of respiration and changes in blood gases and acid base balance. New York, Association for the Aid of Crippled Children, 1966.

45. Evans, R.S., Olver, R.E., Appleyard, W.J., Newman, C.G.H.: Effects of intragastric and intravenous sodium bicarbonate on rate of recovery from postasphyxial acidosis in the neonate. Arch. Dis. Child. **45**:321, 1970.
46. Finberg, L.: Danger to infants caused by changes in osmolal concentration. Pediatrics **40**:1931, 1967.
47. Finberg, L., Kiley, J., Luttvell, C.N.: Mass accidental salt poisoning. JAMA **184**:187, 1963.
48. Fomon, S.J., Harris, D.M., Jensen, R.L. Acidification of the urine by infants fed human milk or whole cows milk. Pediatrics **23**:113, 1958.
49. Gandy, G.M., Adamsons, K., Jr., Cunningham, N., et al.: Thermal environment and acid base homeostasis in human infants during the first few hours of life. J. Clin. Invest. **43**:751, 1964.
50. Gandy, G., Patridge, J.W., Gairdner, D.: Control of acidosis during exchange transfusion with citrated whole blood. Arch. Dis. Child. **43**: 147, 1968.
51. Gibson, J.G., II: International forum. Vox. Sang. **19**:546, 1970.
52. Gluck, L.: Fetal lung development—current concepts. Pediatr. Clin. N. Am. **20**:367, 1973.
53. Gluck, L., Kulovich, M.V., Eidelman, A.I., et al.: Biochemical development of surface activity in mammalian lung. IV Pulmonary lecithin synthesis in human fetus and newborn and etiology of the respiratory distress syndrome. Pediatr. Res. **6**:81, 1972.
54. Goldbenberg, V.E., Wiegenstein, L., Hopkins, G.B.: Hepatic injury associated with tromethamine. JAMA **205**:81, 1968.
55. Goodyear, A.V.N., Eckhardt, W.F., Ostbey, R.H., et al.: Effect of metabolic acidosis and alkalosis on coronary blood flow and myocardial metabolism in the intact dog. Am. J. Physiol. **200**:628, 1961.
56. Hall, R.T., Oliver, T.K., Jr.: Aortic blood pressure in infants admitted to a neonatal intensive care unit. Am. J. Dis. Child. **121**:145, 1971.
57. Harris, R.J.: Plasma non-esterified fatty acid and blood glucose levels in healthy and hypoxemic newborn infants. J. Pediatr. **84**:578, 1974.
58. Hatemi, N., McCance, R.A.: Renal aspects of acid base control in the newborn, III. Response to acidifying drugs. Acta Pediatr. **50**:603, 1961.
59. Haworth, S.G., James, L.S.: Danger of rapid correction of pH following asphyxia (American Pediatric Society (Abs), Atlantic City, 1968), in James, L.S.: Birth Asphyxia and Resuscitation, in Winters, R.W. (ed.): The Body Fluids in Pediatrics. Boston, Little, Brown and Co., 1973.
60. Himwich, H.E., Berstein, A.D., Hernlich, H., et al.: Mechanism for the maintenance of life in the newborn during anoxia. Am. J. Physiol. **135**: 389, 1942.
61. Hoebel, C.J., Oh, W., Hyrarihem, M.A., et al.: Early versus late treatment of neonatal acidosis in low birth weight infants. Relation to respiratory distress syndrome. J. Pediatr. **81**:1178, 1972.
62. Holmadhl, M.H., Nahas, G.G., Hassan, D., Verosky, M.: Acid base changes in the cerobrospinal fluid following rapid changes in the bicarbonate/carbonic acid ratio in the blood. Ann. N.Y. Acad. Sci. **92**:520, 1961.
63. Hutchinson, J.H., Kerr, M.M., Douglas, T.A., et al.: A therapeutic ap-

proach in cases of the respiratory distress syndrome of the newborn infant. Pediatrics, **33**:956, 1964.

64. Jacobson, L., Rooth, G.: Interpretive aspects on the acid base composition and its variation in fetal scalp blood and maternal scalp blood during labor. J. Obstet. Gynaecol. Br. Common. **78**:971, 1971.

65. James, L.S.: Acidosis of the newborn and its relation to birth asphyxia. Acta Pediatr. **49**: (suppl. 122) 17, 1960.

66. Johnson, G.H., Kirshbaum, T.H., Brinkman, C.R., III, Assali, N.S.: Effect of acid base and hypertonicity on fetal and neonatal cardiovascular heomdynamics. Am. J. Phys. Med. **220**:1798, 1971.

67. Kildberg, P.: Disturbances of hydrogen ion balance occurring in premature infants. II. Late metabolic acidosis. Acta Pediatr. **53**:517, 1964.

68. Kjellmer, I., Karlsson, K. Olsson, D., Rosen, K.G.: Cerebral reaction during intrauterine asphyxia in the sheep. I. Circulation and oxygen consumption in the fetal brain. Peditr. Res **8**:50, 1974.

69. Kravath, R.E., Aharon, A.S., Abal, G., Finberg, L.: Clinically significant physiologic changes from rapidly administered hypertonic solutions: acute osmol poisoning. Pediatrics **46**:267, 1970.

70. Kubli, F.W.: Fetal acid base and labor. Clin. Obstet. Gynecol. **11** (1): 168, 1968.

71. Kubli, F.W., Ruttgers, H.: Iatrogenic fetal hypoxia, in Gevers, R.H., and Ruys, J.V. (eds.): Proceeding of the Symposium on Physiology and Pathology in the Neonatal Period, Leiden Holland 1970. Holland, Leiden University Press, 1971.

72. Lusia, J.B.: Clinical aspects of placental insufficiency, in Aladjem, S. and Brown, A.K. (eds.): Clinical Perinatology. St. Louis, C.V. Mosby, 1976.

73. Maisels, M.J.: Bilirubin: on understanding and influencing its metabolism in the newborn infant. Pediatr. Clin. N. Amer. **19**:447, 1972.

74. Makoff, D.L., DaSilva, J.A., Rosenbaum, B.J., and Levy, S.E.: Hypertonic expansion, acid base and electrolyte changes. Am. J. Physiol. **218**: 1201, 1970.

75. McCance, R.A., Von Finck, M.A.: The titratable acidity, pH, ammonia and phosphate in the urines of very young infants. Arch. Dis. Child. **22**: 200, 1947.

76. Melichar, V., Wolf, H.: Postnatal changes in the blood serum content of glycerol and free fatty acids in premature infants. Influence of hypothermia and respiratory distress Biol. Neonate **11**:50, 1967.

77. Merritt, T.A., Farrell, P.M.: Diminished pulmonary lecithin synthesis in acidosis: Experimental findings as related to the respiratory distress syndrome. Pediatrics **57**:32, 1976.

78. Mitchell, R.A., Carman, C.T., Severinghaus, J.W., et al.: Stability of cerebrospinal fluid pH in chronic acid base disturbances in blood. J. Appl. Physiol. **20**:443, 1965.

79. Mitchell, R.A., Singer, M.M.: Respiration and cerebrospinal fluid pH in metabolic acidosis and alkalosis. J. Appl. Physiol. **20**:905, 1965.

20. Mott, J.C.: The ability of young mammals to withstand total oxygen lack: Br. Med. Bull. **17**:144, 1961.

81. Murdock, A.I., Swyer, P.: The contribution to venous admixture by shunt-

ing through the ductus arteriosus in infants with the respiratory distress syndrome of the newborn. Biol. Neonate 13:194, 1968.

82. Myers, R.E.: Two patterns of perinatal brain damage and their conditions of occurrence. Am. J. Obstet. Gynecol. 112:246, 1972.

83. Nahas, G.G., Fink, B.R., Ploski, W.S., Teneick, R.G.: The depressant effect of tris (hydroxymethyl) aminomethane and of mannitol on respiration. Ann. N.Y. Acad. Sci. 109:783, 1963.

84. Nahas, G.G., Manger, W.M., Mittleman, A., Ultmann, J.E.: The use of 2 amino-2hydroxymethyl-1,3 propanediol in the correction of addition acidosis and its effect on sympathoadrenal activity. Ann. N.Y. Acad. Sci. 92:596, 1961.

85. Oliver, T.K., Jr.: The use of THAM buffered ACD blood in high risk infants who require exchange transfusion: J. Pediatr. 67:951, 1965.

86. Oliver, T.K., Jr., Dennis, J.A., Bates, G.D.: Serial blood gas tensions and acid base balance during the first hour of life in human infants. Acta. Pediatr. 50:346, 1961.

87. Opie, L.H.: Cardiac metabolism. The effect of some physiologic, pharmacologic and pathologic influences: Am. Heart J. 69:401, 1965.

88. Opie, L.H., Kadas, I., Gevers, W.: Effect of pH on the function and glucose metabolism of the heart. Lancet 2:551, 1963.

89. Oski, F.A.: The unique fetal red cell and its function. Pediatrics 51:494, 1973.

90. Oski, F.A., Delivoria-Papadopoulos, M.: The red cell 2,3 diphosphoglycerate and tissue oxygen release. J. Pediatr. 77:941, 1970.

91. Ostrea, E.M., Jr., Odell, J.B.: The influence of bicarbonate administration on blood pH in a closed system: clinical implications. J. Pediatr. 80:671, 1972.

92. Pierson, W.E., Barrett, C.T., Oliver, T.K., Jr.: The effect of buffered and non-buffered ACD blood on electrolyte and acid base homeostasis during exchange transfusion. Pediatrics 41:802, 1968.

93. Poseiro, J.J.: Causes of fetal distress in labor. Int. J. Gynaecol. Obstet. 8:913, 1970.

94. Posner, J.B., Plum, F.: Spinal fluid pH and neurologic symptoms in systemic acidosis. N. Engl. J. Med. 277:605, 1967.

95. Posner, J.B., Swanson, A.G., Plum, F.: Acid base balance in cerebrospinal fluid. Arch. Neurol. 12:479, 1965.

96. Povey, M.J.C.: pH changes during exchange transfusions. Lancet 2:339, 1964.

97. Prod'hom, L.S., Levison, H., Cherry, R. B., Smith, C.A.: Adjustment of ventilation, intrapulmonary gas exchange and acid base balance during the first day of life. Infants with early respiratory distress. Pediatrics 35:662, 1965.

98. Ramsey, E.M.: Uteroplacental circulation during labor. Clin. Obstet. Gynecol. 11 (1): 78, 1965.

99. Ramsey, E.M.: Placental circulation in rhesus monkeys and man, in Mack, H. (ed.): Prenatal Life. Detroit, Wayne State University Press, 1970.

100. Reardon, H.S., Bauman, M.L., Haddad, E.J.: Chemical stimuli of respiration in the neonatal period. J. Pediatr. **57**:151, 1960.
101. Rhodes, P.G., Hall, R.T., Hellerstein, S.: The effects of single infusion of hypertonic sodium bicarbonate on body composition in neonates with acidosis. J. Pediatr. **90**:789, 1977.
102. Roberts, M., Linn, S.: Acute and subacute chronic toxicity of 2-amino-2-hydroxy-methyl-1,3-propanediol. Ann. N.Y.: Acad. Sci. **92**:724, 1961.
103. Robertson, N.R.C.: Apnoea after THAM administration in the newborn. Arch. Child. **45**:206, 1970.
104. Rosa, P.: Foetal hypoxia related to uterine motility. J. Int. Fed. Gynecol. Obstet. **5**:65, 1967.
105. Rudolph, A.M., Yuan, S.: Response of the pulmonary vasculature to hypoxia and H^+ ion concentration change. J. Clin. Invest. **45**:399, 1966.
106. Rush, B.F., Jr., Finberg, L., Daviglus, G.F., Cheung, C.S.: Pathological lesions in experimental hypernatremia induced by extrocorporeal dialysis. Surgery **50**:359, 1951.
107. Russel, G., Cotton, E.K.: Effect of sodium bicarbonate by rapid injection and of oxygen in high concentration in respiratory distress syndrome of the newborn. Pediatrics **41**:1063, 1970.
108. Saito, M., Gittleman, I.F., Pincus, J.B., Sobel, A.E.: Plasma proteins patterns in premature infants of varying weights on the first day of life. Pediatrics **17**:657, 1956.
109. Saling, E., Schneider, D.: Biochemical supervision of the foetus during labour. J. Obstet Gynaecol. Br. Common. **79**:799, 1967.
110. Schiff, D., Stern, L., Leduc, J.: Chemical thermogenesis in newborn infants. Catecholamine excretion and the plasma non-esterified fatty response to cold exposure. Pediatrics **37**:577, 1966.
111. Sessler, A.D., Taswell, H.F., Moffitt, E.A., Kirklin, J.W.: Heparinized versus acid citrate dextrose blood for cardiopulmonary bypass. Proc. Mayo Clin. **40**:859, 1965.
112. Shaw, R.S., Grove-Rasmussen, M.: Complications of blood transfusions. Surg. Clin. North Am. **43**:677, 1963.
113. Siegel, S.R., Phelps, D.L., Leake, R.D., Oh, W.: The effect of rapid infusion of hypertonic sodium bicarbonate in infants with respiratory distress. Pediatrics **51**:651, 1973.
114. Simmons, M.A., Adcock, E.W., Bard, H., Battaglia, F.C.: Hypernatremia intracranial hemorrhage and $NaHCO_3$ in neonates. N. Engl. J. Med. **291**:6, 1974.
115. Sinclair, J.C., Engel, K., Scient, M., Silverman, W.A.: Early correction of hypoxemia and acidemia in infants of low birth weight. A controlled trial of oxygen breathing rapid alkali infusion and assisted ventilation. Pediatrics **42**:565, 1968.
116. Singer, R.B., Deering, R.C., Clark, J.K.: The acute effects in man of a rapid intravenous infusion of hypertonic sodium bicarbonate. II Changes in respiration and output of carbon dioxide. J. Clin. Invest. **35**:245, 1956.
117. Stahlman, M., Blankenship, W.J., Shepard, F.M., et al.: Circulatory studies in clinical hyaline membrane disease. Biol. Neonate **20**:300, 1972.

118. Steichen, J.J., Kleinman, L.I.: Studies in acid base balance. I Effect of alkali therapy in newborn dogs with mechanically fixed ventilation. J. Pediatr. **91**:287, 1977.
119. Stephenson, J.M., Du, J.N., Oliver, T.K., Jr.: The effect of cooling on blood gas tensions in newborn infants. J. Pediatr. **76**:848, 1970.
120. Stern, L.: The newborn infant and his thermal environment, in Current Problems in Pediatrics I (I). Chicago, Yearbook Medical Publishers, 1970.
121. Stern, L., Lees, M.H., Leduc, J.: Environmental temperature oxygen consumption and catecholamine excretion in newborn infants. Pediatrics **36**:367, 1965.
122. Strauss, J.: Tris (Hydroxymethyl) amino methane (THAM). A pediatric evaluation. Pediatrics **41**:667, 1968.
123. Sulyok, E., Heim, T.: Assessment of maximal urinary acidification in premature infants. Biol. Neonate **19**:200, 1971.
124. Sureau, C.: The stress of labor, in Aladjem, S., and Brown, A.K. (eds): Clinical Perinatology. St. Louis, C.V. Mosby Co., 1974.
125. Teck, T.W.T.: Respiratory distress syndrome of the newborn in Kandsay Kaban Hospital. J. Singapore Paediatr. Soc. **7**:44, 1965.
126. Thomas, D.B.: Hyperosmolarity and intraventricular hemorrhage in premature babies. Acta Paediatr. Scand. **65**:429, 1976.
127. Towell, M.E.: The influence of labor on the fetus and the newborn. Pediatr. Clin. North Am. **13**:575, 1966.
128. Troelstra, J.A., Jonxis, J.H.P., Visser, H.K.A., Van der Vlugt, J.J.: Metabolism and acid-base regulation in respiratory distress syndrome; treatment with tris-hydroxy-methyl-amino methane (THAM), in Jonxis, J.H.P., et al. (eds.): Nutricia Symposium: The Adaptation of the Newborn Infant to Intrauterine Life. Leiden, Stenfert Kroese, 1964.
129. Turbeville, D.F., Bowen, F.W., Killann, A.P.: Intracranial hemorrhage in kittens: hypernatremia versus hypoxia. J. Pediatr. **89**:294, 1976.
130. Usher, R.: Clinical and therapeutic aspects. The respiratory distress syndrome of prematurity. Pediatr. Clin. North Am. **8**:525, 1961.
131. Usher, R.: Reduction of mortality from respiratory distress syndrome of prematurity with early administration of intravenous glucose and sodium bicarbonate. Pediatrics **32**:966, 1963.
132. Vliet, P.K.J. Van, Gupta, J.M.: THAM v. sodium bicarbonate in idiopathic respiratory distress syndrome. Arch. Dis. Child. **48**:247, 1973.
133. Vorherr, H.: Disorders of uterine function during pregnancy labor and puerperium, in Assali N. (ed.): Pathophysiology of Gestation. I. Maternal Disorders. New York, Academic Press, 1972.
134. Wood, C.: Studies of the human fetus during normal and abnormal labor. Int. J. Gynaecol. Obstet. **8**:850, 1970.
135. Wood, C., Ng, K.H., Hounslow, D., Benning, H.: The influence of differences of birth times upon fetal conditions in normal deliveries. J. Obstet. Gynaecol. Br. Common **80**:289, 1973.
136. Wood, C., Ng, K.H., Hounslow, D., Benning, H.: Time—an important variable in normal delivery. J. Obstet. Gynaecol. Br. Common. **80**:295, 1973.

12
Respiratory Treatment of the Neonate

Elizabeth D. Stein

The respiratory competence of the newborn infant is among the first elements assessed at birth (3). Clearing the airway and assistance with breathing and oxygen supplementation, if indicated, must be undertaken immediately once the need is recognized.

Close observation of the respiratory status of the neonate should continue for the first 48 hours of life. Most conditions that require intervention will manifest themselves within the first few minutes or hours, but certain pathology which is minimal at birth (e.g., pneumonia contracted during delivery) may progress and become symptomatic during the next day or two.

Warning signals that demand further study include abnormality in rate, depth, or rhythm of respiration; persistent cyanosis, other than peripheral; cardiac arrhythmias, especially bradycardia; stridor, grunting, flaring and use of accessory muscles. Auscultation, x-ray examination, and blood gas analysis must be used to determine the cause of any abnormalities in breathing, and the infant in need of ventilatory support must be dealt with on an emergent basis.

The primary pathology in neonatal respiratory insufficiency may be pulmonary or extrapulmonary. Intensity and duration of respiratory support will vary with the specific disease. Central nervous system depression following birth asphyxia or maternal oversedation is usually self-limited, requiring brief ventilatory support. In contrast, neuromuscular disorders in the neonate involve a prolonged course of assisted respiration. Ventilatory inadequacy stemming from pneumonia, aspiration, or idiopathic respiratory distress syndrome will usually require intensive care for several days or weeks. Congenital anomalies such as diaphragmatic hernia, tracheo-esophageal fistula, and lung cysts require surgical correction of the basic deformity before respiratory support can be withdrawn. Prompt restoration of obvious metabolic imbalances (hypoglycemia, hypocalcemia) usually will eliminate associated respiratory dysfunction.

Therapy and prognosis of neonatal respiratory insufficiency vary with the underlying pathology, but there are basic principles applicable to many conditions.

General Principles of Respiratory Support

The development of sophisticated methods of regulating the respiratory status of newborns has been a mixed blessing. Prudent titration of oxygen therapy and other modalities have prevented hypoxic brain damage and acidosis, but they have also fostered the development of a new group of maladies directly due to the therapy. Direct toxicity of oxygen to the pulmonary parenchyma and retinal vessels has been well documented (16, 20, 26, 34, 35). Tracheal stenosis following intubation, and bronchopulmonary dysplasia, a direct result of prolonged mechanical ventilation with high oxygen concentrations, are complications which may themselves become chronic or even fatal (9, 12, 20, 24, 28, 35).

Despite a plethora of studies attempting to establish an absolutely safe maximum inspired oxygen concentration, there are few firm guidelines in this area. In general, the inspired oxygen level should be kept as low as possible while providing arterial oxygenation sufficient to prevent cerebral hypoxia. Although it is generally accepted that arterial oxygen tension (Pao_2) is more important than inspired concentration (F_Io_2) in the development of oxygen toxicity, universal agreement is lacking on this issue (5, 7, 22, 24, 29, 34, 35).

One "absolute" in this area of shifting variables is that any therapy provided for the infant must be accompanied by frequent monitoring of both inspired oxygen concentration and arterial blood gas values. If available, the radial and/or temporal arteries are usually chosen for blood gas sampling; if these routes are unavailable or if a prolonged course of respiratory support is anticipated, cannulation of the umbilical artery may be undertaken (16, 20, 35). This route is not without its complications (see Chapter 13): rigid adherence to sterile technique, radiologic confirmation of the location of the catheter tip, and firm anchoring of the catheter in position by both suture and tape are essential. Arterialized capillary blood is not always satisfactory for accurate evaluation of oxygenation or acid-base status, especially in shock and other conditions characterized by peripheral vasoconstriction (9, 16, 28, 35).

The least invasive or aggressive method of therapy that will correct the disturbance should be used. If blood gas values indicate deficiency in oxygenation alone, with normal or below-normal carbon dioxide tension, a slight to moderate increase in inspired oxygen concentration should be employed as the first mode of therapy. Only if hypoxia fails to improve with inspired fractions up to 50%, or if hypercarbia and resultant acidosis supervene, should more vigorous methods of treatment be used.

Insertion of an artificial airway, regardless of type, does not in itself improve respiratory status unless the basic problem is one of isolated upper airway obstruction (e.g., choanal atresia, nasal mucosal edema in infants of reserpinized mothers, internal or external compromise of the tracheal lumen). Indications for intubation of the neonate (as in any patient) include:

1. Relief of upper airway obstruction;
2. Need for frequent tracheopulmonary toilet;
3. Provision of means for assisted mechanical ventilation;
4. Prevention of soilage of the pulmonary tree (as in a severely depressed infant or one with a high tracheo-esophageal fistula) (9, 12).

Mechanical ventilation should be reserved for instances of complete apnea; for conditions in which pulmonary compliance is so decreased that the work of breathing threatens to exhaust the infant; when arterial carbon dioxide tension ($Paco_2$) cannot be maintained within normal limits by any other means; or when all other modalities of improving oxygenation, including continuous positive airway pressure with 100% oxygen, fail to achieve acceptable oxygenation (16, 20, 28).

Normal Blood Gas Values

Adequate oxygenation of the newborn can be assumed if the arterial oxygen tension is 60 torr or better and pH and hemoglobin provide normal oxygen transport. Hypercarbia of over 50 torr is suggestive of respiratory compromise and a need for careful observation, while a $Paco_2$ of 65 torr or greater indicates the need for prompt and aggressive intervention. Cor-

Table 12.1 Abbreviations and Symbols

F_IO_2	Inspired oxygen concentration
Pao_2	Arterial oxygen tension (pressure)
$Paco_2$	Arterial carbon dioxide tension
RV	Residual volume
FRC	Functional residual capacity
CPAP	Continuous positive airway pressure
PEEP	Positive end-expiratory pressure
IMV	Intermittent mandatory ventilation

rection of acid-base status should be in accordance with both carbon dioxide tension and metabolic considerations (see Chapter 11).

Oxygen Analyzers

Measuring and recording the inspired oxygen concentration (F_IO_2) is not only medically appropriate, it is mandated by law in most state hospital codes. Sampling may be done intermittently (at least every two hours) or constantly; the latter method is more desirable. Most monitors designed for constant use have both audible and visual alarm systems which may be set by the operator to warn of either increase or decrease beyond desired levels. The analyzer itself should be checked and calibrated against gas mixtures of known oxygen concentrations (e.g., 21% and 100%) at least once a day (2, 7, 16, 28, 33).

Humidification and Warming

One of the major functions of the normal intact respiratory tract is the humidification and warming of inspired air so that it is fully saturated with water vapor at body temperature when it reaches the alveoli. In the neonate requiring ventilatory support, the introduction of cool, dry gas with a relative humidity of zero imposes a considerable burden in terms of heat and water loss, one which the sick infant cannot support. Energy in the form of heat must be expended to warm the inspired gas mixture; loss of water from the tracheobronchial mucosa may result in a significant fluid deficit. Prolonged dehydration of the respiratory mucosa results in loss of ciliary motility with drying, crusting, and inspissation of secretions. It is essential that both heat and moisture be added to any inspired gas mixture utilized in the care of the newborn (2, 9, 12, 14, 16, 28, 32).

Moisture is added to inspired gas by nebulizers and humidifiers. The *nebulizer* uses a vibrating crystal or a system of baffles to break a stream of water into an aerosol of tiny droplets, which are then injected into the inspiratory stream. Since the nebulizer injects particulate water and other particulate matter. (such as bacteria) into the inspired atmosphere, such complications as "rain-out" in the tubing, fluid overload, and bacterial infection are not uncommon and the problem of heat loss remains (9, 14, 16, 32, 33, 35).

The *humidifier* passes the inspired gases through a water bath where it picks up water as vapor. Most humidifiers in use today incorporate a heating unit, thus solving both problems simultaneously. The only major hazard in the use of the heated humidifier is the danger of overheating if the thermostat malfunctions; use of a temperature probe in the proximal airway is essential in guarding against this possibility (14, 33).

In general, a humidifier is adequate for neonatal use if it is capable of delivering 60 to 80% relative humidity at a temperature of 32° to 34°C (9, 14, 16, 33, 35).

Care of Artificial Airways

Since the presence of an endotracheal tube prevents glottic closure and interferes with the normal cough mechanism, periodic aspiration of secretions is essential to maintain the airways free of obstructing secretions. The effectiveness of suctioning is greatly enhanced when it is preceded by gentle percussion of the chest and by postural drainage to aid in movement of secretions toward the carina where they will be accessible to the suction catheter (9, 12, 16).

Suctioning is inherently traumatic. Excessive vacuum may strip and denude tracheal mucosa, leading to bleeding and facilitating the establishment of infection. Prolonged aspiration can induce atelectasis and significant hypoxia. Suctioning should be performed only when indicated, as by noisy respirations or decreased compliance, and not at regular, fixed intervals. Adherence to a rational, stepwise procedure is mandatory (7, 9, 12, 16, 30).

First the infant should be hyperventilated with 100% oxygen for two to three minutes. The vacuum to be applied to the suction catheter should be set between 50 and 80 cm H_2O. A sterile glove should be donned and a fresh, sterile catheter taken up and lubricated in sterile water; only then should the infant be disconnected from the respirator or T-piece. The catheter is inserted into the airway *with the side port open;* occlusion of the port is accomplished only after withdrawal has begun. The entire time interval between insertion and withdrawal of the catheter must not exceed 10 seconds. Bradycardia is an early signal of prolonged suctioning. The patient's lungs should be reinflated with a manual resuscitator or mechanical ventilator before suctioning is undertaken again. The mouth and nose should be suctioned last, and the catheter then discarded (7, 9, 12, 16).

The instillation of 0.5 to 1 ml of sterile saline prior to suctioning may be helpful in loosening thick, viscid secretions, although adequate humidification usually makes this unnecessary (9, 16, 30, 35).

Rigid adherence to sterile technique is essential whenever manipulation of the airway is undertaken.

Techniques of Supporting Ventilation

Oxygen Therapy

Mild respiratory dysfunction such as is seen with a small pneumothorax, aspiration other than meconium, or pneumonia, may be treated conservatively with supplemental oxygen alone.

Oxygen may be administered to newborns of any size by means of an incubator or an oxygen hood or head-box. The incubator provides a completely isolated environment for the infant, with close control of oxygen concentration, temperature, and humidity. (It also provides full visibility for the staff caring for the baby.) Oxygen concentrations up to 80% may be achieved. Commercially available models provide side ports for easy access to the infant as well as orifices for intravenous tubing, temperature monitoring, and oxygen sampling devices. The major disadvantage of the incubator is that the oxygen concentration drops drastically each time the ports are opened, and may take up to 15 minutes to restabilize (2, 33, 35).

Hoods or head-boxes are designed to sit over the infant's head, providing a micro-environment of oxygen-enriched, warmed, humidified air. A large opening around the infant's neck affords an exit for expired gases. The head-box can deliver oxygen in concentrations up to 85%. It affords easier access to the baby than does the incubator, but used alone it fails to provide a total environment. A radiant heater may be placed above the patient to offset the heat loss occasioned by exposure, or the head-box may be used inside an incubator to provide the advantages of both devices; in this case, a constant oxygen concentration up to 97% may be attained (2, 16, 28, 35).

If the degree of respiratory insufficiency is mild to moderate and can be remedied by an increase in inspired oxygen concentration alone, either of these devices is suitable. Face masks and nasal cannulas, which may be appropriate for older children, have met with little success when dealing with neonates (35).

Electrical equipment which has not been "approved for use in hazardous environments" must not be used in the oxygen-enriched atmosphere. All such equipment must be periodically inspected by a qualified biomedical technician to insure that leakage current is within acceptable limits, that all contacts are secure, and that the device is still safe for the use for which it was intended.

Continuous Positive Airway Pressure (CPAP)

The use of continuous positive airway pressure (CPAP) in the spontaneously breathing infant was introduced in the early 1970s, and has significantly reduced the morbidity and mortality of the infant respiratory distress syndrome. The system as originally described maintained airway and alveolar pressure above atmospheric throughout all phases of the respiratory cycle. It used either an endotracheal tube or sealed head-box, with the expiratory circuit connected to an anesthesia bag whose partially occluded "tail" afforded a variable resistance to expiration (see Fig. 12.1). Beneficial effects of CPAP include prevention of small airway collapse, improvement in right-to-left shunt, and increase of both residual volume

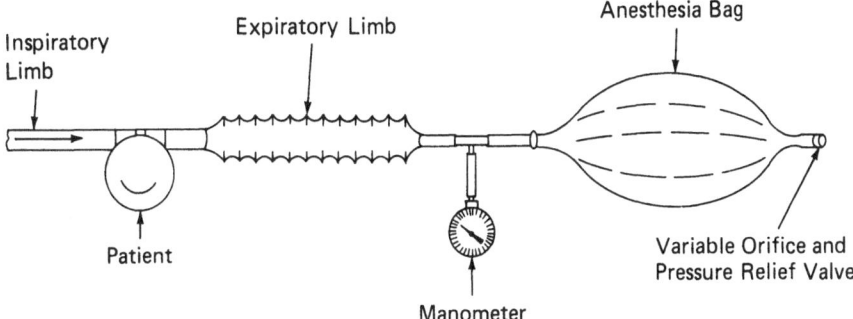

Fig. 12.1 Expiratory side of the CPAP circuit. End-expiratory pressure is reflected on the manometer and may be altered by adjustment of the variable orifice on the end of the anesthesia bag.

(RV), and functional residual capacity (FRC) (9, 16, 17, 18, 23, 24). Since its introduction, CPAP has proved valuable in a variety of conditions which formerly would have necessitated mechanical ventilation.

Indications for the Institution of CPAP

In addition to its use in treatment for respiratory distress syndrome, CPAP has become the method of choice for conditions in which atelectasis, low compliance, and significant ventilation-perfusion mismatching contribute to the disease state.

Methods of Administration

Essentials of the CPAP system are constant. The *inspiratory limb* begins with a gas source (preferably an air-oxygen blender) whereby gas with a predetermined oxygen concentration passes through a flowmeter and small-bore connecting tubing into a heated humidifier. From the humidifier a large-bore corrugated tubing leads into the device chosen for application to the infant, the patient connecting device (see below); in this inspiratory portion of the circuit are incorporated instruments for measuring both oxygen concentration and temperature of the inspired gas mixture.

The *expiratory limb* consists of a short length of corrugated tubing with a sensing device indicating end-expiratory pressure and leading to a 0.5 liter reservoir bag for maintaining pressure, with a pressure relief valve for escape of expired gases into the atmosphere. End-expiratory pressure is adjusted either by altering the pressure at which the relief valve opens or by changing the inspiratory flow rate. End-expiratory pressure is usually maintained at levels between 5 and 10 cm of water, but may be increased to 15 cm in cases of severe alveolar-arterial oxygen gradient.

The *patient connecting device* may be an endotracheal tube, a commercially available nasal mask that allows for custom fit and snug application, double nasal airways or modified nasal "prongs," or a plastic head-box that provides a tight seal around the infant's neck to maintain constant positive pressure within the box. The nasal mask or prong techniques seem to be the most popular. All devices except the head-box require some degree of ingenuity in attaching the two limbs of the circuit securely, but weightlessly, to the infant's face (8, 16, 17, 18, 22).

Discontinuing CPAP

CPAP may be maintained as long as a severe alveolar-arterial oxygen gradient exists. When the infant has an acceptable arterial oxygen tension (>70 torr) on an inspired concentration of 40% or less, weaning from CPAP may be instituted in steps of 2 cm H_2O at a time. Stepwise decreases in pressure are continued at two-hour intervals, with blood gas determinations before and after each change, until zero pressure is attained. The infant should be observed for at least four hours without CPAP, with appropriate blood gas sampling, before he can be assumed to be safely independent of this modality (21, 22, 31).

Mechanical Ventilation

The decision to intubate and mechanically ventilate a newborn is not made easily; if indicated, it must be done expeditiously. If severe hypoxemia and/or hypercarbia, with resultant respiratory acidosis, fail to respond to other methods of therapy (including CPAP with over 60% oxygen), mechanical ventilation with its inherent risks must be undertaken.

Absolute indications for mechanical ventilation include:

1. Pao_2 less than 60 torr in 60% O_2 and 10 cm CPAP;
2. $Paco_2$ greater than 60 torr;
3. pH less than 7.2 after correction of metabolic acidosis;
4. Frequent apneic episodes (9, 10, 16, 33, 35).

Characteristics of an Ideal Ventilator

The perfect ventilator for neonatal use must offer precise control of *tidal volumes* over a wide range; even a few milliliters of error can have significant consequences in an infant with a normal tidal volume of only 10 ml. It must be capable of delivering this preset volume at *rates* of 20 to 60 breaths per minute with no alteration in *inspiratory:expiratory (I:E) ratio*. The ventilator should be capable of serving as an assistor, assistor-controller, or pure controller. When used in the assist or assist-control modes, its *response time* should be minimal (less than 0.2 seconds) with maximum *sensitivity* (0.05 to 0.1 cm water). Inspiratory *flow rates* should be adjustable to less than 2 liters/minute for ventilation of very small infants. A fail-safe *pressure relief valve* must be incorporated into the circuit to prevent generation of excessive intra-alveolar pressures in the face of partial airway obstruction or changes in compliance. Both audible and visual battery-powered *alarms* should quickly alert the clinician to any pressure drop in the system (indicative of power failure, leak, or patient disconnect), excess pressure needed to achieve preset volume, or changes in oxygen concentration above or below preset limits. The *volume* of the system and hence its *internal compliance* should be low enough to allow for precise estimation of very small tidal volumes. A *heated humidifier* with a means of monitoring inspired gas temperature should be incorporated into the system. The patient circuit should be easy to change and sterilize. Such features as CPAP, PEEP, and IMV should be built into it, and it should lend itself to easy modification with commercially available parts.

Finally, it would be desirable if such a versatile and sophisticated machine were simple to understand and operate, and small enough to be unobtrusive in the typically overcrowded area immediately surrounding the very sick neonate (9, 19, 20, 22).

Unfortunately, no one perfect machine is yet available commercially. It is necessary, therefore, for the clinician to be aware of these criteria and to be thoroughly familiar with the ventilator(s) in use in his (her) own unit, with an eye to compensating for any shortcomings.

The machines most commonly used for neonatal ventilation are the Bourns Pediatric Ventilator, the Bennett MA-1 with infant circuit, the Amsterdam Infant Ventilator, the Puritan-Bennett PR-2, the Bird Mark 14 and the Babybird. Lack of adequate alarm systems limits the usefulness of the last four models (9, 20, 27, 28, 30, 33, 35).

Setting the Ventilator

The following suggestions for ventilator settings are merely guidelines. The real test of adequate ventilation is in normalization of blood gas values, and these must be analyzed as frequently as conditions warrant. Changes in ventilator settings should usually be made one at a time, lest the clinician be left at a loss to determine which of three or four variables was really responsible for a sudden change (9, 22).

Tidal Volume

A tidal volume of 6 to 7 ml/kg is an appropriate initial setting, although use of the Radford or other nomogram allows for more precise estimation of ideal values. Arterial carbon dioxide tension is the ultimate determinant of adequacy of volume; the $Paco_2$ should be kept above 24 and below 40 torr. Allowance must be made for the internal compliance factor of each individual ventilator and circuit—usually 3 to 5 ml/cm of water pressure —and this volume must be added to the desired tidal volume (9, 20, 25, 33).

Rate

If the infant is allowed to set his own rate (i.e., the ventilator is in the "assist" mode), alteration of tidal volume is the physician's only means of regulating carbon dioxide tension. If, however, the respiratory rate is controlled, which may be advisable in cases of extreme tachypnea or severely decreased compliance, both rate and volume may be adjusted to correct hyper- or hypocarbia. It is usually convenient to choose a ventilator rate near the normal value for the infant's weight and gestational age, but deliberate slowing of this rate may prove beneficial in cases of severe diffusion defect or low compliance states. Such a decrease in rate may require the use of sedatives or muscle relaxants to keep the child "in phase" with the ventilator. In such instances, attending personnel must be doubly vigilant, since the patient is now totally ventilator dependent (19, 20, 22, 35).

Inspired Oxygen Concentration

The lowest possible F_IO_2 compatible with adequate tissue oxygenation should be employed. An arterial oxygen tension between 60 and 90 torr is the primary criterion for determining inspired concentration; it may sometimes be necessary to maintain a high F_IO_2 for a day or more in order to insure adequate oxygenation. The Pao_2 should be monitored frequently, at least every four hours, in such cases, and the F_IO_2 reduced appropriately as soon as improvement is noted. We prefer to reduce F_IO_2 in decrements of 5% at a time, to guard against an unexpectedly large drop in Pao_2 with concomitant hypoxia. Obviously, arterial oxygenation must be checked 10 to 15 minutes after each decrement in inspired concentration. Such modalities as PEEP and CPAP may and should be utilized, when appropriate, to improve oxygenation at an acceptable F_IO_2 (20, 22, 31).

Inspiratory:Expiratory (I:E) Ratio

The normal I:E ratio lies between 1:2 and 1:3 and produces minimal interference with cardiovascular function. In conditions with markedly reduced compliance or with increased resistance to air flow, it may be helpful to prolong inspiration to allow for attainment of adequate volume. Reverse I:E ratios of 3:1 or even 4:1 may be necessary (19, 20, 22).

Sighing is an added feature of many ventilators. This periodic extra-deep breath is said to help prevent microatelectasis of peripheral alveoli, although its efficacy has been questioned recently. If it is used, the sigh volume should be set at one and a half times the normal tidal volume; the frequency may be varied from once every two to three minutes to six times an hour (7, 20, 22).

Pressure

Even with a built-in pressure relief valve (usually set at 40 to 60 cm H_2O), most volume ventilators give the operator a choice of pressure limits considered appropriate for a normal tidal volume in the individual patient. The pressure limit should be set about 10 cm higher than the peak inspiratory pressure indicated on the manometer. If patient resistance, airway obstruction, or a sudden change in compliance makes a higher pressure necessary for delivery of the preset volume, the pressure alarm will be activated to warn of changing conditions, although the excess pressure will be applied in order to maintain constant volume. It is incumbent upon the individual caring for the patient to respond immediately to this warning signal. The need for suctioning of the airway is the most common cause of sudden pressure increase, although more serious conditions such as tension pneumothorax may first present in this way (7, 19, 20, 27, 28, 33).

Positive End-Expiratory Pressure (PEEP)

Positive end-expiratory pressure is a means of maintaining constant positive airway pressure in a patient whose respirations are controlled by a ventilator. PEEP is differentiated from CPAP, in which the patient is breathing spontaneously. Even at the end of expiration, airway pressure never returns to atmospheric. This technique often improves arterial oxygenation by 20 to 30 torr, and sometimes even by 100 torr at a given F_IO_2; hence it is a valuable means of reducing the risks inherent in oxygen therapy. PEEP improves ventilation-perfusion mismatching, increases FRC and RV, and is especially useful in low-compliance states with atelectasis and/or small airway collapse. Because mean intrathoracic pressure never returns to zero, PEEP may interfere with cardiac output by reducing venous return; this is more likely in hypovolemic than in normovolemic states. Thus it is recommended that PEEP should be instituted gradually, 2 to 4 cm H_2O at a time, with careful observation of cardiovascular response after each increment (21, 22, 24).

Most effective PEEP is established when maximum increase in PaO_2 at a given F_IO_2 is achieved; in newborns, this value usually lies between 5 and 10 cm H_2O positive pressure, although higher values (15 to 20 cm) are sometimes required. Other than cardiovascular compromise, the most serious potential hazard of PEEP is the development of pneumothorax due to pulmonary overdistension, with rupture of a bleb or other weakened area.

The clinician must be aware of this possibility and must respond immediately in case of sudden deterioration in an infant who was previously well ventilated. If physical examination reveals a shift in the mediastinum with hyperresonance and absent or decreased breath sounds on the side opposite the direction of shift, PEEP must be discontinued immediately and x-ray confirmation of the diagnosis obtained. A significant pneumothorax in an infant dependent on positive pressure ventilation must be treated with a chest tube connected to constant vacuum and underwater seal (11, 20, 23, 24, 35).

Discontinuing PEEP

Like CPAP, PEEP may be continued as long as alveolar-arterial oxygen differences warrant its use. The hazards of high inspired oxygen concentrations almost always outweigh those of PEEP. When arterial oxygenation is adequate at an F_IO_2 of 40% or less, PEEP may be gradually discontinued in decrements of 2 to 4 cm H_2O at a time. If, after four hours without PEEP, the infant is able to maintain stable vital signs and blood gases, he may be considered PEEP-independent, and the next phase in the weaning process can be undertaken as indicated (21, 31).

Intermittent Mandatory Ventilation (IMV)

Intermittent mandatory ventilation may prove to be one of the most significant advances in mechanical ventilation during the 1970s. It was originally introduced as a technique for accelerating the weaning process, but in many centers it has now become a primary mode of therapy. By adding a modified T-piece circuit to the standard ventilator circuit, IMV allows the patient who needs mechanical ventilation to breathe spontaneously some of the time, with the ventilator delivering an additional, preset optimum tidal volume at regular intervals. The period between assisted respirations may vary from every other breath to once every two minutes, depending on individual needs and the capability of the ventilator. The primary advantage of intermittent mandatory ventilation lies in insuring adequate minute ventilation while allowing the patient to exercise his own respiratory muscles at least part of the time, and to establish his own $Paco_2$; it may also offer less interference with cardiac function (4, 13, 15, 21, 24, 31, 33). Many of the newer ventilators used for neonates have incorporated an IMV mode, with the capability of using PEEP or CPAP simultaneously with IMV; older models can be modified with disposable circuits.

Intermittent mandatory ventilation is an effective method of mechanical ventilation. In many cases its use significantly eases the weaning process. It is somewhat doubtful that it will ever (as its more enthusiastic proponents claim) become the only way of administering mechanical ventilation. Its proper place in the therapeutic regimen remains to be established (24).

Weaning from Mechanical Ventilation

If therapy is successful, there comes a time at which the question of discontinuing therapy becomes appropriate. In general, no attempt at discontinuing mechanical ventilation should be made until the patient can maintain an adequate arterial oxygen tension at an F_IO_2 of 0.5 or less, with a $Paco_2$ of less than 60 torr. Other general criteria for assessing readiness for weaning are: general improvement in clinical condition; hematocrit $>40\%$; stable vital signs; good spontaneous inspiratory effort (>20 cm H_2O negative pressure on occlusion of the airway); and absent or clearing pulmonary pathology on x-ray (16, 21, 24, 31).

When the patient is judged ready, weaning may be started in one of two ways. The ventilator may be set to the IMV mode with the respirator frequency set at two-thirds of the patient's spontaneous rate and the sensitivity decreased so that the machine will not respond to the baby's inspiratory efforts. If the patient tolerates this decrease in mechanical assistance with no significant alteration in vital signs or blood gas values over a half-hour period, continued decrements of two to four breaths per minute may be made every half hour until the baby is breathing essentially unaided. Depending on the lowest machine frequency attainable (i.e., one breath every two minutes up to six breaths per minute, depending on the machine used), it is advisable to change to a T-piece for a period of two to four hours before considering extubation. If the baby can tolerate four hours on a T-piece at an F_IO_2 no more than 10% higher than the concentration on the ventilator, he probably can be extubated safely with oxygen supplementation by hood or incubator (21, 28, 31).

The second method of weaning to be used, if IMV is impracticable or if the baby has been ventilated for less than 24 hours (with little opportunity to become ventilator-dependent), is the classical T-piece technique. The baby is removed from the ventilator and connected to a T-piece with an F_IO_2 10% higher than that of the ventilator. After an uneventful 10 minutes on the T-piece, blood gases are drawn and the infant is reconnected to the ventilator. If tachypnea, tachycardia, retractions, cyanosis, or other evidence of respiratory insufficiency become manifest in less than 10 minutes, the patient must be reconnected to the ventilator and further attempts at weaning abandoned until conditions improve. If he tolerates it well, intervals on the ventilator may be shortened progressively until the baby is able to tolerate a total absence of ventilatory assistance for four hours, at which point extubation may be considered (16, 21, 28, 31).

Continuous positive airway pressure (CPAP) is a major aid to successful weaning; it helps counteract the tendency toward microatelectasis and reduces the effort necessary to keep the airways open. Periodic hyperinflation with a self-inflating bag (a technique which can be continued even after extubation), also aids in preventing atelectasis with subsequent "failure to wean" (16, 17).

Extubation

Removal of the endotracheal tube should be performed after the patient is thoroughly suctioned and the lungs are reinflated with 100% oxygen. Gentle positive pressure on the breathing bag while the tube is withdrawn reduces the likelihood of pooled secretions dropping downward into the lungs as the tip of the tube passes through the cords.

Some pediatricians elect to administer a single intravenous dose of corticosteroid 15 to 30 minutes before extubation to reduce laryngeal edema resulting from tube trauma; others prefer to withhold steroids unless specifically indicated, as by the development of stridor (1, 6, 8, 19, 30, 35). Inhalation of racemic epinephrine may be helpful in mild postextubation croup; maintenance of a high-humidity environment is essential to preservation of a patent airway after extubation (28, 30, 35).

Two points about extubation merit special emphasis:

1. No patient should be extubated unless equipment and personnel for reintubation are at the bedside. Sudden laryngospasm or obstruction by a dislodged mucous plug may make rapid reintubation a lifesaving procedure; a "STAT" page for reintubation heralds potential tragedy. Postextubation croup usually manifests itself within three hours; the patient requires very careful observation during this interval.
2. Elective withdrawal of full respiratory support should never occur during the hours of darkness. Major changes are best accomplished when a full complement of alert personnel, both in the nursery and in the support areas such as Respiratory Therapy and the blood gas laboratory, is available to help monitor the baby and give support in case of deterioration (9, 16).

Conclusion

In discussing respiratory care of the newborn, it has been convenient to pretend that the cardiopulmonary system is a separate entity, independent of the rest of the organism. Treatment of respiratory insufficiency is often symptomatic, designed to protect the patient from permanent hypoxic damage until the underlying disease can be identified accurately and treated appropriately. Maintenance of adequate nutrition, augmentation of hemoglobin and oxygen-carrying capacity, surgical correction of anatomic anomalies, restoration of fluid and electrolyte balance, and antibiotic therapy of infection must be accomplished before the respiratory component can be successfully resolved.

References

1. Adair, J.C., Ring, W.H.: Management of epiglottitis in children. Anesth. Analg. **54**:622, 1975.
2. Ahlgren, E.W.: Environmental control of the neonate receiving intensive care. Int. Anesthesiol. Clin. **12**:173, 1974.
3. Apgar, V.: A proposal for a new method of evaluation of the newborn infant. Anesth. Analg. **32**:260, 1953.
4. Banner, M.J., Clark, J.R.: IMV: innovation in long-term ventilation. Respir. Ther. **4**:83, 1974.
5. Barber, R.E., Lee, J., Hamilton, W.K.: Oxygen toxicity in man. A prospective study in patients with irreversible brain damage. N. Engl. J. Med. **283**:1473, 1970.
6. Bass, B.: Steroids. Clin. Anesth. **10**:249, 1973.
7. Bendixen, H.H., Egbert, L.D., Hedley-Whyte, J., et al: Respiratory Care. St. Louis, C. V. Mosby Co., 1965.
8. Case History Number 79: Steroid therapy for post-intubation respiratory obstruction. Anesth. Analg. **53**:588, 1974.
9. Cox, J.M.: Techniques in neonatal ventilation. Int. Anesthesiol. Clin. **12**: 111, 1974.
10. Daily, W.J.R., Meyer, H.B.P., Sunshine, P., Smith, P.C.: Mechanical ventilation of newborn infants, III: Historical comments and development of a scoring system for selection of infants. Anesthesiology **34**:119, 1971.
11. Daily, W.J.R., Sunshine, P., Smith, P.C.: Mechanical ventilation of newborn infants, V: Five years experience. Anesthesiology **34**:132, 1971.
12. Davenport, H.T.: Prolonged endotracheal intubation in children—a perspective. Int. Anesthesiol. Clin. **8**:909, 1970.
13. Desautels, D., Bartlett, J.L.: Methods of administering intermittent mandatory ventilation (IMV). Respir. Care **19**:187, 1974.
14. Dick, W.: Aspects of humidification: requirements and techniques. Int. Anesthesiol. Clin. **12**:217, 1974.
15. Downs, J.B., Klein, E.F., Jr., Desautels, D., et al: Intermittent mandatory ventilation: A new approach to weaning patients from ventilators. Chest **64**:331, 1973.
16. Gregory, G.A.: Respiratory care of newborn infants. Pediatr. Clin. North Am. **19**:311, 1971.
17. Gregory, G.A., Kitterman, J.A., Phibbs, R.H., et al: Treatment of the idiopathic respiratory distress syndrome with continuous positive airway pressure. N. Engl. J. Med. **284**:1333, 1971.
18. Hunsinger, D.L., Lisnerski, K.J., Maurizi, J.J., Phillips, M.L.: Respiratory Technology: A Procedure Manual (2nd Ed.). Reston, Va., Reston Publishing Company, 1976.

19. Keuskamp, D.G.H.: Ventilation of premature and newborn infants. Int. Anesthesiol. Clin. **12**:281, 1974.
20. Lough, M.D., Doershuk, C.F., Stern, R.C. (eds.): Pediatric Respiratory Therapy. Chicago, Year Book Medical Publishers, 1974.
21. McNabb, T.G., and Hall, S.V.: Weaning from respiratory support. Int. Anesthesiol. Clin. **14**:214, 1976.
22. Meyer, H.B.P., Griffin, B.E., Sedaghatian, M.R., et al: Ventilatory support of the newborn infant with respiratory distress syndrome and respiratory failure. Int. Anesthesiol. Clin. **12**:81, 1974.
23. Oliver, T.K.: Positive transpulmonary airway pressure. Pediatrics **48**:175, 1971.
24. Pontoppidan, H., Wilson, R.S., Rie, M.A., Schneider, R.C.: Respiratory intensive care. Anesthesiology **47**:96, 1977.
25. Radford, E.P., Jr.: Ventilation standards for use in artificial respiration. J. Appl. Physiol. **7**:451, 1955.
26. Rudolph, A.M., Barnett, H.L., Einhorn, A.H. (eds.): Pediatrics, 16th Ed., Chapter 6. New York, Appleton-Century-Crofts, 1977.
27. Shapiro, B.L., Harrison, R.A., Trout, C.A.: Clinical Application of Respiratory Care. Chicago, Year Book Medical Publishers, 1975.
28. Slonim, M.B., Schneider, S.N., Weng, T.R., and Fields, L.J.: Pediatric Respiratory Therapy. Monsey, N.Y., Glenn Educational Medical Services, Inc., 1974.
29. Singer, M.M., Wright, F., Stanley, L.K., et al: Oxygen toxicity in man. A prospective study in patients after open-heart surgery. N. Engl. J. Med. **283**:1473, 1970.
30. Verhoog-Bloembergen, M.P.J., Leader, G.L.: Long-term nasotracheal intubation. Int. Anesthesiol. Clin. **12**:241, 1974.
31. Vidyasagar, D., Wai, W.: Respiratory weaning of the newborn: some practical considerations. Crit. Care Med. **3**:16, 1975.
32. Welsh, B.E., Conn, A.W.: Humidity and mist therapy: devices and principles. Int. Anesthesiol. Clin. **8**:569, 1970.
33. Williams, T.J., Hill, J.W.: Handbook of Neonatal Care. Riverside, Cal., Bourns, Inc., 1974.
34. Winter, P.M., Smith, G.: The toxicity of oxygen. Anesthesiology **37**:210, 1972.
35. Wolfsdorf, J.: The acute care of respiratory problems in the neonate, infant, and child. Int. Anesthesiol. Clin. **13**:73, 1975.

13
Exchange Transfusion of the Newborn Infant

Ermelando V. Cosmi

The first successful exchange transfusions were performed by Robertson (99, 100) in 1921 and by Hart (57) in 1925 for treatment of carbon monoxide poisoning and of erythroblastosis fetalis, respectively. However, exchange transfusion (ET) did not become widely used until Wallerstein (119) in 1946 and Diamond (40) in 1947 described its efficacy in the therapy of hemolytic disease of the newborn infant (HDN). The procedure is now applied as a routine treatment of HDN as well as for hyperbilirubinemia from other causes and has been effective in preventing kernicterus. ET has been employed also as a basic supportive measure in the therapy of various other diseases (12).

The objective of ET is to correct the severe anemia of erythroblastosis, to treat actual hyperbilirubinemia, and to prevent potential hyperbilirubinemia (by removing antibody-coated red cells).

Indications for ET

Neonatal Hyperbilirubinemia

It has long been accepted that a relationship exists between the occurrence of kernicterus and the serum level of free (unionized, lipid-soluble, unconjugated) bilirubin, the only form capable of crossing the blood-brain barrier (79, 80). Kernicterus and resultant brain damage have appeared in infants with serum unconjugated bilirubin levels of 12 mg/dl especially if preterm

(1, 55, 112), and the incidence of these complications is greatly increased with levels above 15 mg/dl, particularly when the duration of exposure to such high bilirubin levels is prolonged. Most bilirubin in blood is hydrophobically bound to albumin and is not available for diffusion into the tissues. However, when binding sites on albumin become saturated, the excess, unbound bilirubin may be taken up by cells to produce kernicterus. Binding of bilirubin to serum protein has been documented by many methods, and 1 M of albumin has been found to bind 2 M of bilirubin (102). Thus, excess free bilirubin may result either from high total bilirubin or from insufficient albumin.

Under normal conditions, the newborn infant produces an average of 8.5 mg/kg of bilirubin per day (73) which is more than twice the rate of normal production in the adult (3.8 to 4.0 mg/kg/day) (11). The increased amount of bilirubin in the neonate is due to three factors: a higher circulating red cell volume per kg body weight (76), a shorter mean red cell life span (73, 128), and sources of heme other than breakdown of hemoglobin (116). While an elevated bilirubin load can be handled easily by the adult liver, the less efficient hepatic clearance of the newborn may exaggerate the effect of even small increases in bilirubin production (71). This is particularly evident in premature infants in whom lower serum binding capacity allows higher concentrations of bilirubin. Finally, dissociation of bilirubin from its albumin bond may be induced by certain conditions such as hypoxia and acidosis (81, 102), high free fatty acid levels (95), exogenously administered anions and other complications (Table 13.1).

An etiologic classification of neonatal hyperbilirubinemia is shown in Table 13.2, and the more frequently occurring syndromes will be described.

Increased Production

The most dangerous type of hyperbilirubinemia is that due to an increased production secondary to hemolytic disease or to breakdown of hemoglobin originating from extravasated blood into skin or viscera. Hemolytic disease from *Rh alloimmunization* (especially anti-D) presents serious problems,

Table 13.1   Factors Increasing the Risk from Hyperbilirubinemia

1. Birth weight (<1500 g)	6. Hypothermia ($<35°$C)
2. Low serum protein (≥ 5 g/100 ml)	7. Signs of clinical or CNS deterioration
3. Starvation-hypoglycemia	8. Competing drugs (sulfonamides, salicylates, diazepam, procaine, bupivacaine, etc.)
4. Perinatal asphyxia	
5. Respiratory distress	9. Infection
	10. Male sex (?)

Modified from Brown, A.K.: Neonatal hyperbilirubinemia, in Behrman, R.E. (ed.): Neonatology Diseases of the Fetus and Infant. St. Louis, C.V. Mosby Co., 1973.

Table 13.2   Etiologic Classification of Neonatal Hyperbilirubinemia

INCREASED PRODUCTION	DECREASED CLEARANCE
Hemolytic diseases	Physiologic jaundice
Rh or ABO incompatibility	Hypothyroidism
Inherited red cell defects: sphero-	Crigler-Najjar syndrome
cytosis, enzyme deficiencies (G-6-	
PD, PK, etc.)	INHIBITION OF CONJUGATION
Hemoglobinopathies	
	Maternal serum and milk steroids
Prenatal infections	(pregnanediol)
Rubella, cytomegalic inclusion dis-	Novobiocin
ease (CID), hepatitis, herpes virus	Oxytocin, prostaglandin E_2 (?)
hominis (HVH), toxoplasmosis,	
syphilis or other bacterial diseases	DISPLACEMENT OF BILIRUBIN FROM ALBUMIN
Drugs	sulfonamides
Vitamin K analogues, naphthalene	salicylates
or aniline dyes	diazepam (sodium benzoate)
	procaine (PABA), bupivacaine (?)
Large hematomata (cephalohematoma)	

From Carapella, E., and Cosmi, E.V. (25).

not only because of rapidly increasing levels of bilirubinemia, but also because hemolysis may develop *in utero*. Therefore, the infant may be born with a marked degree of anemia accompanied by cardiac failure, edema and/or hydrops, and ET is indicated for the correction of both hyperbilirubinemia and anemia (75, 84, 118, 123). In the treatment of the latter, the aim is to provide red blood cells without increasing blood volume.

In recent years, routine Rh typing of all pregnant women, routine antibody surveillance, fetal red cell screening of Rh-negative mothers, and the administration of Rh immunoglobulin have significantly decreased the incidence of Rh isoimmunization, although prophylaxis is unlikely to eliminate sensitization. Amniocentesis, spectrophotometric and biochemical analysis of amniotic fluid, and proper timing of delivery have reduced the severity of Rh hemolytic disease.

Intrauterine intraperitoneal transfusion of fresh (<24 h) Group O, Rh-negative, packed cells, cross-matched against maternal serum, together with early delivery of the fetus, have been employed in an attempt to arrest the progress of hemolysis and lower the incidence of hydrops. Intraperitoneal transfusion of adult hemoglobin might be beneficial to the hypoxic fetus, as the decreased oxygen affinity of adult hemoglobin (due to increased 2,3-DPG) facilitates the release of oxygen to fetal tissues. However, it has become apparent that early management of the severely affected newborn with respiratory assistance, correction of acidosis, and immediate ET yields better overall results than intrauterine transfusion (30, 46, 68, 85).

Infants born after intrauterine transfusion are, in general, critically affected and have high cord blood levels of bilirubin (117), reflecting the severity of hemolysis and its effect on the liver. They deserve particular care, not only because of their prematurity and resultant cardiorespiratory distress, but because their anemia (usually proportional to the hyperbilirubinemia) is masked to a great degree by the intrauterine transfusion. In some infants, the cord blood hemoglobin value may be almost normal, with negative direct Coombs reaction and predominantly nonfetal red cells; nevertheless, most develop marked jaundice and require multiple ETs (78).

In hemolytic disease due to ABO incompatibility, neonatal jaundice (icterus precox) is the main problem; anemia is rarely severe enough to constitute a threat to survival. However, spherocytosis, reticulocytosis, homologous serum antibodies (by indirect antiglobulin tests), and decreased erythrocyte acetylcholinesterase activity may occur (62).

Among the *genetic diseases*, glucose-6-phosphate dehydrogenase (G-6-PD) and pyruvate kinase (PK) deficiencies are the most common enzymatic defects. Of the many types of G-6-PD deficiencies, which are all linked to the X-chromosome, but have different clinical implications, the "Mediterranean" and the "African" varieties are the most frequent. The "Mediterranean" gene is responsible for the massive hemolytic response to fava bean ingestion in afflicted persons (Favism). The possibility of G-6-PD deficiency contributing to severe hyperbilirubinemia and kernicterus is now recognized as a definite clinical entity, noted predominantly in male Caucasian infants (74, 86, 88, 108). In contrast to the jaundice caused by Rh or ABO blood group incompatibility, peak levels of bilirubin are found toward the end of the first week of life. Not all G-6-PD deficient newborns become icteric, although the incidence of low birthweight is high (88). However, hemolysis and hyperbilirubinemia are easily precipitated by various complicating factors such as infection or certain oxidant drugs and their metabolites (42, 88).

Hyperbilirubinemia may also be a complication of some autosomal recessive metabolic diseases such as alpha$_1$-antitrypsin deficiency, galactosemia, hereditary fructose intolerance, and tyrosinemia (111). However, because the excess bilirubin is of a direct-reacting type and effective methods of treatment are available, kernicterus is not of serious concern.

A number of *drugs and chemicals*, such as vitamin K analogues (16), naphthalene, and aniline dyes (29) have been implicated in the development of hyperbilirubinemia and hemolysis, but unequivocal relationships have seldom been substantiated. Prenatal and intrapartum *infections* may also cause bilirubin overload. Particularly in bacterial infections, the excess bilirubin may be indirect reacting initially, changing later to a direct-reacting type (101). In many instances, there is a fall in hemoglobin, signifying hemolysis (39).

Decreased Clearance

Dangerous levels of indirect bilirubin may be attained when hepatic clearance is insufficient as in the following conditions: reduced uptake by cytoplasmic proteins Y and Z in the liver (33, 66, 71); impaired conjugation, e.g., Crigler-Najjar syndrome due to a congenital deficit of glucuronyl transferase (6, 31); and decreased excretion (50) or increased reabsorption of bilirubin from the gastrointestinal tract (17, 96). This mechanism accounts for the so-called physiologic jaundice as well as the icterus associated with hypothyroidism.

Inhibition of Conjugation

Conjugation of bilirubin may be inhibited by breast feeding (7, 56) or the administration of certain drugs, e.g., novobiocin (55, 113). Neonatal jaundice linked to maternal milk has been reported by numerous investigators (7, 45, 49, 56). Gartner and Arias (49) have attributed this hyperbilirubinemia to the transmission in human milk of a thermo-stable factor, 3α, 20β-pregnanediol. The inhibitory activity, which is maximal after storage of milk at $+4°C$ for 96 hours and is destroyed by heating at $56°C$ for 15 minutes, is linked to increased lipolytic action with release of nonesterified fatty acids which compete with bilirubin for hepatic Z protein, thus reducing the conjugation substrate (45).

Administration of oxytocin and of prostaglandin E_2 to induce or accelerate labor was thought to cause an increased incidence of neonatal jaundice (10, 22, 42, 52). However, no relationship between these drugs and the development of hyperbilirubinemia could be established. Instead, the high postnatal serum bilirubin levels have been attributed to the artificial rupture of membranes rather than the direct effect of oxytocin, with resultant lack of the normal hormonal surge of spontaneous labor that stimulates hepatic enzyme induction and, hence, bilirubin metabolism (22, 28). Although, in these cases, clinical consequences have been minimal and ET never necessary (10, 42), the use of oxytocin or prostaglandins should be of concern when the fetus is otherwise at risk of hyperbilirubinemia.

Displacement from Binding Sites

Uncoupling of bilirubin from albumin has been found following the administration to the newborn of sulfonamides (107), salicylates (80), or diazepam (whose buffer, sodium benzoate, displaces bilirubin) (10, 42, 105). A case of neonatal "intoxication" requiring ET occurred after the intravenous injection of 120 mg of diazepam to the mother for treatment of severe preeclampsia (114). However, clinical doses of diazepam given to the mother are unlikely to interfere with fetal serum bilirubin-binding capacity, as sodium benzoate is readily metabolized and excreted in the urine (mostly as hippuric acid). A metabolite of procaine, para-aminobenzoic acid (which has been recovered from the fetal circulation) (115), also competes with bilirubin for albumin binding sites. Another local anesthetic, bupivacaine, which is characterized by a high degree of albumin binding, may reduce the available binding sites (67). However, the physicochemical properties of both agents prevent them from crossing the placenta to any appreciable degree.

Non-Bilirubin-Related Complications

Recently, ET has been proposed as treatment of a variety of unrelated neonatal problems.

Low–Birth–Weight Infants with Respiratory Distress Syndrome

The rationale for the use of ET as an adjunct to conventional therapeutic measures in the management of low-birth-weight infants, particularly those affected with respiratory distress syndrome (RDS) (35–37, 53), is based on the following factors: (1) Infants with severe RDS suffer from impaired tissue oxygenation, hypovolemia, reduced serum protein and plasma oncotic pressure, and decreased levels of plasminogen and of antithrombin III (3, 13, 19, 26, 70). (2) Neonatal blood possesses a higher affinity for oxygen because the oxygen-hemoglobin dissociation curve is shifted to the left (mainly as a result of failure to bind 2,3-DPG to the same degree as adult hemoglobin) (38). Oxygen-hemoglobin affinity is even greater in premature infants, especially in the presence of RDS, and the P_{50} (partial pressure of oxygen at which hemoglobin is 50% saturated) is lower than that of normal term infants. Thus, the less mature the newborn, the greater the shift to the left of the oxygen-hemoglobin dissociation curve and, consequently, the lower the average capillary and tissue oxygen tensions (37, 38, 53). Therefore, ET using fresh adult blood with its higher 2,3-DPG content, i.e., decreased affinity of hemoglobin for oxygen, will improve the release of oxygen to the tissues at an equivalent or even higher Po_2 despite the decreased blood oxygen saturation. ET will also reduce ventilation/perfusion ratio disturbances by supplying plasma constituents, e.g., serum protein, as well as by removing toxic substances, e.g., vasoactive agents such as vasopressin and prostaglandin $F_{2\alpha}$ which are known to produce pulmonary hypoperfusion (37, 53). Another beneficial effect of ET in these infants is the correction of coagulation abnormalities as reflected by a prolongation of the partial thromboplastin time (35). The survival rate of infants with severe RDS has been significantly increased when ET was employed in addition to conventional therapy (36, 37, 53).

Neonatal Septicemia

In the therapy of neonatal septicemia, ET has been recommended to re-move bacteria or bacterial toxins, to enhance humoral and cellular defense mechanisms, and to replace the infant's blood, which has a high oxygen affinity, with adult blood, which has a lower oxygen affinity, thus produc-ing better oxygen delivery to the tissues (98, 125).

Intoxication with Local Anesthetics

ET was used successfully in newborn infants who had been poisoned by a local anesthetic agent injected accidentally into the fetal scalp during at-tempted caudal block of the mother during labor (110).

Neonatal Myasthenia

Recently, ET has been employed for the treatment of neonatal myasthenia, particularly when complicated by hyperbilirubinemia due to ABO incom-patibility (44). Neonatal myasthenia occurs during the first 24 to 48 hours of life in about 10% of infants born to mothers with myasthenia gravis.

Laboratory Determinations

In documented or suspected jaundice, routine tests such as ABO-Rh type, direct Coombs, hemoglobin concentration, reticulocyte and nucleated red cell levels, and serum bilirubin levels should be undertaken at birth, pref-erably in the blood obtained from the umbilical cord.

At birth, the normal cord hemoglobin level is approximately 16–18 g/dl and the normal hematocrit value is about 60%. During the first few hours of life, hemoglobin concentration may change rapidly (75); capillary or venous samples taken postnatally have higher values than cord blood be-cause of a shift of fluid out of the vascular compartment (84). Thus, cord hemoglobin concentration is the only reliable index of the severity of hemolytic disease at birth. Increases in reticulocytes (>15%) and nu-cleated red cell levels are indicative of the intensity of the bone marrow's compensatory response to hemolytic anemia.

Various laboratory methods have been developed to characterize the type of hyperbilirubinemia, to assess the risk of kernicterus, and to serve as a guide to rational management (ET, phototherapy, enzyme induction) (see Fig. 13.1). The Sephadex G-25 gel filtration test for determination of free bilirubin (60, 61, 63, 87, 106, 127) is based on the ability of the heavier, bound fraction of bilirubin to pass through the column more

TIME   FROM   BIRTH (hours)

Bilirubin mg/100ml	< 24	24 - 48	49 - 72	> 72
< 5				
5 - 9	PHOTOTHERAPY			
10 - 14	EXCHANGE TRANSFUSION	PHOTOTHERAPY		
15 - 19	EXCHANGE TRANSFUSION		PHOTOTHERAPY	
≥ 20	EXCHANGE TRANSFUSION			

Fig. 13.1   Guidelines for the management of hyperbilirubinemia during the first few days of life, with consideration of the age of the infant and the level of serum bilirubin. [Modified from Brown, A.K. (18).]

quickly so that the free portion is left in the Sephadex. This provides a quantitative assessment of the reserve bilirubin capacity, i.e., the amount of increase in unconjugated bilirubin that a given infant can tolerate prior to complete saturation of albumin-binding sites. Although the method presents certain limitations, such as insensitivity to low concentrations of free bilirubin, it appears to be a useful tool. A more simple and rapid microfluorometric method utilizing a fluorescent dye and Sephadex G-200 also has been developed for quantitation of albumin-bilirubin binding capacity (65).

A recently developed enzymatic method for measurements of low concentrations of unbound bilirubin is based on the observation that unbound bilirubin is oxidized to colorless compounds by hydrogen peroxide in the presence of horseradish peroxidase, whereas albumin-bound bilirubin is protected from oxidation. Therefore, both binding affinity and binding capacity can be determined (59). A spectropolarimetric method for quantitation of unbound bilirubin using circular dichroism and optical rotatory dispersion has been reported (54). Finally, a technique has been described which determines the reserve albumin-binding capacity of serum by measuring the amount of phenolsulfonphthalein (PSP) taken up by the albumin (97, 120); a more rapid micromethod utilizes the dye 2-(4-hydroxybezeneazo)benzoic acid (HBABA). The presence of a reserve binding capacity of more than 50 μg PSP/ml serum (HBABA binding 20 to 25%) indicates that nearly all the serum bilirubin is safely bound to albumin although serum bilirubin concentration may exceed 20 mg/dl.

Table 13.3 Criteria for Exchange Transfusion (E.T.) of the Newborn

	IMMEDIATE E.T.	EARLY E.T.
Cord Hemoglobin	<8 gm/100 ml	Cord Hemoglobin <13 gm/100 ml
	>8 gm/100 ml complicated by severe edema and/or hydrops	Cord bilirubin >4 mg/100 ml
		Bilirubin increment >0.5 mg/h on the first day

From Carapella, E., and Cosmi, E.V. (25).

Criteria for ET and Basic Management

The major concern in the newborn with positive direct Coombs test is whether to perform an immediate or early ET; this decision should be based on cord blood hemoglobin and indirect bilirubin levels (118, 123) (Table 13.3). In most instances, amniotic fluid findings will suggest the severity of the disease to be anticipated at birth (47). Infants requiring immediate ET, i.e., within the first few hours, often present a number of disturbances demanding special treatment such as removal of ascitic fluid, correction of acidosis, therapy of respiratory distress syndrome, and maintenance of body temperature (18). The guidelines for immediate ET are listed in Table 13.4.

Some of these infants may have an elevated central venous pressure secondary to peripheral (and pulmonary?) vasoconstriction in the face of normal blood volume (89, 90). The exchange should then be performed with deficit, i.e., each time a volume of blood approximately double that infused should be taken out until venous pressure approaches normal values. A deficit of 40 to 80 ml may be indicated (84). The total volume of this first critical exchange varies according to the condition of the newborn. If im-

Table 13.4 Guidelines for Immediate Exchange Transfusion of the Newborn with Severe Anemia and Cardiac Failure

Packed cells—Group O, Rh negative—Fresh (<24 hours)	
1. Anticoagulated	CPD or ACD
2. Prewarmed for 1–2 hours	Water bath (37°C)
3. Thermally regulated during ET	—
4. Exchanged with deficit (until venous pressure is normal)	Infuse 5–10 ml, remove 10–20 ml (up to a deficit of 40–80 ml)
5. Volume exchange	≈90 ml/kg

provement occurs during the initial stages of the transfusion, an exchange of 90 ml/kg is completed (84, 118).

When immediate ET is not deemed necessary, serum bilirubin concentration and bilirubin-binding capacity must be determined at regular intervals to follow the rate of change. In general, ET should be initiated earlier in preterm newborns, as compared with full-term infants, because of their lower bilirubin-binding capacity and impaired clearance capacity.

Phototherapy is an adjunct to treatment used to reduce the need for repeat ET or to avoid the necessity for ET when hemolysis is mild (69, 126). However, the question of whether light-induced reduction in serum bilirubin decreases the risk of later neurologic and psychologic defects has not been answered as yet. Therefore, phototherapy should never be used as a substitute for ET.

The guidelines for the management of hyperbilirubinemia in hemolytic disease *not* complicated by severe anemia or cardiac failure are presented in Fig. 13.1 and Table 13.5.

Whole blood is preferred to provide plasma containing an ample supply of bilirubin-free albumin. Thus, as the exchange proceeds, bilirubin from the extravascular space is drawn into the plasma; at the same time, antibody-coated red cells are removed (71, 75). The volume of exchange should be approximately twice the infant's anticipated blood volume (per kg body weight) (94).

Salt-poor albumin is useful in selected cases to increase the amount of bilirubin removed by ET (83, 121). In hydropic infants, who frequently

Table 13.5 Guidelines for the Management of Hyperbilirubinemia by Exchange Transfusion

1. Whole blood anticoagulated with CPD (or ACD under 3–4 days)	Anti-Rh(D)hemolytic disease: same ABO group or group O, Rh negative ABO hemolytic disease: group O (no hemolysin), same Rh type Other types of H.D. (anti-c, E, K, etc.): selected by cross-matching Jaundice from other causes: same ABO-Rh type
2. Cross-matched against maternal serum (indirect Coombs test)	Advisable Mandatory in presence of alloantibodies (c, E, K, etc.)
3. Correction of acidosis	Seldom necessary
4. Warmed (left at room temperature for 3–4 hrs)	
5. Volume exchange	170–200 ml/kg b.w. in term newborns
6. Salt-poor albumin	1 g/kg b.w. (not mandatory)
7. Calcium gluconate (?)	

Table 13.6   Basic Requirements for Exchange Transfusion

1. Aspiration of gastric contents	6. Careful umbilical vein catheterization
2. Suction and resuscitation apparatus	7. Proper localization of catheter by x-ray
3. Prevention of hypothermia	8. Volume exchange: 10–20 ml
4. Evaluation of cardiopulmonary function	9. Rate of infusion: 400 ml/hr in term infants; 100–120 ml/kg/hr in preterm and very sick babies
5. Asepis	

have hypoalbuminemia but are not hypervolemic (89, 91), the addition of albumin to donor blood aids in the removal of edema fluid. However, salt-poor albumin is contraindicated in severely anemic newborns because of the risk of increasing plasma volume and, thus, precipitating or aggravating congestive heart failure (83, 121).

Conduct of ET

ET should be performed with the infant placed under an open source of radiant heat for maintenance of a neutral thermal environment (i.e., temperature at which oxygen consumption is minimal but sufficient to keep body temperature normal) and under a blue fluorescent light for phototherapy. Plastic disposable ET kits have simplified the procedure greatly (2, 25, 65, 75, 82, 92, 94). The umbilical vein, identified as the largest of three vessels in the cord, is the usual site of catheterization; should this prove impossible, catheterization of the great saphenous vein in the groin may be considered. A detailed description of the procedure is beyond the scope of this book, but a variety of publications is recommended for the interested reader (5, 8, 24, 25, 43, 58, 64, 92, 93, 122, 123).

Stomach contents should be removed by suction prior to ET to prevent inhalation during the procedure. Resuscitation equipment and means for recording ECG and blood pressure and for measurements of hematocrit, blood gas tensions, and acid-base status must be available. The basic requirements for ET are listed in Table 13.6.

Careful monitoring of color, respiratory and circulatory parameters, and core temperature must be carried out all through the procedure. Biochemical determinations should be repeated at frequent intervals depending on the infant's condition and the number of therapeutic measures.

The time required for an ET is controversial. Too rapid and too slow exchanges are equally undesirable since the infant needs time to adjust to the changing volume and to metabolize the citrate of donor blood. An uncomplicated ET takes approximately one hour. Restlessness is usually a warning sign that the exchange proceeds too rapidly. The last sample of blood should be used for determinations of serum bilirubin and hemoglobin levels as well as for blood culture.

Selection of Donor Blood

Newborns with anti-Rh hemolytic disease must be exchanged with ABO-specific, Rh-negative blood compatible with the mother's serum as determined by the Coombs cross-match method. As the infant does not actively produce blood group antibodies at birth, antibodies, if present, reach higher concentrations in maternal than in neonatal serum (Table 13.5). Furthermore, neonatal red cells which are coated with Rh antibodies will often appear to be Rh-negative. Therefore, a direct Coombs test will identify the Rh-positive infant.

In ABO-incompatibility, the mother's blood is O but the infant's is either group A or group B. The donor's blood should be group O with low anti-A and anti-B antibody titers, but the Rh type should be the same as that of the infant (Table 13.5). For the management of hyperbilirubinemia from other causes and the treatment of neonates with severe RDS, the donor blood should be of the same ABO-Rh type as the newborn's.

Blood anticoagulated with citrate-phosphate-dextrose (CPD) has the advantage of preserving pH and 2,3-DPG better than acid-citrate-dextrose (ACD) blood (20, 34). Acidosis consequent to the use of ACD blood seldom requires correction, since citrate administered as citric acid or as sodium citrate is metabolized, mole for mole, to bicarbonate. This may, in fact, produce a state of alkalosis (23, 58, 124) which may be marked for a few hours post-exchange (93) and may persist for 1 to 2 days (23). A recent study revealed no change in acid-base status due to ET with unbuffered ACD blood in newborns who were mature and whose exchange was undertaken more than 24 hours after birth (58). In contrast, preterm or asphyxiated infants developed acidosis, especially when ET was performed within the first 24 hours. Therefore, buffering each unit of ACD blood with 10 mM of 1.2M THAM or of 0.9 M sodium bicarbonate (1.8 mEq/dl) has been advocated for ET in preterm and/or acidotic neonates (9, 14, 15, 77, 93). The advantages of THAM over bicarbonate are discussed in Chapter 11.

Heparinized blood presents two disadvantages: (1) its storage time is short and (2) protamine sulfate may be required post-exchange to counteract the anticoagulant effect of heparin (93) as well as to reduce the stimulation of plasma FFA (free fatty acids) release by heparin (secondary to activation of lipoprotein lipase) (32). It should also be recalled that FFA can displace bilirubin from albumin (95, 103).

Following ET the infant should be maintained on an infusion of 10% glucose in water (65 ml/kg/day) to reduce the risk of hypoglycemia, a complication seen particularly in infants transfused with ACD blood (104). When heparinized blood is employed, glucose will aid in diminishing FFA levels.

Potential Hazards of ET

ET presents potential hazards. Some of these have been described in detail (82) and are presented in Table 13.7.

Catheterization of the umbilical vein is relatively simple. Nevertheless, trauma and malposition with subsequent visceral perforation have been reported (109, 122). In addition, the catheter may coil or be misdirected into the left portal vein, especially when the umbilical vein outlet and the ductus venosus inlet are not perfectly aligned on opposite sides of the left portal vein.

Spontaneous perforation of the intestine, most frequently the colon, is thought to be due to cannulation of the portal vein, causing venous thrombosis and transient hypertension with consequent hemorrhagic infarction of the bowel (27).

Air embolism may develop during central venous pressure measurements, particularly when the infant coughs, thereby producing a negative intra-abdominal pressure.

The most common side-effects involve the circulatory system. The incidence of anemia can be reduced by allowing the donor blood to settle before transfusion. However, anemia may also result from "undershooting" the volume of transfused blood. Conversely, "overshooting" may induce car-

Table 13.7   Potential Hazards of Exchange Transfusion

Vascular	Air and clot embolism Thrombosis Hemorrhagic infarction of colon Anemia	Clotting	Thrombocytopenia Overheparinization
		Infections	Bacteremia Serum hepatitis
Cardiac	Arrhythmias Arrest Volume overload	Miscellaneous	Perforation of vessels Hypothermia Mechanical injury to donor cells
Metabolic	Hypernatremia Hyperkalemia Hypocalcemia Hypomagnesemia Acidosis Hypoglycemia		Retrolental fibroplasia

Modified from Odell, G.B., et al. (82).

diac failure. In order to avoid overloading, therapy should be guided by frequent measurements of its effect on aortic and central venous pressures. Cardiac arrhythmias and even arrest may ensue from advancing the catheter into the right atrium, especially if the blood is cold, or from hyperkalemia, if the blood is old. Hypernatremia and hypocalcemia may develop secondary to the use of ACD blood. Hypernatremia may be responsible for subependidymal and intraventricular hemorrhages, primarily in low-birth-weight infants (41), while hypocalcemia may lead to tetany. It has been recommended to slowly inject calcium gluconate (0.5 to 1.0 ml of a 10% solution) after each 100 ml of blood exchanged to prevent hypocalcemia (94). However, the value of this is doubtful, since calcium gluconate elevates the level of total calcium, not that of ionized calcium (72).

Other hazards include post-exchange bleeding at the umbilical stump, elevated venous pressure, transient reactions from minor blood incompatibilities and retrolental fibroplasia (4, 21, 53). Finally, it should be stressed that erythropoiesis is markedly depressed following ET, probably as a result of abnormally high hemoglobin A concentrations (48).

Conclusion

ET is a well-established procedure for the treatment of severe anemia and of hyperbilirubinemia from any cause. It has significantly reduced the morbidity and mortality of hemolytic disease of the newborn. It is additionally a valuable modality for the removal of toxic substances from the infant's circulation. Finally, ET can be of benefit to newborns with severe respiratory distress syndrome in whom oxygen delivery is impaired by hypoxia, anemia, and alterations in blood flow.

Acknowledgment

This work was supported in part by Consiglio Nazionale delle Ricerche, Rome, Italy, Grant Nos. 78.00578.83, 78.01853.65.

References

1. Ackerman, B.D., Dyer, G.Y., Leydrof, M.M.: Hyperbilirubinemia and kernicterus in small premature infants. Pediatrics 45:918, 1970.
2. Agostino, R., Nodari, S.: Unpublished data.
3. Ambrus, C.M., Weintraub, D.H., Ambrus, J.L.: Studies on hyaline membrane disease. III. Therapeutic trial of urokinase-activated human plasmin. Pediatrics 38:231, 1966.

4. Aranda, J.V., Clark, T.E., Maniello, R., Outerbridge, E.W.: Blood transfusion: Possible potentiating risk factor in retrolental fibroplasia. Pediatr. Res. (Abstract) 9:633, 1975.

5. Aranda, J.V., Sweet, A.Y.: Hemodynamic alterations during slow and fast exchange transfusion. Pediatr. Res. 7:399, 1973.

6. Arias, I.M., Gartner, L.M., Cohen, M., Ben Ezzer, J., Levi, A.J.: Chronic non-hemolytic unconjugated hyperbilirubinemia with glucuronyl transferase deficiency. Clinical, biochemical, pharmacologic and genetic evidence for heterogeneity. Am. J. Med. 47:395, 1969.

7. Arias, I.M., Gartner, L.M., Seifter, S., Furman, M.: Prolonged neonatal unconjugated hyperbilirubinemia associated with breast feeding and a steroid, pregnane, -3(alpha), 20(beta)-diol, in maternal milk that inhibits glucuronide formation in vitro. J. Clin. Invest. 43:2037, 1964.

8. Ata, M., Holman, C.A.: Simultaneous umbilical arteriovenous exchange transfusion. Br. Med. J. 2:743, 1966.

9. Barrie, H.: Acid-base control during exchange transfusion. Lancet 2:712, 1965.

10. Beazley, J.M., Alderman, B.: Neonatal hyperbilirubinaemia following the use of oxytocin in labour. Br. J. Obstet. Gynaecol. 82:265, 1975.

11. Berk, P.D., Howe, R.B., Bloomer, J.R., Berlin, N.I.: Studies of bilirubin kinetics in normal adults. J. Clin. Invest. 48:2176, 1969.

12. Bessis, M.: Use of replacement transfusion in diseases other than hemolytic disease of newborn. Blood 4:324, 1949.

13. Bland, R.D.: Cord total protein level as a screening aid for the idiopathic respiratory distress syndrome. N. Engl. J. Med. 287:9, 1972.

14. Bleich, H.L., Schwartz, W.B.: Tris buffer (THAM). An appraisal of its physiologic effects and clinical usefulness. N. Engl. J. Med. 274:782, 1966.

15. Boda, D., Muranji, L., Toth, G., Eck, E.: Acid-base and electrolyte changes during exchange transfusions. Acta Paediatr. Scand. 56:217, 1966.

16. Bound, J.P., Talfer, T.P.: Effect of vitamine K dosage on plasma-bilirubin levels in premature infants. Lancet 1:720, 1956.

17. Brodersen, R., Hermann, L.S.: Intestinal re-absorption of unconjugated bilirubin. A possible contributing factor in neonatal jaundice. Lancet 1: 1242, 1963.

18. Brown, A.K.: Neonatal hyperbilirubinemia, in Behrman, R.E. (ed.): Neonatology Diseases of the Fetus and Infant. St. Louis, C. V. Mosby Co., 1973, p. 218.

19. Brown, E.G., Krouskop, R.W., McDonnell, F.E., Sweet, A.Y.: Blood volume and blood pressure in infants with respiratory distress. J. Pediatr. 87:1133, 1975.

20. Bursaux, E., Freminet, A., Brossard, Y., Poyart, C.F.: Exchange transfusion in the neonate with ACD or CPD stored blood. Biol. Neonate 23: 123, 1973.

21. Bustamente, S.A., Scott, K.E.: Failure of exchange transfusion to alter course or outcome of RDS and very low birth weight infants. Pediatr. Res. 9:639, 1975 (abstract).

22. Calder, A.A., Ounsted, M. K., Moar, V.A., Turnbull, A.C.: Increased bilirubin levels in neonates after induction of labour by intravenous prostaglandin E_2 or oxytocin. Lancet 2:1339, 1974.
23. Calladine, M., Gairdner, D., Naidoo, B.T., Orrell, D.H.: Acid-base changes following exchange transfusion with citrated blood. Arch. Dis. Child. 40:626, 1965.
24. Carapella, E.: La terapia trasfusionale del neonato. Prospect. Pediatr. (Italian) 14:149, 1974.
25. Carapella, E., Cosmi, E.V.: Exchange transfusion, in Conseiller, C. et al. (eds.): Le Sang en Anésthesie et en Réanimation. Paris, Librairie Arnette, 1976, p. 261.
26. Cassady, G.: Plasma volume studies in low birth weight infants. Pediatrics 38:1020, 1966.
27. Castor, W.R.: Spontaneous perforation of the bowel in the newborn following exchange transfusion. Can. Med. Assoc. J. 99:934, 1968.
28. Chew, W.C., Swann, I.L.: Influence of simultaneous low amniotomy and oxytocin infusion and other maternal factors on neonatal jaundice: a prospective study. Br. Med. J. 1:72, 1977.
29. Cock, T.C.: Acute hemolytic anemia in the neonatal period. Am. J. Dis. Child. 94:77, 1957.
30. Cosmi, E.V., Freda, V.J.: Trasfusioni fetali nelle gravidanze con isoimmunizzazione al fattore Rh-Nota I: Trasfusione col metodo percutaneo intraperitoneale. Riv. Ostet. Ginec. (Italian) 21:538, 1966.
31. Crigler, J.F., Jr., Najjar, V.A.: Congenital familial nonhemolytic jaundice with kernicterns. Pediatrics 10:169, 1952.
32. Cser, A., Milner, R.D.G.: Metabolic and hormonal changes during and after exchange transfusion with heparinized or ACD blood. Arch. Dis. Child. 49:940, 1974.
33. Davis, D.R., Yeary, R.A.: Bilirubin binding to hepatic Y and Z protein (LIGANDIN): Tissue bilirubin concentrations in phenobarbital treated gunn rats (38466). Proc. Soc. Exp. Biol. Med. 148:9, 1975.
34. Dawson, R.B., Jr., Kocholaty, W.F., Gray, J.L.: Hemoglobin function and 2,3-DPG levels of blood stored at 4°C in ACD and CPD. pH effect. Transfusion 10:299, 1970.
35. De Lemos, R.A., McLaughlin, G.W., Koch, H.F., Diserens, H.W.: Abnormal partial thromboplastin time and survival in RDS: Effect of exchange transfusion. Pediatr. Res. 7:168, 1973.
36. Delivoria-Papadopoulos, M., Miller, R.D., Branca, P.A., Foster, R.E., Oski, F.A.: Effect of exchange transfusion on altering mortality in: 1) infants weighing less than 1,250 grams at birth and 2) infants with severe respiratory distress (RDS). Pediatr. Res. 7:291, 1973.
37. Delivoria-Papadopoulos, M., Miller, L.D., Forster, R.E., Oski, F.A.: The role of exchange transfusion in the management of low-birth-weight infants with and without severe respiratory distress syndrome. I. Initial observations. J. Pediatr. 89: 273, 1976.
38. Delivoria-Papadopoulos, M., Roncevic, N.P., Oski, F.A.: Postnatal changes in oxygen transport of term, premature, and sick infants: The

role of red cell 2,3-diphosphoglycerate and adult hemoglobin. Pediatr. Res. **5**:235, 1971.

39. Dent, P.B., Finkel, A.: Intrauterine infection and cord immunoglobulin M: III. Serological analysis of infants with elevated cord serum immunoglobulin M. Can. Med. Assoc. J. **110**:1354, 1974.

40. Diamond, L.K.: Erythroblastosis fetalis or hemolytic disease of the newborn. Proc. R. Soc. Med. **40**:546, 1947.

41. Doyle, P.E., Lee, K., Gartner, L.M.: Hypernatremia and exchange transfusion associated with intracranial hemorrhage in very-low-birth-weight (VLBW) infants. (Abstract). 2nd Annual Scientific Symposium. New York Metropolitan Perinatal Society, 1977, p. 7.

42. Drew, J.H., Kitchen, W.H.: The effect of maternally administered drugs on bilirubin concentrations in the newborn infant. J. Pediatr. **89**:657, 1976.

43. Dunn, P.M.: Localization of the umbilical catheter by post-mortem measurements. Arch. Dis. Child. **41**:69, 1966.

44. Dunn, J.M.: Neonatal myasthenia. Am. J. Obstet. Gynecol. **125**:265, 1976.

45. Foliot, A., Ploussard, J.P., Housset, E., Christoforov, B.: Breast milk jaundice: In vitro inhibition of rat liver bilirubin-uridine diphosphate glucuronyltransferase activity and Z protein-bromosulfophthalein binding by human breast milk. Pediatr. Res. **10**:594, 1976.

46. Fong, S.W., Margolis, A.J., Westberg, J.A., Johnson, P.: Intrauterine transfusion: fetal outcome and complications. Pediatrics **45**:576, 1970.

47. Freda, V.J., Cosmi, E.V.: Alcuni recenti sviluppi nel trattamento del problema Rh in ostetricia e il particolare valore dell'analisi spettrofotometrica del liquido amniotico. Riv. Ostet. Ginec. (Italian) **21**:513, 1966.

48. Gahr, M., Jentsch, E., Schröter, W.: Imbalance of globin chain synthesis in newborn infants with hemolytic disease after exchange transfusion. Pediatr. Res. **11**:9, 1977.

49. Gartner, L.M., Arias, I.M.: Studies of prolonged neonatal jaundice in the breast-fed infant. J. Pediatr. **68**:54, 1966.

50. Gartner, L.M., Lane, D.: Hepatic metabolism and transport of bilirubin during physiologic jaundice in the newborn Rhesus monkey. Pediatr. Res. **5**:413, 1971.

51. Gartner, L.M., Snyder, R.N., Chabon, R.S., Bernstein, J.: Kernicterus: high incidence in premature infants with low serum bilirubin concentrations. Pediatrics **45**:906, 1970.

52. Ghosh, A., Hudson, F.P.: Oxytocic agents and neonatal hyperbilirubinemia. Lancet **2**:823, 1972

53. Gottuso, M.A., Williams, M.L., Oski, F.A.: The role of exchange transfusions in the management of low-birth-weight infants with and without severe respiratory distress syndrome. II. Further observations and studies of mechanisms of action. J. Pediatr. **89**:279, 1976.

54. Grahnén, A., Sjöholm, I., Michaëlsson, M.: A new method for the determination of unconjugated bilirubin in human serum by spectropolarimetry. Clin. Chim. Acta **52**:187, 1974.

55. Hargreaves, T., Holton, J.B.: Jaundice of the newborn due to novobiocin. Lancet 1:839, 1972.
56. Hargreaves, T., Piper, R.F.: Breast milk jaundice. Effect of inhibitory breast milk and 3α,20β-pregnanediol on glucuronyl transferase. Arch. Dis. Child. 46:195, 1971.
57. Hart, A.P.: Familial icterus gravis of the newborn and its treatment. Can. Med. Assoc. J. 15:1008, 1925.
58. Hervei, S., Malik, T., Rötfalusy, M.: Acid-base changes of mature and premature neonates following exchange transfusion. Biol. Neonate 29: 323, 1976.
59. Jacobsen, J., Wennberg, R.P.: Determination of unbound bilirubin in the serum of newborns. Clin. Chem. 20:783, 1974.
60. Jirsová, V., Jirsa, M., Heringová, A., Koldovsky, O., Weirichová, J.: The use and possible diagnostic significance of Sephadex gel filtration of serum from icteric newborn. Biol. Neonate 11:204, 1967.
61. Kapitulnik, J., Valaes, T., Kaufmann, N.A., Blondheim, S.H.: Clinical evaluation of Sephadex gel filtration in estimation of bilirubin binding in serum in neonatal jaundice. Arch. Dis. Child. 49:886, 1974.
62. Kaplan, E., Herz, F., Scheye, E.: ABO hemolytic disease of the newborn, without hyperbilirubinemia. Am. J. Hematol. 1:279, 1976.
63. Kaufmann, N.A., Kapitulnick, M.S., Blondheim, S.H.: The adsorption of bilirubin by Sephadex and its relationship to the criteria for exchange transfusion. Pediatrics 44:543, 1969.
64. Kitterman, J.A., Phibbs, R.H., Tooley, W.H.: Catheterization of umbilical vessels in newborn infants. Pediatr. Clin. N. Am. 17:895, 1970.
65. Lee, K., Gartner, L.M., Zarafu, I.: Fluorescent dye method for determination of the bilirubin-binding capacity of serum albumin. J. Pediatr. 86: 200, 1975.
66. Levi, A.J., Gatmaitan, Z., Arias, I.M.: Two hepatic cytoplasmic protein fractions, Y and Z, and their possible role in the hepatic uptake of bilirubin, sulfobromophthalein and other anions. J. Clin. Invest. 48:2156, 1969.
67. Levinson, G., Shnider, S.M.: Placental transfer of local anesthetics: clinical implications, in Clinical Anesthesia Series: G.F. Marx (ed.): "Parturition and Perinatology. Philadelphia, F.A. Davis Co., 1973, p. 175.
68. Lucey, J.F.: Intrauterine transfusion and erythroblastosis fetalis. Report of the 53rd Ross Conference on Pediatric Research. Columbus, Ross Laboratories, 1966.
69. Lucey, J.F.: Neonatal jaundice and phototherapy. Pediatr. Clin. N. Am. 19:827, 1972.
70. Mahasandana, C., Hathaway, W.E.: Circulating anticoagulants in the newborn: Relation to hypercoagulability and the idiopathic respiratory distress syndrome. Pediatr. Res. 7:670, 1973.
71. Maisels, M.J.: Bilirubin. On understanding and influencing its metabolism in the newborn infant. Pediatr. Clin. N. Amer. 19:447, 1972.
72. Maisels, M.J., Li, T.K., Piechocki, J.T., Werthman, M.V.: Effect of exchange transfusion on serum ionized calcium. Pediatr. Res. 5:412, 1971.
73. Maisels, M.J., Pathak, A., Nelson, N.M., Natham, D.G., Smith, C.A.:

Endogenous production of carbon monoxide in normal and erythroblastotic newborn infants. J. Clin. Invest. **50**:1, 1971.

74. Milbauer, B., Peled, N., Svirsky, S.: Neonatal hyperbilirubinemia and glucose-6-phosphate dehydrogenase deficiency. Isr. J. Med. Sci. **9**:1547, 1973.

75. Mollison, P.L.: Blood Transfusion in Clinical Medicine, Oxford, 5th Ed., Blackwell Scientific Publishers, 1972, p. 615.

76. Mollison, P.L., Veall, N., Cutbursh, M.: Red cell and plasma volume in newborn infants. Arch. Dis. Child. **25**:242, 1950.

77. Nahas, G.G., Manger, W.M., Ultmann, J.E.: Transfusion acidosis. Proc. 9th Con. Int. Soc. Blood Trans., Mexico 1962, p. 610, 1964.

78. Naiman, J.L.: Current management of hemolytic disease of the newborn infant. J. Pediatr. **80**:1049, 1972.

79. Nakamura, H., Lardinois, R.: Unbound bilirubin in icteric newborns. Biol. Neonate **21**:400, 1972

80. Odell, G.B.: Studies in kernicterus. I. The protein binding of bilirubin. J. Clin. Invest. **38**:823, 1959.

81. Odell, G.B.: Influence of pH on the distribution of bilirubin between albumin and mitochondria. Proc. Soc. Exp. Biol. Med. **120**:352, 1965.

82. Odell, G.B., Bryan, W.B., Richmond, M.D.: Exchange transfusion. Pediatr. Clin. N. Am. **9**:605, 1962.

83. Odell, G.B., Cohen, S.N., Gordes, E.H.: Administration of albumin in the management of hyperbilirubinemia by exchange transfusion. Pediatrics **30**:613, 1962.

84. Oski, F.A., Naiman, J.L.: Hematologic Problems in the Newborn, 2nd Ed. Philadelphia, W.B. Saunders Co., 1972.

85. Palmer, A., Gordon, R.R.: A critical review of intrauterine fetal transfusion. Br. J. Obstet. Gynaecol. **83**:688, 1976.

86. Panizon, F.: Erythrocyte enzyme deficiency in unexplained kernicterus. Lancet **2**:1093, 1960.

87. Pearlman, F.C., Lee, R.T.Y.: Detection and measurement of total bilirubin in serum, with use of surfactants as solubilizing agents. Clin. Chem. **20**:447, 1974.

88. Perkins, R.P.: The significance of glucose-7-phosphate dehydrogenase deficiency in pregnancy. Am. J. Obstet. Gynecol. **125**:215, 1976.

89. Phibbs, R.H., Johnson, P., Kitterman, J.A., Gregory, G.A., Tooley, W.H., Schlueter, M.: Cardiorespiratory status of erythroblastotic newborn infants. III. Intravascular pressures during the first hours of life. Pediatrics **48**:484, 1976.

90. Phibbs, R., Johnson, P., Tooley, W.H.: Circulatory changes in newborn with erythroblastosis fetalis. Pediatr. Res. **1**:321, 1967.

91. Phibbs, R.H., Johnson, P., Tooley, W.H.: Cardiorespiratory status of erythroblastotic newborn infants: II. Blood volume, hematocrit, and serum albumin concentration in relation to hydrops fetalis. Pediatrics **53**:13, 1974.

92. Philpott, M.G., Banerjee, A.: Automated method for exchange transfusion. Arch. Dis. Child. **47**:815, 1972.

93. Pierson, W.E., Barrett, C.T., Oliver, T.K., Jr.: The effect of buffered and

non-buffered ACD blood on electrolyte and acid-base homeostasis during exchange transfusion. Pediatrics 41:802, 1968.

94. Pochedly, C.: The exchange transfusion. Newer concepts and advances in technic. Clin. Pediatr. (Phila.) 7:383, 1968.

95. Polacek, K., Novak, M., Melichar, V.: Influence of free fatty acids on the distribution of bilirubin and its clinical significance in the newborn. Rev. Czech. Med. 11:161, 1965.

96. Poland, R.D., Odell, G.B.: Physiologic jaundice: The enterohepatic circulation of bilirubin. N. Engl. J. Med. 284:1, 1971.

97. Porter, E.G., Waters, W.J.: A rapid micromethod for measuring the reserve albumin binding capacity in serum from newborn infants with hyperbilirubinemia. J. Lab. Clin. Med. 67:660, 1966.

98. Prod'hom, L.S., Choffat, J.M., Frenck, N., Mazoumi, M., Relier, J.P.: Care of the seriously ill neonate with hyaline membrane disease and with sepsis (sclerema neonatorum). Pediatrics 53:170, 1974.

99. Robertson, L.B.: Blood transfusion in severe burns in infants and young children: preliminary report of treatment of toxic shock by blood transfusion with or without preceding exsanguination. Can. Med. Assoc. J. 11:744, 1921.

100. Robertson, L.B.: Exsanguination-transfusion: new therapeutic measurement treatment of severe toxemias. Arch. Surg. 9:1, 1924.

101. Sass-Kortsak, A.: Management of young infants presenting with direct-reacting hyperbilirubinemia. Pediatr. Clin. N. Am. 21:777, 1974.

102. Sawitsky, A., Cheung, W.H., Seifter, E.: The effect of pH on the distribution of bilirubin in peripheral blood, cerebrospinal fluid, and fat tissues. Pediatr. Pharmacol. Ther. 72:700, 1968.

103. Schiff, D., Aranda, J.V., Chan, G., Colle, E., Stern, L.: Metabolic effects of exchange transfusion. I. Effect of citrated and of heparinized blood on glucose, non-esterified fatty acids, 2-(4 hydroxy-benzeneazo) benzoic acid binding and insulin. J. Pediatr. 78:603, 1971.

104. Schiff, D., Aranda, J.V., Colle, E., Stern, L.: Metabolic effects of exchange transfusion. II. Delayed hypoglycemia following exchange transfusion with citrated blood. J. Pediatr. 79:589, 1971.

105. Schiff, D., Chan, G., Stern, L.: Fixed drug combinations and the displacement of bilirubin from albumin. Pediatrics 48:139, 1971.

106. Schiff, D., Chan, G., Stern, L.: Sephadex G-25 quantitative estimation of free bilirubin potential in jaundiced newborn infants' sera: A guide to the prevention of kernicterus. J. Lab. Clin. Med. 80:455, 1972.

107. Silverman, W.A., Andersen, D.H., Blanc, W.A., Crozier, D.N.: A difference in mortality rate and incidence of kernicterus among premature infants allotted to two prophylactic antibacterial regiments. Pediatrics 18:614, 1956

108. Silverstein, E., Roadman, C., Byers, R.H., Kitay, D.Z.: Hematologic problems in pregnancy. III. Glucose-6-phosphate dehydrogenase deficiency. J. Reprod. Med. 12:153, 1974.

109. Simpson, J.S.: Misdiagnosis complicating umbilical vessel catheterization. A small omphalocele containing intestine is accidentally transected. Clin. Pediatr. (Phila.) 14:727, 1975.

110. Sinclair, J.C., Fox, H.A., Lentz, J.F., Fuld, G.L., Murphy, J.: Intoxication of the fetus by a local anesthetic. A newly recognized complication of maternal caudal anesthesia. N. Engl. J. Med. **273**:1173, 1965.
111. Stanbury, J.B., Wyngaarden, J.B., Fredrickson, D.S.: The Metabolic Basis of Inherited Disease. New York, McGraw-Hill Book Co., 1972.
112. Stern, L., Denton, R.L.: Kernicterus in small premature infants. Pediatrics **35**:483, 1965.
113. Sutherland, J.M., Keller, W.H.: Novobiocin and neonatal hyperbilirubinemia. Am. J. Dis. Child. **101**:447, 1961.
114. Thearle, M.J., Dunn, P.M., Hailey, D.M.: Exchange transfusion for diazepam intoxication at birth followed by jejunal stenosis. Proc. R. Soc. Med. **66**:349, 1973.
115. Usubiaca, J.A., Juppa, M.L., Moya, F., Wikinski, J.A., Velazco, R.: Passage of procaine hydrochloride and para-aminobenzoic acid across the human placenta. Am. J. Obstet. Gynecol. **100**:918, 1968.
116. Vest, M., Strebel, L., Hauenstein, D.: The extent of "shunt" bilirubin and erythrocyte survival in the newborn infant measured by the administration of (15N) glycine. Biochem. J. **95**:11c, 1965.
117. Walker, W.: Pediatric aspects of intrauterine transfusion, in Robertson, J.G., and Dambrosio, F. (eds.): Proc. Int. Symp. "Management of the Rh Problem," Milano, 1969. Annali Ostet. Ginec. (Ital.), Special No., 1970, p. 196.
118. Walker, W.: Haemolytic disease of the newborn, in Gairdner, D., and Hull, D. (eds.): Recent Advances in Pediatrics, 4th Ed. London, J. & A. Churchill Publ., 1971, p. 119.
119. Wallerstein, H.: Treatment of severe erythroblastosis by simultaneous removal and replacement of blood of newborn infant. Science **105**:583, 1946.
120. Waters, W.J., Porter, E.G.: Dye-binding capacity of serum albumin in hemolytic disease of the newborn. Am. J. Dis. Child. **102**:807, 1961.
121. Waters, W.J., Porter, E.G.: Indications for exchange transfusion based upon the role of albumin in the treatment of hemolytic disease of the newborn. Pediatrics **33**:749, 1964.
122. Weber, A.L., DeLuca, S., Shannon, D.C.: Normal and abnormal position of the umbilical artery and venous catheter on the roentgenogram and review of complications. Am. J. Roent. Radium Ther. Nucl. Med. **120**:361, 1974.
123. Wu, P.Y.K., Oh, W.: Management of the newborn, in Charles, A.G., and Friedman, E.A. (eds.): Rh Isoimmunization and Erythroblastosis Foetalis. London, Butterworths Publ., 1969, p. 179.
124. Xanthou, M., Ceconomopoulis, P., Nicolopoulis, D., Patathanassion, P., Matsaniotis, N.: The acid-base balance of the newborn during and after exchange transfusion. Clin. Pediatr. (Phila.) **13**:759, 1974.
125. Xanthou, M., Xypolyta, A., Anagnostakis, D., Economou-Mavrow, C., Matsaniotis, N.: Exchange transfusion in severe neonatal infection with sclerema. Arch. Dis. Child. **50**:901, 1975.
126. Zachman, R.D.: Alternate phototherapy in neonatal hyperbilirubinemia. Biol. Neonate **25**:283, 1974.

127. Zamet, P., Nakamura, H., Perez-Robles, S., Larroche, J.C., Minkowski, A.: The use of critical levels of birth weight and "free bilirubin" as an approach for prevention of kernicterus. Biol. Neonate **26**:274, 1975.
128. Zipursky, A.: The erythrocytes of the newborn infant. Semin. Hematol. **2**:167, 1965.

14
The Newborn
of the Drug-Dependent Mother

Stephen R. Kandall

The problem of drug abuse and drug addiction has achieved major social and medical significance in recent years. Although accurate data are not available, it is felt that at least 500,000 addicts live in the United States, approximately half of them in the metropolitan New York area. In 1970, it was estimated that in New York at least 3.5 million dollars per day were spent by heroin-dependent persons for maintenance of their habits (54). Drug abuse is not restricted to the urban areas, however, and few regions of this country remain untouched by this epidemic problem. Since many drug-abusing women are in the childbearing age group, and since these drugs freely cross the placenta, it is not surprising that experience with passively addicted neonates has steadily grown.

Many abused drugs have been reported to affect fetal growth and development or produce physical dependency in the newborn period. Most studies have focused on the effects of maternal heroin and methadone usage, but other such agents include alcohol, amphetamines, barbiturates, codeine, ethchlorvynol (Placidyl), meperidine (Demerol), morphine, pentazocine (Talwin), and propoxyphene hydrochloride (Darvon). Use or abuse of these drugs is extremely widespread. Based on one epidemiologic study (8) involving 30,000 personal interviews in the United States, it was projected that there were 4,500,000 regular users of barbiturates, 350,000 regular users of nonbarbiturate sedatives, 5,000,000 users of minor tranquilizers, 500,000 users of antidepressants, over 2,000,000 users of amphetamines, almost 4,000,000 users of nonnarcotic analgesics, and 18,-000,000 heavy users of alcohol. "Polydrug abuse," or abuse of multiple controlled substances, may significantly alter maternal, fetal, and neonatal

222 Stephen R. Kandall

effects ascribed to a single agent. In general, however, overall patterns of drug abuse in the past five to ten years reflect a decline in the importance of heroin and an increase in methadone usage, both licit and illicit. In our study (27), during the years 1971 to 1974 at the Bronx Municipal Hospital Center, heroin-associated neonatal withdrawal fell from 55% to 16% of total recognized cases, while methadone-associated withdrawal rose from 14% to 46% of the cases. This chapter will therefore deal primarily with effects of heroin and methadone use on the mother, fetus, newborn, and young infant.

Drugs and Pregnancy

Heroin Abuse

Problems in the identification of the pregnant addict have changed in recent years. When heroin is the sole or major drug used, recognition of maternal drug abuse is often quite difficult. Fear of legal punitive action frequently leads to the mother's concealment of active drug abuse despite serious life-threatening illness in her newborn infant. In such cases, a detailed history is directed toward uncovering drug abuse; this is aided by the recognized association of heroin abuse with known disease states. Menstrual abnormalities, including amenorrhea and anovulation, as well as infertility, are extremely common. Gastrointestinal effects of opiate usage include vague abdominal pains, constipation, fecal impaction, and hemorrhoids. Heroin addiction of greater than two years' duration is often associated with a large number of dental caries, especially of frontal incisors. Infectious diseases prevalent among heroin addicts include hepatitis, tetanus, and malaria. The incidence of venereal disease, acquired by needle sharing or sexual contact, is also high. Skin and vascular complications of heroin abuse include abscesses, lymphangitis, cellulitis, and thrombophlebitis. Pulmonary complications, including pulmonary edema, emboli, infarctions, abscesses, and pneumonia, account for significant mortality and morbidity in adult heroin addicts. Bacterial endocarditis due to *Staphylococcus aureus, Candida, Klebsiella,* and *Pseudomonas* may reflect delay or neglect in seeking medical attention despite obvious illness. Severe medical or surgical illness, or deterioration in the life style associated with heroin abuse, may result in general debilitation and malnutrition.

When maternal heroin abuse is suspected, clues should also be sought in other areas. Lack of prenatal care should always be noted with suspicion. Our own study (27) revealed that 53% of heroin addicts received no prenatal care, while only 8% received consistent care. Twenty-seven percent of women with active habits of both heroin and methadone received no prenatal care, while only 13% of such women had seven or more clinic visits during pregnancy. Past delivery of a mother's infants at different hospitals should arouse suspicion of concealed drug abuse. Diminished response to obstetric analgesia, bizarre conduct while in the hospital, and insistence on early discharge from the hospital should always be regarded with suspicion.

Physical examination of the mother should be comprehensive, with particular attention paid to those diseases mentioned above. Evidence of needle tracking should be carefully sought, not only over major vessels, but also in the interdigital spaces. Skin ulcerations and tattoos should be noted, since they often obscure needle marks.

Despite the value of a complete history and physical examination, determination of drug-taking patterns must rest heavily on urine assays of drug metabolites. Ideally one would like access to all urine specimens obtained during pregnancy. Since this is often impossible, urinalyses should be done at the time of entry into the hospital. These tests are of limited value, however, since they only reflect drug-taking patterns during the preceding few days. Although thin-layer chromatography is used for mass screening, more accurate qualitative or quantitative testing, such as gas-liquid chromatography, radioimmunoassay, or spectral analysis may reveal unsuspected drug abuse. Studies from the Odyssey House in New York (4) indicate that 25 to 50% of drug-using women abuse multiple drugs during pregnancy. Although the patterns were variable, the study did suggest that heroin users had the greatest tendency to abuse multiple drugs.

Methadone and Pregnancy

The introduction of methadone maintenance and its widespread use during pregnancy has significantly altered the impact of drug addiction during this period. Registration in an approved drug treatment program has made concealment of drug usage less of a problem. Availability of methadone maintenance and other drug treatment programs has led to a reduction in punitive measures, since the period surrounding the birth of a baby may be marked by high parental motivation and is generally regarded as a favorable time for psychosocial intervention (4, 7).

Within methadone programs, however, polydrug abuse is a serious problem, reducing the effectiveness of this therapeutic modality (4). Despite faithful attendance in a treatment program, therefore, urinalyses for drug metabolites should be screened in this population. Alcohol abuse also appears to be common, as is the practice of "topping off" with "street methadone" to supplement medically regulated methadone dosages (4). Despite these problems, methadone administration in "blocking" dosages can effectively combat the desire for heroin. Clinical stabilization through methadone maintenance should then be used to provide a network of psychosocial supports in an effort to restructure the patient's life style. The daily oral administration of methadone should eliminate medical problems related to the use of unsterile needles (hepatitis, pulmonary disease, phlebitis, etc.). Representative studies have documented marked improvement in the general health of pregnant populations while receiving methadone maintenance (6, 10). Methadone administration also affords the opportunity to ensure prenatal care on a regular basis. Our data, for example, showed that significantly more prenatal care was received in the methadone group compared with the heroin group ($p < 0.05$) (27).

Although methadone maintenance is an accepted substitution therapy for heroin addiction, regulation of methadone dosages during pregnancy remain controversial. Some workers have suggested that maintenance of dosages over 100 mg per day during pregnancy stabilize the patient and reduce the incidence of polydrug abuse (2). Supporters of this regimen have pointed to studies indicating no relationship between maternal dosage and severity of neonatal withdrawal (38, 47). Other studies, however, have found that severity of neonatal withdrawal is directly related to the amount of maternal methadone, i.e. the higher the dosage, the more severe the withdrawal (9, 39). This would imply that proper management should be based on gradual reduction of dosage during the pregnancy, attempting to achieve a drug-free state before delivery. Although clinical trials with longer-acting methadone preparations are in progress, there are no studies on their effects during pregnancy.

Methadone maintenance also appears to have reduced fetal wastage and neonatal death rates. Reports have noted fetal death in association with withdrawal in heroin-using mothers (45, 53). Our own study (27) found that each of the four drug-associated stillbirths occurred in fetuses of mothers abusing either heroin alone or heroin-methadone combinations; there were no stillbirths in the methadone maintenance group. It seems reasonable that fetal exposure to heroin would be variable in time and amount; withdrawal, if severe, might lead to passage of meconium and subsequent pulmonary aspiration, leading to intrauterine death (45). Fetal exposure to methadone would be expected to be more regular, even in those cases of dosage reduction during pregnancy. It should be noted, however, that Blinick et al. (1) found poor correlation between maternal methadone dosage and amount of methadone measured in biofluids (maternal serum, breast milk, amniotic fluid, cord blood, fetal urine), implying the existence of a complex mechanism of biotransformation in the human.

Fetal Growth and Development

Effects of maternal drug use on fetal growth and development have been recognized for many years. Heroin appears to have a direct adverse effect on fetal growth, causing intrauterine growth retardation out of proportion to the reduction in gestational length (30, 52). In our study (28), mean birth weights were no different between the heroin group (2490 g) and the heroin-methadone group (2535 g); mean gestational ages were 38.0 and 38.3 weeks, respectively. Low mean birth weight (2615 g) was also observed in those infants born to mothers who had abused heroin in the past but not during the current pregnancy. This suggests that the effect of heroin on birth weight may persist long after the period of addiction. Infants born to mothers on methadone maintenance had a significantly higher mean birth weight of 2961 g ($p < 0.01$); mean gestational age was 39.4 weeks. All drug groups, however, had lower mean weights than the control group weight of 3176 g ($p < 0.01$). Our study also found a significant relationship between maternal methadone dosage in the first trimester and birth weight, i.e., the higher the dosage, the larger the infant ($p < 0.01$). No correlation was seen between birth weight and second or third trimester dosage. We estimated that 25% of the variance in birth weight among the methadone-addicted infants could be accounted for by methadone dosage. The mechanism for heroin-associated fetal growth reduction is not known. Postmortem data on heroin-exposed fetuses led Naeye et al. (35) to suggest that significant reductions in organ cell number may limit intrauterine growth. Methadone may correct this fetal growth retardation in a dose-related fashion. Speculation might also be directed towards fetal carbohydrate homeostasis and endocrine regulatory mechanisms in explaining these observations.

Congenital anomalies have not been reported to occur with increased frequency in association with maternal heroin or methadone usage. Other nonnarcotic agents, however, such as phenobarbital (51), alcohol (25, 40), and LSD (22) have been implicated in fetal malformation syndromes.

Transitional Period

Transition from intrauterine to extrauterine life is accomplished without difficulty in the majority of infants born to drug-using mothers. In our study (27), there were no differences between drug groups and controls in one-minute Apgar scores (7.9 versus 8.1) or five-minute Apgar scores (9.2 versus 9.4).

Despite this, care in the delivery room for mother and child may be complicated by maternal drug abuse. Maternal withdrawal may become apparent, requiring acute treatment for stabilization. This may be confusing if maternal symptoms are compatible with withdrawal but the mother denies drug intake. Regimens for acute management under these conditions have not been well standardized. Obstetricians may elect to titrate methadone dosage on the basis of maternal symptoms, beginning with one-quarter the mother's maintenance dosage and repeating that dosage at intervals based on objective signs or subjective maternal discomfort. Alternatively, obstetricians may choose to control maternal withdrawal with meperidine, usually in the range of 50 to 100 mg intravenously. Once large doses of meperidine are given to control maternal withdrawal or promote obstetric analgesia, the possibility of respiratory and neurologic depression in the newborn must be faced. Naloxone (Narcan) should not be administered to the mother prior to delivery since its effect on fetal and neonatal withdrawal will be unpredictable. If naloxone treatment to reverse acute narcotic depression is considered advisable for the infant, neonatal withdrawal will often begin immediately in the delivery room.

Meconium staining of the amniotic fluid, representing passage of fetal intestinal contents prior to delivery, represents a hazard for the fetus and newborn. Should fetal asphyxia result in gasping, severe intrauterine asphyxia may result in fetal death (45). In our study (27), meconium passage prior to birth occurred with greater frequency in the heroin and heroin-methadone groups compared to methadone and control groups ($p < 0.02$). This increased incidence was not associated with clinical evidence of meconium aspiration or reduction in Apgar scores, suggesting that intrauterine withdrawal, rather than fetal hypoxia, was responsible for evacuation of fetal stool. Should meconium aspiration occur, however, immediate care in the delivery room is essential (see Chapter 10).

Previous reports have suggested that heroin accelerates lung maturation in the preterm infant. Glass et al. (14) noted no cases of respiratory distress syndrome in 33 premature infants of 32 to 37 weeks gestation born to heroin-addicted mothers. We could not confirm this observation, although eight of our twelve infants with RDS were of less than 32-weeks gestation (27). These data suggest that a stage of pulmonary maturation must be present for heroin to promote lung stability. Although chronic morphine administration to pregnant rabbits did not influence lung maturation in their fetuses (46), acceleration of lung development did occur after injections directly into rabbit fetuses (55). Studies attempting to link lowered incidence of RDS with increased cord levels of hemoglobin A and 2,3-diphosphoglycerate have also been reported (13).

Another reported physiologic effect of heroin, perhaps beneficial to fetus and newborn, is the accelerated maturation of hepatic bilirubin conjugating systems, with subsequent reduction of serum levels of unconjugated bilirubin (36). This effect of enzyme induction has not been reported for methadone.

Neonatal Drug Withdrawal

Drug Withdrawal Signs

Signs of neonatal drug withdrawal may be subtle or obvious, and can be divided into four main groups: central nervous system, gastrointestinal, respiratory, and autonomic nervous system signs.

Central nervous system signs

These are the most common manifestation of neonatal withdrawal, occurring in about 90% of symptomatic neonates. Most often, the infants
present with marked irritability, excessive crying which may be high-
pitched and "cerebral," and lack of consolability. Most of the infants show
hyperreflexia and exaggeration of flexor tone. Tremors both of the high
frequency, low amplitude, and coarser higher amplitude types are extremely
common; these may progress to seizures. Convulsions associated with drug
withdrawal have been reported to occur in about 1 to 2% of heroin-
addicted newborns and about 5 to 10% of methadone-addicted newborns (58). In our own study (20), seizures occurred in 7.8% of the
methadone group and 1.2% of the heroin group. Mean day of seizure
onset in our 17 patients was 9.5 ± 7.8 days. Convulsions classified as
"myoclonic" on "tonic-clonic" were the most common types seen, and
almost all of the infants were being treated with specific medication at the
time of the seizure. Compared with passively addicted newborns without
seizures, this group had more severe symptomatology and needed specific
medication at higher dosages prior to the seizures. Convulsions occurred
more commonly when diazepam rather than camphorated tincture of opium
(paregoric) was used to control early symptoms of withdrawal. Electro-
encephalograms, read as abnormal during the seizure, reverted to normal
in the postictal period in all but one of 13 tracings obtained. Since abnormal EEGs were also seen in the "myoclonic" type of seizure, we would
suggest that rhythmic myoclonic spasms seen in association with neonatal
withdrawal should be regarded as true seizures.

Illustrative Case History

> *A 2750-g male infant was born to a 22-year-old mother after
> a term gestation. The mother had taken 20 mg of methadone
> a day for the entire pregnancy. Labor and delivery were un-
> eventful. The infant became jittery and irritable within the
> first day of life, and paregoric 0.25 cc every three hours was
> started. The dosage was gradually increased to 0.5 cc every
> three hours because of increasing jitteriness. When an attempt
> was made to reduce the paregoric dosage on the 25th day of
> life, multiple myoclonic jerks were noted. Laboratory workup
> for neonatal seizures was unrevealing. The electroencephalo-
> gram revealed unifocal paroxysmal activity at the time of the
> myoclonic jerks. Phenobarbital 7 mg/kg/day was added to
> the therapeutic regimen and the episodes ceased. Phenobar-
> bital was discontinued on the 30th day, while paregoric was
> maintained at a dosage of 0.5 cc every three hours. On the
> 40th day, a series of myoclonic jerks was noted, but no further
> episodes occurred. Paregoric was discontinued on the 65th*

day. Developmental examination at eleven months of age was completely normal.

More subtle effects of maternal narcotic usage on neonatal neuroadaptive behavior have been reported by Kron et al. (31), who have shown abnormal sucking behavior shortly after birth. Although these infants often have voracious appetites and are frequently noted to have an increased sucking need, their suck is dysrhythmic and "chomping," often interfering with proper nutrition. Kron also noted that sucking behavior was more depressed in infants born to mothers on methadone maintenance than in those born to "street addicts." The same authors found that paregoric restored sucking behavior to normal significantly better than phenobarbital or diazepam.

Abnormalities in electroencephalographic patterns of neonates born to drug-using women have also been noted. Schulman (50) reported disorganization of normal sleep patterns in such infants, and Lodge et al. (33) noted "high frequency dysynchronous activity suggestive of CNS irritability." In another study of passively addicted infants (3), 16 of 37 EEGs were considered to manifest paroxysmal abnormalities.

Gastrointestinal Symptoms

Most common gastrointestinal symptoms include diarrhea and vomiting, occurring in about 30% of affected infants in our series (27). Although gastrointestinal symptoms contributed to the high mortality once associated with this condition, these symptoms can usually be easily controlled with paregoric and now only rarely progress to significant electrolyte and water loss.

Common Respiratory Signs

Tachypnea or hyperpnea, with a resulting mild respiratory alkalosis are among the common signs (15). More serious respiratory symptoms, including cyanosis and apnea, are not commonly seen with early institution of specific therapy.

Autonomic Nervous System Signs

These may include sneezing, yawning, lacrimation, and sweating. Temperature elevations to 99 to 100°F are common, and untreated infants who become more hypermetabolic may reach much higher temperatures (21).

Although signs referable to the autonomic nervous system have the greatest *relative* specificity, none of the above signs can be considered *diagnostic* for neonatal drug withdrawal. Narcotic withdrawal syndrome may be mistaken for a number of metabolic disturbances (hypoglycemia, adrenal collapse, thyrotoxicosis, etc.), infection (sepsis, meningitis), and intracranial hemorrhage, among other serious conditions. Even the knowledge of drug usage by the mother, in the presence of characteristic neonatal withdrawal symptoms, should not lead physicians to regard withdrawal as the *only* possible diagnosis. In certain situations, therefore, it may be wise to screen such infants with tests such as blood glucose, serum calcium and electrolytes, blood acid-base studies, lumbar puncture and cultures of blood, stool, urine, and cerebrospinal fluid. Clinical response to opiate (paregoric) administration may occasionally help in the differential diagnosis of nonspecific symptoms.

Most studies indicate that severity of symptoms appear to be worse in methadone withdrawal than that attributable to heroin (9, 43, 59). Our own study (27) found that about 80% of infants exposed to maternal narcotics became symptomatic in the newborn period. Individual symptoms, except for seizures, were seen with similar frequency in the heroin, methadone, and heroin-methadone groups. Symptoms appeared to be more severe, however, in the methadone group, based on need for specific treatment, maximal dose of medication needed to control symptoms, and days of hospital treatment required for control of symptoms.

Controversy still surrounds the relationship of maternal dosage to onset and severity of neonatal symptoms. As noted earlier, some studies have not been able to correlate severity of neonatal symptoms with maternal methadone dosage (27, 47), while others have found a correlation between the two factors (9, 39). Variability of symptoms is poorly understood, and may be a result of complex interaction of maternal metabolism, placental transfer and metabolism, and fetal metabolism and disposal. One study found that a plasma methadone level of $\geqslant 0.06$ $\mu g/ml$ protected the infant against withdrawal; a decline below this level was followed shortly by withdrawal symptoms (47). Although mean time of symptom onset was the same in all three of our study groups (2 to 3 days), the methadone group showed considerably more variability in the onset and pattern of withdrawal, necessitating closer observation in the hospital and after discharge (27).

Management of Neonatal Drug Withdrawal

Recognition and prompt treatment of neonatal withdrawal has substantially reduced the mortality associated with this condition. Whereas early studies noted a mortality of 34 to 93% (5, 17), death associated with acute neonatal withdrawal has become a rare occurrence in recent years. Proper management can be divided into *general* and *specific* measures. *General* measures comprise those elements of care afforded "high-risk" patients, with attention to the specific problems of withdrawal. Newborns undergoing withdrawal should be considered "high-risk," and observed in a special care unit with a high nurse:patient ratio. Vital signs should be taken frequently, fluid and caloric intake charted accurately, and development and progression of symptoms assessed by trained observers. Generous amounts of fluids and calories should be provided for those symptomatic infants who are considered to be hypermetabolic. Weighing infants once or twice daily will identify those infants who are losing an excessive amount of weight. Unnecessary handling should be minimized since these infants often respond to stimuli with increased irritability. Observation of these patients may be accomplished in an enclosed isolette or in an open bassinette. Irritability can often be reduced if the infants are swaddled, kept prone, and placed in a quiet, dimly lit environment. If infants are treated under these environmental conditions, however, extremely close observation is essential, since symptoms, especially seizures, may go unrecognized.

Specific treatment involves the control of withdrawal symptoms by pharmacologic agents. At the present time, four drugs are widely used: camphorated tincture of opium (paregoric), phenobarbital, diazepam, and chlorpromazine. The use of paregoric in the treatment of withdrawal has been based on the concept that intrauterine opiate dependency should be treated with another opiate, with subsequent gradual reduction in dosage under strict observation and control. The other three agents are sedatives, and although less specific in their action, these are also effective in controlling withdrawal symptoms.

Paregoric is probably the most widely used agent for control of neonatal drug-related symptoms. Paregoric is administered orally and has very few side effects, but obstipation may result if dosages are excessive. Treatment is begun at 0.25 cc every three hours; if symptoms are not well controlled, each subsequent dosage is increased by 0.05 cc until a stabilizing dosage is reached. In severe cases of withdrawal, in which dosages exceed 0.75 cc, a second medication should be added and the paregoric dosage reduced. Once the infant has been clinically stable for at least five days, gradual reduction of the paregoric dosage may be started. As the dosage is lowered, mild withdrawal symptomatology may be noticed, but continued dosage reduction should proceed unless symptoms are severe. Beneficial effects of paregoric include its superior prevention and control of seizures (20), and rapid normalization of neonatal sucking behavior (31).

Phenobarbital has also been shown to be effective in treatment of neonatal drug withdrawal (26, 43). It is usually administered in a dosage of 5 to 10 mg/kg/day, first intramuscularly until the baby is clinically stable, and then orally. Phenobarbital is the treatment of choice in barbiturate withdrawal, a syndrome which may first appear at or later than 5 to 7 days of life and may be associated with a high incidence of seizures (11). Excessive dosages of phenobarbital administered for narcotic withdrawal may produce lethargy and poor feeding, preventing adequate intake of fluid and calories.

Diazepam (Valium), although reportedly effective in heroin withdrawal (37), has not been well studied in neonatal methadone or polydrug withdrawal. Diazepam is administered every eight hours intramuscularly in a dosage of 1 mg for mild, 1.5 mg for moderate, and 2 mg for severe withdrawal. In many cases of withdrawal, dosages of the medication may be lowered rapidly, with shortening of the infant's hospital stay. In some patients, however, symptoms have recurred once diazepam has been discontinued; this may reflect progression of symptoms until about two weeks of age, or incomplete treatment of withdrawal. Recurrence of severe symptoms requires rehospitalization of the infant. Vital signs should be monitored frequently, since bradycardia and respiratory depression have been noted after intramuscular injection of diazepam.

Chlorpromazine also appears to be effective in management of neonatal drug withdrawal; a large series of infants treated with this agent was reported by Zelson and co-workers (60). Chlorpromazine is usually given in a dosage of 2.3 to 3 mg/kg/day orally or intramuscularly in four divided doses. The drug is known to have widespread effects on the cardiovascular, endocrine, and central and autonomic nervous systems in adults, but little such data is available on neonates.

Treatment should be individualized as much as possible, since marked variability exists between babies in response to treatment. Infants born to different mothers taking equal amounts of methadone may show quite different presentations, ranging from absence of symptoms to severe symptoms with convulsions. Some of this unpredictability may be caused by inaccurate assessment of maternal methadone dosage due to "topping off" with illicit methadone, or alternatively, to polydrug abuse. Qualitative urine analyses for toxic metabolites, performed both on mother and child, are therefore of great help in determining specific treatment. Whereas paregoric is extremely effective in the treatment of opiate withdrawal, it may be less effective than one of the other agents if the major part of the withdrawal is not opiate related. Although it is preferable to use one pharmacologic agent in the treatment of withdrawal, a poor clinical response to adequate dosages of a drug should lead clinicians to consider the use of another agent.

It would be desirable to encourage breast feeding to foster development of mother-infant bonding; however, the unpredictable excretion of maternal drugs into breast milk (1) has led most workers to discourage the practice of using breast feeding to treat neonatal withdrawal.

Treatment of newborns undergoing withdrawal has generally been confined to the hospital setting. In the past, this has been necessary for close observation of the withdrawal syndrome, and to provide protective agencies the opportunity to ensure infant safety after discharge. The development of methadone maintenance and other treatment modalities has led some workers to try home treatment of infant withdrawal once acute symptoms have been controlled and reduction of the medication has begun (48). This approach has the obvious advantages of shortening hospital stays and allowing closer parent-child interaction in the first few weeks of life. It should only be considered, however, for those mothers who are in registered drug treatment programs and who have fulfilled strict reliability criteria established jointly by the hospital and treatment program. The mother must not be a polydrug user, and must have easy accessibility by phone. She also must know how to administer medication to the baby, and must be willing to make frequent hospital visits, since examinations by a competent, trained physician should be performed often during the period of medication reduction.

Later Complications of Neonatal Drug Dependency

Although the neonatal withdrawal syndrome has generally been regarded as acute and clinically manifest within the first few days of life, concern has been increasing over delayed or prolonged effects attributable to maternal drug-taking.

Delayed Drug Withdrawal

The great majority of infants exhibiting drug withdrawal will develop symptoms within the first three days of life, but withdrawal from methadone appears to be more variable in its onset. In our initial study (29), seven infants were described who showed initial or major symptomatology beyond 12 days of age. In all cases, methadone, either alone or in combination with other drugs, was taken by the mother during the pregnancy.

Illustrative Case History

> *This 2030-g female infant was born to a 25-year-old primigravida after a 36-week gestation. The mother had abused heroin for seven years, but was enrolled in a methadone maintenance program during the pregnancy, and was maintained on 10 mg of methadone twice a day. Urine analyses during the last month of pregnancy showed only methadone. Labor and delivery were normal, and the baby's Apgar scores were 5 at one minute and 10 at 5 minutes. The infant's initial course was marked by respiratory distress, requiring assisted ventilation. At 12 days of age, after resolution of the respiratory problem, the baby developed jitteriness, sneezing and diarrhea. Laboratory studies were all within normal limits, and symptoms were controlled with 0.1 cc of paregoric every three*

hours. The paregoric was gradually discontinued during the next week and the remainder of the hospital stay was uneventful. At 22 months of age, the child's physical and developmental examinations were normal.

Prominent central nervous system manifestations were seen in all of our patients, and three of the seven experienced convulsions. In all seven infants, recognizable metabolic causes (hypoglycemia, hypocalcemia, electrolyte imbalance), infectious causes, and central nervous system hemorrhage or malformation were ruled out. One patient died on the 23rd day of life after progressively severe withdrawal at home. Five of the seven infants had not been treated in the immediate neonatal period; the remaining two had been treated with diazepam. Since paregoric is much more widely used than diazepam in that institution as treatment for withdrawal, it is noteworthy that major delayed symptoms did not occur when paregoric was initially used.

The mechanism for this delayed onset of major symptoms is not clear. It has been known for some time that in adults withdrawal from methadone is more severe than from heroin (23). Methadone is reported to accumulate in various body tissues, including lung, liver, kidney, and spleen (12). It seems reasonable that fetal storage and delayed metabolism and excretion of the drug are responsible for delayed onset of withdrawal. Variability in these metabolic processes may determine the rate of fall of drug levels in neonatal serum as well as the length of time to reach a critical level for onset of symptoms (47).

Although only about 5 to 10% of methadone-addicted infants will present with delayed withdrawal symptoms, others will have exacerbations of previously controlled symptoms at 12 to 21 days of age (27). It is therefore imperative that such infants be kept under observation for a prolonged period of time. If infants show no withdrawal or only minor symptoms, provisions for follow-up must be carefully made through a supervisory agency. Physicians and allied health personnel caring for such infants should be aware of the potential seriousness of the condition and should readmit the baby to the hospital for observation and possible treatment.

Subacute Withdrawal

The syndrome of "subacute withdrawal," described by Wilson et al. (57) in heroin-addicted babies, is characterized by persistence for four to six months of restlessness, agitation, irritability, hypertonicity, and poor socialization. In some infants, severity of symptoms may lead to rehospitalization. Lipsitz and Blatman (32) have also noted withdrawal persisting for up to 12 weeks in infants of methadone-maintained women. The following case is drawn from our hospital records:

> *The baby was born to a 19-year-old primigravida after a full-term pregnancy marked by abuse of opiates, LSD, and alcohol in unknown amounts. Delivery was uneventful, and the Apgar scores were 9 at one minute and 10 at 5 minutes. The infant weighed 2480 g and showed physical evidence of intrauterine growth retardation. During the first day of life the infant was jittery, fed poorly, and showed poor coordination of sucking and swallowing. Laboratory workup for marked hypertonicity and irritability was unremarkable, and the baby was treated with diazepam for seven days, with symptomatic improvement. The infant was discharged with a normal neurologic examination, but was readmitted at one month of age with increasing tremulousness, clonus, and irritability. Treatment with phenobarbital led to clinical improvement. Follow-up in the out-patient department showed persistence of symptoms for four to five months, during which time the mother discontinued administration of phenobarbital. Subsequent neurologic examinations and attainment of developmental milestones have been normal.*

Although these persistent symptoms are probably due to intrauterine drug exposure, similar symptoms may be associated with intrauterine growth retardation, often a feature of maternal drug usage (see section on Fetal Growth and Development).

Recognition of this syndrome should significantly influence the follow-up care of drug-using mothers and their infants. Since drug usage imposes an impediment to normal parenting behavior (7), parental feelings of inadequacy and rejection could develop when the infant displays stiffness, irritability, poor feeding, and abnormal socialization. Counseling should be supportive, and parents should be told not to interpret infant behavior of this type as a rejection of care-taking efforts. Counselors should also assure parents that symptoms tend to improve at about four to six months of age. Lack of sensitive intervention might contribute to emotional deprivation of children, reportedly more common in families marked by drug usage (4).

Sudden Infant Death Syndrome: (SIDS)

The frequency of sudden infant death syndrome (SIDS) in the United States is reported to be two to three per 1000 live births (56), making it the leading cause of death between one month and one year of age. Reports from two centers have suggested a possible association between SIDS and maternal drug usage (19, 41). Review of data (44) accumulated between 1972 to 1974 at Lincoln Hospital and Bronx Municipal Hospital Center has also suggested an increased incidence of SIDS in infants born to drug-using mothers.

Illustrative Case History

> The infant was a 3000-g male born to a 24-year-old unmarried Hispanic female after a term pregnancy. The mother had been on methadone maintenance at a dosage of 70 mg per day for six years. The baby's perinatal course was uneventful and no drug withdrawal was noted. The infant was discharged on the seventh day of life and was reported by the Visiting Nurse Service to be doing well, without evidence of withdrawal at home. On the twenty-first day of life at 1:00 p.m., the infant was fed and put to bed; he was found lifeless in his crib at 5:00 p.m. Autopsy revealed no external abuse and no obvious cause of death. Toxicologic analysis failed to reveal drugs in the infant.

Previous reports have linked SIDS with varying patterns of maternal drug ingestion (heroin, methadone, heroin and methadone, pentacozine) (16, 41). In our study (44) of eight cases, four of the mothers were in registered methadone programs, while the remaining four admitted to methadone and heroin abuse during the pregnancy. Common features between our study group and SIDS in the general population include male predominance, occurrence within sibships, increased incidence of low birth weight, age at death (21 to 113 days), diurnal pattern (more in early morning), and seasonal distribution (more in winter). These features suggest that drug-associated SIDS may be a relevant study model for SIDS in the general population.

Although the etiology of SIDS is not known, major interest now focuses on the relationship of sudden death and respiratory patterns during sleep (18). It has been known for many years that morphine and related narcotics reduce brain stem responsiveness to carbon dioxide and depress pontine and medullary centers which control respiratory rhythmicity (24). These effects are more prominent during sleep (24), and have been shown to persist for up to 30 weeks in adults (34). These physiologic aberrations have also been confirmed following methadone administration in adults (42). We would postulate that intrauterine exposure to narcotics, perhaps at a critical developmental stage, may adversely affect central regulatory centers controlling respirations. Further studies may determine whether maternal drug usage should be added to the contingency list for predisposition of young infants to SIDS.

Follow-up of Passively Addicted Infants

Follow-up studies on passively addicted infants are preliminary at the present time. Well-designed studies have been hampered by difficulty in maintaining contact with a patient population after discharge from the hospital, as well as the lack of a suitable control group. This control group should be similar to the study group in weight, gestational age, perinatal events, and socioeconomic factors, but should be free of intrauterine drug exposure. Wilson et al. (57), in their study of subacute withdrawal, noted persistence for up to 24 months of neurologic dysfunction and behavioral abnormalities in infants born to heroin addicts. In another study (49) of 17 Danish infants born to mothers with varying drug histories, evaluation of the children at a mean age of 18 months revealed normal physical and psychologic development. Lipsitz, in another preliminary study (32), found no evidence of neurologic disability in follow-up of 100 methadone-addicted neonates despite persistance of withdrawal for up to 12 weeks in some babies. In all of these reports, however, no separation was made between neurobehavioral effects due to maternal drug usage and possible long-term effects of specific agents used to treat neonatal withdrawal.

Social disposition of passively addicted neonates has also been incompletely studied. Our data (27) showed that of 215 surviving infants born to drug-using mothers, placement of the infant in foster care occurred significantly more frequently when mothers abused heroin. Release of the infant to the mother, on the other hand, was more frequent in the methadone group compared with the heroin and heroin-methadone groups. This reflects the willingness of hospitals and protective agencies to release the infant to the mother when she is enrolled in an approved drug treatment program. Under such circumstances, however, it is still essential that liaison with the drug treatment program be established and maintained to ensure surveillance over parents, children, and their interaction.

Conclusion

Narcotic usage during pregnancy and the resultant neonatal withdrawal syndrome have become problems of major importance in our society. Replacement of heroin abuse with medically supervised methadone maintenance has led to improvement in maternal health during pregnancy and an increase in prenatal care. Methadone also appears to be more compatible with normal fetal growth and development, resulting in lower fetal wastage rates and higher birth weights. Although affected infants usually make the transition from intrauterine to extrauterine life without difficulty, delivery room management may be complicated by maternal withdrawal.

Despite the confusion introduced by "topping off" with methadone and by polydrug abuse, neonatal withdrawal from methadone appears to be worse than that from heroin. Management based on proper supportive care and specific pharmacologic treatment, however, will control withdrawal without difficulty in the majority of cases. Recent observations documenting persistence of neurologic dysfunction and delayed withdrawal, as well as suggesting a possible link to sudden infant death, have broadened our concept of "neonatal withdrawal." Despite the increase in knowledge about effects of maternal drug usage, obvious subjects in need of research include: maternal, placental, and fetal metabolism of heroin and methadone, effects of treatment regimens during pregnancy on neonatal withdrawal, and many aspects of neurobehavioral and physical development of passively addicted neonates.

References

1. Blinick, G., Inturrisi, C.E., Wallach, R.C.: Methadone assays in pregnant women and progeny. Am. J. Obstet. Gynecol. 121:617, 1975
2. Blinick, G., Jerez, E., Wallach, R.C.: Methadone maintenance, pregnancy, and progeny. J.A.M.A. 225:477, 1973
3. Bosch, V., Cracco, J., Shin, K., Yoon, J., Cracco, R.: The neonatal electroencephalogram in infants of addicted mothers. Read at the 30th annual meeting of the American Electroencephalographic Society (Dearborn, Michigan), Sept. 29–Oct. 1, 1976.
4. Carr, J.N.: Drug patterns among drug-addicted mothers. Pediatr. Ann. 4:408, 1975.
5. Cobrinik, R.W., Hood, R.T., Jr., Chusid, E., Slobody, L.B.: The effects of maternal narcotic addiction on the newborn. Am. J. Dis. Child. 92:504, 1956.
6. Connaughton, J.F., Jr., Finnegan, L.P., Schut, J., Emich, J.P.: Current concepts in the management of the pregnant opiate addict. Addict. Dis. 2:21, 1975.
7. Coppolillo, H.P.: Drug impediments to mothering behavior. Addict. Dis. 2:201, 1975.
8. Chambers, C.D., Griffey, M.S.: Use of legal substance within the general population: the sex and age variables. Addict. Dis. 2:7, 1975.
9. Davis, M.M., Brown, B.S., Glendinning, S.T.: Neonatal effects of heroin addiction and methadone-treated pregnancies: preliminary report on 70 live births, in 1973 Proceedings of Fifth National Conference on Methadone Treatment. New York, National Association for the Prevention of Addiction to Narcotics, 1973, p. 1153.
10. Davis, R.C., Chappel, J.N., Mejia-Zelaya, A., Madden, J.: Clinical observations on methadone-maintained pregnancies. Addict. Dis. 2:101, 1975.
11. Desmond, M.M., Schwanecke, R.P., Wilson, G.S., et al: Maternal barbiturate utilization and neonatal withdrawal symptoms. J. Pediatr. 80:190, 1972.
12. Dole, V.P., Kreek, M.J.: Methadone plasma level: sustained by a reservoir of drug in tissue. Proc. Natl. Acad. Sci. U.S.A. 70:10, 1973.
13. Finnegan, L.P., Shouraie, Z., Emich, J.P., et al: Alterations of the oxygen hemoglobin equilibrium curve and red cell 2,3-diphosphoglycerate (2,3-

DPG) in cord blood of infants born to opiate-dependent women. Pediatr. Res. **8**:363, 1974.

14. Glass, L., Rajegowda, B.K., Evans, H.E.: Absence of respiratory distress syndrome in premature infants of heroin-addicted mothers. Lancet **2**:685, 1971.
15. Glass, L., Rajegowda, B.K., Kahn, E.J., Floyd, M.V.: Effect of heroin withdrawal on respiratory rate and acid-base status in the newborn. N. Engl. J. Med. **286**:746, 1972.
16. Goetz, R.L., Bain, R.V.: Neonatal withdrawal symptoms associated with maternal use of pentacozine. J. Pediatr. **84**:887, 1974.
17. Goodfriend, M.J., Shey, I.A., Klein, M.D.: The effects of maternal narcotic addiction on the newborn. Am. J. Obstet. Gynecol. **71**:29, 1956.
18. Guilleminault, C., Peraita, R., Souquet, M., Dement, W.C.: Apneas during sleep in infants: possible relationship with sudden infant death syndrome. Science **190**:677, 1975.
19. Harper, R.G., Concepcion, G.S., Blenman, S.: Observations on the sudden death of infants born to addicted mothers, in Proceedings of Fifth National Conference on Methadone Treatment. New York, National Association for the Prevention of Addiction to Narcotics, 1973, p. 1122.
20. Herzlinger, R.A., Kandall, S.R., Vaughan, H.G.: Neonatal withdrawal seizures. Pediatr. Res. **10**:176, 1976.
21. Hill, R.N., Desmond, M.M.: Management of the narcotic withdrawal syndrome in the neonate. Pediatr. Clin. North Am. **10**:67, 1963.
22. Hsu, L.Y., Strauss, L., Hirschhorn, K.: Chromosome abnormality in offspring of LSD users. D Trisomy with D/D translocation. J.A.M.A. **211**:987, 1970.
23. Isbell, H., Vogel, V.H.: The addiction liability of methadone (amidone, dolophine, 10820) and its use in the treatment of the morphine abstinence syndrome. Am. J. Psychol. **105**:909, 1949.
24. Jaffee, J.H.: Narcotic Analgesics, in Goodman, L.S., and Gilman, A. (eds.): The Pharmacological Basis of Therapeutics. New York, Macmillan Co., 1970, p. 243.
25. Jones, K.L., Smith, D.W., Vuleland, C.N., Streissguth, A.P.: Pattern of malformation in offspring of alcoholic mothers. Lancet **1**:1267, 1973.
26. Kahn, E.J., Neumann, L.L., Polk, G.: The course of the heroin withdrawal syndrome in newborn infants treated with phenobarbital or chlorpromazine. J. Pediatr. **75**:495, 1969.
27. Kandall, S.R., Albin, S., Gartner, L.M., et al: The addicted mother: fetal and neonatal consequences. Early Human Development **1**:159–169, 1977.
28. Kandall, S.R., Albin, S., Lowinson, J., et al: Differential effects of maternal heroin and methadone use on birthweight. Pediatrics **58**:681, 1976.
29. Kandall, S.R., Gartner, L.M.: Late presentation of drug withdrawal symptoms in newborns. Am. J. Dis. Child. **127**:58, 1974.
30. Krause, S.O., Murray, P.M., Holmes, J.B., Burch, R.E.: Heroin addiction among pregnant women and their newborn babies. Am. J. Obstet. Gynecol. **75**:754, 1958.
31. Kron, R.E., Litt, M., Phoenix, M.D., Finnegan, L.P.: Neonatal narcotic

abstinence: effects of pharmacotherapeutic agents and maternal drug usage on nutritive sucking behavior. J. Pediatr. **88**:637, 1976.

32. Lipsitz, P.J., Blatman, S.: Newborn infants of mothers on methadone maintenance. N.Y. State J. Med. **74**:994, 1974.

33. Lodge, A., Marcus, M.M., Ramer, C.M.: Behavioral and electrophysiological characteristics of the addicted neonate. Addict. Dis. **2**:235, 1975.

34. Martin, W.R., Jasinski, D.R., Sapira, J.D., et al: The respiratory effects of morphine during a cycle of dependence. J. Pharmacol. Exp. Ther. **62**:182, 1967.

35. Naeye, R.L., Blanc, W., LeBlanc, W., Khatamee, M.A.: Fetal complications of maternal heroin addiction: abnormal growth, infections, and episodes of stress. J. Pediatr. **83**:1055, 1973.

36. Nathenson, G., Cohen, M.I., Litt, I.F., McNamara, H.: The effect of maternal heroin addiction on neonatal jaundice. J. Pediatr. **81**:899, 1972.

37. Nathenson, G., Golden, G.S., Litt, I.F.: Diazepam in the management of the neonatal narcotic withdrawal syndrome. Pediatrics **48**:523, 1971.

38. Newman, R.G.: Pregnancies of methadone patients. N.Y. State J. Med. **74**:52, 1974.

39. Ostrea, E.M., Jr., Chavez, C.J., Strauss, M.E.: A study of factors that influence the severity of neonatal narcotic withdrawal. J. Pediatr. **88**:642, 1976.

40. Palmer, R.H., Ouellette, E.M., Warner, L., Leichtman, S.R.: Congenital malformations in offspring of a chronic alcoholic mother. Pediatrics **53**:490, 1974.

41. Pierson, P.S., Howard, P., Kleber, H.D.: Sudden deaths in infants born to methadone-maintained addicts. J.A.M.A. **220**:1733, 1972.

42. Prescott, F., Ransom, S.G., Thorp, R.H., Wilson, A.: Effects of analgesics on respiratory response to carbon dioxide in man. Lancet **1**:340, 1949.

43. Rajegowda, B.K., Glass, L., Evans, H.E., et al: Methadone withdrawal in newborn infants. J. Pediatr. **81**:532, 1972.

44. Rajegowda, B.K., Kandall, S.R., Falciglia, H.: Sudden unexpected death in infants of narcotic-dependent mothers. Early Human Development **2/3**:219–225, 1978.

45. Rementeria, J.L., Nunag, N.N.: Narcotic withdrawal in pregnancy: stillbirth incidence with a case report. Am. J. Obstet. Gynecol. **116**:1152, 1973.

46. Roloff, D.W., Howatt, W.F.: The effect of chronic morphine administration on lung development and growth of fetal rabbits. Pediatr. Res. **7**:321, 1973.

47. Rosen, T.S., Pippenger, C.E.: Pharmacologic observations on the neonatal withdrawal syndrome. J. Pediatr. **88**:1044, 1976.

48. Rothstein, P., Gould, J.B.: Natural history of infants born to drug dependent women. Read at 14th Annual Meeting of the Ambulatory Pediatric Association, Washington, D.C., April 29–30, 1974.

49. Sardemann, H., Madsen, K.S., Friis-Hansen, B.: Follow-up of children of drug-addicted mothers. Arch. Dis. Child. **51**:131, 1976.

50. Schulman, C.A.: Alterations of the sleep cycle in heroin-addicted and "suspect" newborns. Neuropaediatric **1**:89, 1969.

51. Seip, M.: Growth retardation, dysmorphic facies, and minor malformations

following massive exposure to phenobarbitone in utero. Acta Paediatr. Scand. **65**:617, 1976.

52. Statzer, D.E., Wardell, J.N.: Heroin addiction during pregnancy. Am. J. Obstet. Gynecol. **113**:273, 1972.

53. Stern, R.: The pregnant addict: a case study of 66 case histories, 1950–1959. Am. J. Obstet. Gynecol. **94**:253, 1966.

54. Stimmel, B.: The socioeconomics of heroin dependency. N. Engl. J. Med. **287**:1275, 1972.

55. Taeusch, H.W., Jr., Carson, S.H., Wang, N.S., Avery, M.E.: Heroin induction of lung maturation and growth retardation in fetal rabbits. J. Pediatr. **82**:869, 1973.

56. Valdes-Dapena, M.A.: Sudden and unexpected death in infancy: a review of the world literature, 1954–1966. Pediatrics **39**:123, 1967.

57. Wilson, G.S., Desmond, M.M., Verniaud, W.M.: Early development of infants of heroin-addicted mothers. Am. J. Dis. Child. **126**:457, 1973.

58. Zelson, C.: Infant of the addicted mother. N. Engl. J. Med. **288**:1393, 1973.

59. Zelson, C., Lee, S.J., Casalino, M.: Neonatal narcotic addiction: Comparative effects of maternal intake of heroin and methadone. N. Engl. J. Med. **289**:1216, 1973.

60. Zelson, C., Rubio, E., Wasserman, E.: Neonatal narcotic addiction: 10 year observation. Pediatrics **48**:178, 1971.

15
Maternal and Perinatal Mortality

Jean Pakter, Morton A. Schiffer, and
Frieda Nelson

A distinct decline has been evident in both maternal and perinatal mortality rates in New York City over the last decade, particularly in the latter half (i.e., since 1970). This phenomenon was noted nationally as well as in New York City.

We felt that an analysis of these favorable trends by time periods, starting with 1960, would help bring into focus the factors that were instrumental in reducing mortality and that served as deterrents in achieving further declines.

A variety and number of programs, many of which were federally sponsored and supported, grew up in the 1960s. Among these were the Maternity, Infant Care–Family Planning Projects launched in 1964, designed to reach out to women of chilbearing age who were considered high risk or potentially at risk, in order to offer early and complete prenatal services. These services were located in areas with a high proportion of deprivation and associated high risk. Also during this time, programs were under development in the City to reach out to teen-age expectant mothers. The aim of the Maternity, Infant Care–Family Planning Projects and related programs was to introduce programs or complete prenatal services, which would bring pregnant women to term safely and reduce the likelihood of premature births, the chief factor in infant mortality.

Another important development was the rise of family planning facilities which began to become available from 1965 on, in hospitals and clinics that heretofore had not offered these services. Prior to that time, family planning was limited to private physicians and to a voluntary organization—Planned Parenthood. Essentially, this deprived patients who were dependent on clinic and ward services of hospitals of contraceptive counselling even if they wished it.

A heightened awareness of the unfulfilled sociomedical needs pertaining to women of childbearing age, especially among the deprived, led to a variety of community services, neighborhood clinics under the aegis of public health and welfare organizations with federal assistance. These clinics (some storefront type) supplemented prenatal and family planning services and helped to reach women through neighborhood counsellors, who were often their peers.

Concern for the prematurely born infant led to development of a program of specialized hospital centers in New York City, initiated as far back as November 1948 and expanded to a full complement of citywide centers to which those infants could be transferred to receive the care not available to them at the hospital of birth. The centers were the beginnings of regionalized care for the prematurely born as well as other infants at high risk. The premature center program accounted in great measure for the advances in care these babies received. The development of neonatologists as an important specialty among pediatricians, and specially trained pediatric nurses, was made possible by the 16 centers.

Advances in obstetrics were occurring particularly in the latter half of the 1960s; notable among these were sonography and fetal monitoring for management of labor and delivery. There was a greater awareness and understanding of the effects on the fetus (and on the mother) of analgesic and anesthetic drugs, especially in those institutions where obstetric anesthesiologists were available.

This past decade has been notable for medical advances and measures through legislation aimed at extending care especially to the poor and high-risk patients who had not been able to get such services previously. Notably, the change in the New York State Law in July 1970 regarding abortions made it possible for women at all socioeconomic levels to receive terminations of pregnancy medically under relatively safe circumstances. Prior to that time, an abortion could be performed legally only if the woman's life was endangered. Practically, this meant that a woman, especially the poor one, would endanger her life by seeking an abortion through unqualified auspices or her own desperate, dangerous attempts. Since January 1973, the Supreme Court of the United States has made abortion legal for all states through 24 weeks of pregnancy.

It would be difficult to assess to what extent any one of the foregoing factors contributed to the decline in maternal and perinatal mortality, since many of these programs and advances were taking place concurrently. Nevertheless, data concerning births and maternal and perinatal mortality have been placed in a framework of three periods: (1) prior to 1965, (2) 1966 to 1970, (3) 1971 to 1975, with the recognition that along with advances in obstetrics and neonatology, the availability of family planning in the second period and of legalized abortions in the third period, co-existing influences in the social and economic spheres could be exerting an effect in altering trends in births and perinatal and maternal mortality.

Methodology

The information for this review was based on (1) birth certificates, which yielded birth characteristics such as mother's age, parity, ethnic group, service, or private patient category (an approximate reflection of the socio-economic status), marital status, and outcome of pregnancy in terms of live-birth-weight groupings; (2) census reports for 1960 and 1970 for New York City for the numbers of women of childbearing age (15 to 44 years) by specific age and ethnic groupings; (3) birth certificate and census popu-lation data, which provided the necessary data for the determination of fertility rates which are age-specific birth rates; (4) death certificates for infants born alive and dying in the first year of life, for two postnatal periods, i.e. from birth through 27 days of age and from 28 days to one year of age. (These were matched with birth certificates of surviving in-fants and grouped by characteristics such as birth weight, ethnic group, mother's age, parity and marital status); (5) fetal death certificates, which were the source for data on fetal deaths (28 weeks and over gestation). In combination with infant deaths occurring in the first seven days of life, these data provided the perinatal mortality rates, which are computed as follows:

$$\text{Perinatal mortality rate} = \frac{\text{Infant deaths (under 7 days)} + \text{fetal deaths (28 weeks and over)}}{\text{Live births} + \text{fetal deaths (28 weeks and over)}} \times 1000$$

(6) maternal death certificates, where deaths are classified as associated with pregnancy, childbirth, or the puerperium; (7) termination of preg-nancy certificates, which were the source for data on induced terminations of pregnancy including an analysis by age, parity, and ethnic group.

Results

Births and Birth Patterns

In the period encompassed by this review, births, rather than increasing as had been predicted by some demographers, declined in New York City. More specifically, however, prior to 1970 the white group of births was primarily responsible for the drop. It was only after 1969 that a distinct decline occurred in all ethnic groups and within each age group among women of childbearing age. In fact, prior to 1970, births to teenagers had been increasing. Thus, from 1962 to 1965 the number of births decreased by only 3.9% and from 1966 to 1969, by 4.6%, but from 1970 on the decline was much sharper, with a distinct drop of 11.6% in the year following legalization of abortions (law went into effect in July 1970 in New York State) and a further reduction of 17.1% through 1975 for all ethnic groups combined.

Family planning may well have influenced the pattern of births in varying measure for each ethnic group and age subgroup in the latter half of the 1960s, thus reversing the upward trend in births which might have prevailed because of the increase in the numbers of women of childbearing age in the population. The census count showed an increase from 1.6 million in 1960 to 1.7 million in 1970 in New York City (almost 5%). The increase was accounted for entirely by the Puerto Rican and nonwhite group, especially the latter.

The ethnic composition of the childbearing age population in New York City has been changing as reflected by a rise in the proportion of nonwhite women of childbearing age from 17% in 1960 to 27% in 1970, a rise among Puerto Rican women from 10% in 1960 to 12% in 1970, while the proportion of white women in this age group dropped from 73% in 1960 to 61% in 1970.

Fertility rates for the nonwhite and Puerto Rican groups consistently were found to be substantially higher than those of the white groups. With the increasing proportion of those groups of women associated with higher fertility rates, it would not have been surprising to witness an increase in births in the city. However, their fertility rates, though still relatively higher than that of white women, had declined sufficiently to effect an overall drop in fertility for the total childbearing population. The fertility rate of 1960 of 101.7 dropped to 87.0 in 1970, by 1971 to 77.0, and in 1975 further down to 63.8.

The fertility rates for the white population by 1971 had decreased to 68.7 and by 1975 to 54.3, from 90.8 in 1960, the nonwhite group to 85.2 in 1971 and 84.5 in 1975 from 120.5 in 1960, and the Puerto Rican women to 100.0 in 1971 and 65.9 in 1975 from 149.4 in 1960.

Detailed analysis disclosed that it was not until the late 1960s that the decline in fertility rates for all ethnic groups became substantial enough to counterbalance the higher proportions of nonwhite and Puerto Rican groups with their relatively high fertility rates compared with that of the white population.

It was estimated that if the fertility rates in New York City had remained at the level of the early 1960s, births would indeed have approached an unprecedented number of 181,000 in 1975.

At the national level, fertility rates also declined from 118.0 in 1960 to 66.7 by 1975.

Births by Age and by Parity of Mother

When birth patterns were analyzed for the time period in terms of age and parity of the mothers, it was noted that teenage births, which had been on the increase through 1969, began to decline after 1970 (the year legalized abortions became available). Evidently, family planning services, which were readily available to teenagers as to the more mature age groups, had little impact on teenage birth trends. However, legalized abortions did have a distinct effect on births to the teenager.

Among women in their 20s, the decline in births also became more apparent after 1970. In fact, the nonwhite Puerto Rican group in their 20s had continued to show slight increases in the period 1966 to 1969.

The most noticeable declines in births occurred among the older age groups. The drop in births for women 35 and over was noted earlier, in the 1960s, undoubtedly influenced by availability of family planning services and further by the legalized abortions. With the shifting proportion from older to younger age groups, the average age of mothers in 1963 was 26.7 and in 1975, 26.1.

The percent of births to women 35 and over dropped from 10.3% in 1963 to 7.0% in 1975, while the percent of women in their 20s dropped from 62.8% in 1963 to 62.5% in 1975. The percent of teenage mothers rose from 10.3% in 1963 to 14.4% in 1975.

The trends in number of previous births to mothers revealed a rise in the proportion of births to Para 1 and Para 2 (the groups with the most favorable outcome of pregnancy generally) with a concomitant fall in the proportion of high parity births. Thus, in 1963, 61% of all births were Para 1 and Para 2 and by 1975 that proportion rose to 74.6%. On the other hand, the proportion of Para 5 and Para 6 births, which constituted 11.7% in 1963, declined to only 5.8% by 1975.

Comparing the ethnic groups, the Puerto Rican mothers in 1975 maintained the greatest proportion of high parity—four or more—births at 18.5%; nonwhite mothers were second, with 14.2%; white mothers were third, with 8.6% having four or more births.

The average parity for all births declined from 2.5 births in 1963 to 2.1 in 1971 and further down to 2.0 in 1975, with each ethnic group sharing in the decline, but the Puerto Rican women still showing the highest parity relatively.

Births by Marital Status

A steady rise in the number of out-of-wedlock births has been evident in New York City. Whereas, in 1962, 9.9% of births were to unmarried women, by 1965 it was 13.2%, by 1969, 20.1%, and by 1970, 21.4%, with a concomitant increase in number. It was only after 1970 that a change occurred with a decline in 1971 in the total number. Availability of abortions evidently had an effect. However, more recently the number of out-of-wedlock births again began to increase, although not at the previous rate. In 1975, 28.9% of births were out of wedlock and numbered 31,627. Whereas in-wedlock births declined by 25%, out-of-wedlock births increased by 12.6% from 1971 to 1975 following a transient decline from 1970 to 1971. (Since out-of-wedlock births are associated with higher infant mortality rates, increasing proportions of out-of-wedlock births would serve as deterrents to the decline in infant mortality.)

The rise in out-of-wedlock births has occurred despite the fact that two-thirds of the abortions have been among the unmarried and that the ratio of abortions to births among residents was approximately 1 : 2, with an even higher ratio for the teenage population (3). One can postulate that were it not for the large number of terminations, out-of-wedlock births would have been almost double the actual number.

Births and Socioeconomic Status

Since socioeconomic status appears to exert an influence on outcome of pregnancy, with a high infant mortality generally associated with low socioeconomic status, it was pertinent to review the trends among births in terms of private and general hospital services as an approximate measure of economic status. Of the total births in 1963, 54.5% births were on private services and 43.5% on general service. In 1975, the proportion was slightly lower for private service births and higher for general services. When reviewed by ethnic group, the proportion for nonwhite patients on private services was twice that of 1967, with one-third of this group on private services. Likewise, among Puerto Rican women the proportion rose from 9.9% in 1967 to 25.9% on private services in 1975. The findings must be interpreted with a degree of caution since a proportion of patients covered by Medicaid received care on private services yet had limited means. Nevertheless, the significant rise in proportion of nonwhite and Puerto Rican private births would suggest that, on the whole, economic improvement had occurred among the minority groups.

Another indicator was the rise in median annual income from 1960 to 1970. These income data were not restricted to the childbearing population, but were based on income of population of all ages and thus were of limited value in interpretation. Nevertheless, it was observed that the median annual income rose for each ethnic group, with the white income rising from $6627 in 1959 to $11,183 in 1969, the nonwhite income, from $4437 to $7150, and Puerto Rican income, from $3811 to $5575. These gains have undoubtedly been offset to a considerable extent by inflation and the increased cost of living (2). Unless a reversal in the economic situation occurs, the gains may not only be destroyed, but the situation may be worsened with a predictably adverse impact on outcome of pregnancy.

Births to women on welfare rolls had been increasing steadily up until the time family planning and legalized abortions became available. Then, in 1972, a significant decline in these births occurred with 72 per 1000 and further down to 67 per 1000 in 1973, compared with 115 per 1000 in 1969. However, after 1973 an upturn was noted again, reflecting the worsening of the socioeconomic climate of the city, and by 1975 the rate of births on public assistance was 90 per 1000 monthly average cases with indications of a further rise to 95 per 1000 for 1976 (4).

Births to Women Receiving Early Prenatal Care

It has long been observed and noted that women who received early and continued prenatal care had the best pregnancy outcome. In contrast, women who had received little or no prenatal care had the poorest outcome.

According to birth certificate data in 1975, more than 72% of women received early and intermediate prenatal care. This is a very conservative estimate in view of the fact that if the woman received prenatal care elsewhere, the birth certificate might not contain this information. Among patients receiving prenatal care through federally funded projects, the Maternity and Infant Care-Family Planning Projects in New York City, almost one-third registered for care in the first trimester (1). Without a doubt, the special project and outreach programs have increased the availability of prenatal care.

Changes in Number of Live Births in New York City by Weight and Ethnic Group

Prior to 1965, the number of infants born weighing less than 2501 g increased. However, in succeeding years, 1966 to 1969, the number of low-birth-weight babies decreased for each ethnic group, with an overall distinct decrease which became even more evident after 1970. The downturn in numbers noted for all weight groupings was particularly significant in that the very lowest birth-weight groups shared in the decline. Since infants under 1500 g have a much higher risk of dying, the drop in their number should have a beneficial effect on infant mortality. Altogether, the numerical decline among the low-birth-weight groups was proportionately greater than that for infants of normal and optimal birth weight. Thus, the changing distribution of births by weight groups was more favorable for survival.

This change, coupled with the distinct decrease in mortality rates noted for each weight group through the past decade, resulted in a significant decline in infant mortality.

Decline in Neonatal Mortality

In 1962, infants born under 1000 g had an 87.5% mortality. In 1975, the rate had dropped to 75.3. For the group, weighing 1001 to 1500 g, the mortality declined from 45% to 31.2%, and for the 1501 to 2000 g infants, from 14.4% down to 8.0%. For those weighing 2001 to 2500 g, the mortality decreased from 3.2% to 1.7%. For babies born over 2500 g, a reduction in mortality also occurred from 0.5% to 0.4%. Altogether, for infants of all weight groupings, a 25% decline in neonatal infant mortality was effected in this study period. Each ethnic group shared in the decline.

The decline in infant mortality rates was apparent even among the out-of-wedlock births, which have been associated with about twice the mortality of births among the married. This was true for each ethnic group and for the various age groups of the mothers. However, despite the declines, the disparity in mortality rates was still apparent. Prior to 1960, the period 1955 to 1959, the infant mortality rate for the in-wedlock was 23.9/1000, while among the out-of-wedlock it was 48.2. By 1966 to 1967, the in-wedlock group had a mortality rate of 19.4 compared with 37.1 for the out-of-wedlock. In 1971, a further drop in infant mortality occurred for both groups, with the in-wedlock down to 15.4 and the out-of-wedlock to 31.7. By 1975, the mortality rates further declined to 13.5/1000 for the in-wedlock and 26.3/1000 for the out-of-wedlock—almost twice that of the in-wedlock. Within each ethnic group, the impact of marital status on mortality rates was distinct.

Another feature associated with outcome of pregnancy is the age and parity of the mother. It has been observed for many years that the extremes of ages (young teen-agers and older mothers) were more likely to have an adverse outcome—particularly the teen-age group. The greatest risks, as far as infant survival was concerned, were among births of high parity order to the younger mothers. Here, too, declines in infant mortality have occurred in recent years for all these groups, with the differences in mortality rates persisting for each group. For example, among the 25 to 29 year-old Para 1 and 2, the infant mortality rate of 16.5, noted in 1963 to 1965, dropped to 13.3 in 1971, while births to those under 20 or Para 4, which were associated with a mortality rate of 71.6/1000 in 1963 to 1965, declined to 42.6/1000 in 1971. However, the disparity in mortality rates was still striking.

By 1975, high parity births had diminished to such a degree that too few had occurred to compute a mortality rate for Para 3 or more among teen-age mothers. Likewise, births among older women, 40 and over, had declined so much that infant mortality rates could not be computed. In 1975, the lowest infant mortality rate of 5.8/1000 was found among Para 2 births to women 25 to 29 years of age. Every age group and birth order shared in the declining mortality rates. The mortality in the group of birth order of two or more exhibited the greatest decrease in 1975, as compared with the preceding years.

Trends in Perinatal Mortality

The decline in perinatal mortality (fetal deaths 28 weeks and over and infant deaths under seven days) was apparent for each ethnic group. Whereas in 1960, the overall rate in New York City was 31.6, with the nonwhite group highest at 47.7, the Puerto Rican at 36.4, and the white at 25.4, a gradual decline was noted through the 1960's. In 1970, the perinatal mortality rate for New York City was 26.5, with the nonwhite still highest relatively with a rate of 34.1, the Puerto Rican next with 25.8, and the white, 22.4. By 1975, the rate for New York City had dropped to 22.8, with a range of 26.3 for the nonwhite, 22.2 for the Puerto Rican group, and 20.6 for the white.

The distinctly improved survival rates for all birth-weight categories can be attributed to the advances that have occurred in perinatology. The reduction in the numbers of low-birth-weight infants born since 1970 has also contributed to the decline in infant mortality. Other factors that have been a positive influence in improving survival of infants include the more favorable distribution by age and parity of the mother and particularly the significant reduction in births of high parity (birth order five or more).

Decline in Infant Mortality in the United States

The trends noted in New York City were evident for the United States as well. In 1960, the infant mortality rate of the United States was 26.0 per 1000 live births and 24.7 in 1965, further down to 20.0 in 1970, reaching a new low by 1975 with a rate of 16.1. The decline in infant mortality was noted for both the white and nonwhite populations. However, the infant mortality in the nonwhite group still remained at a higher level than the white, viz., 22.9/1000 live births (for nonwhite) versus 14.4 (for the white).

Causes of Death Among Infants

In 1975, the leading causes of infant deaths were congenital malformations, immaturity, respiratory distress, hyaline membrane disease, postnatal asphyxia and atelectasis. Almost two-thirds of infant deaths occurred in the first seven days of life and three-fourths in the neonatal period.

It is apparent that the greatest avenue for reducing infant mortality lies in the prevention of premature births and the associated hazards, which predominate in this group, of respiratory distress and hyaline membrane disease. The growing knowledge of factors contributing to congenital malformations, though limited at present, may yield more insights and lead to a significant reduction of this group.

Congenital malformations related to rubella in the pregnant woman constitute one example of a correlation established a little over a decade ago in this country. The role of other viral infections, and exposure to drugs and environmental contaminants, will undoubtedly be expanded in the foreseeable future.

Maternal Mortality

A dramatic decline occurred in maternal deaths in New York City, as well as the United States, in this period under review. After 1970, the drop was steep, establishing a record low for both the entire country and New York City. For the United States, the maternal mortality was 37.1/100,000 live births in 1960, dropping to 31.6/100,000 live births in 1965, and further down to 21.5/100,000 live births in 1970, with a relatively steeper decrease halving the rate to 12.8/100,000 live births by 1975.

In New York City maternal mortality rates, which have been consistently higher than that of the United States, declined to 65.5/100,000 in 1965, further down to 45.6/100,000 in 1970, and to a new low of 23.7/100,000 in 1975.

Family planning facilities currently available to all women desirous of utilizing the services, regardless of their socioeconomic status, have enabled women to plan pregnancies and curtail the number of births, as well as to space the intervals between pregnancies. Special programs such as the Maternity Infant Care Project, community outreach, and nutrition programs with federal subsidies, such as WIC have been important in improving prenatal care for women.

Advances in Obstetric and Perinatal Management

The past decade has been remarkable for advances in prenatal and obstetric diagnostic techniques. Sonography, estriol determinations, amniocentesis, determination of lecithin-sphingomyelin ratios are illustrative of aids in assessing the maturity of the fetus. The sonogram is important in ascertaining placental location, fetal position, cephalic size, and multiple pregnancy. Fetal monitoring (both external and internal) has a vital function in the management of labor to detect fetal distress promptly and enables the obstetrician to improve the course of labor and delivery by anticipatory approaches.

The judicious use of cesarean section has helped eliminate excessively long traumatic labor and delivery and diminished the use of instrumental deliveries, breech extractions or versions, particularly where cephalopelvic disproportion is diagnosed. In 1960, 5.7% of all live births were cesarean sections, in 1965, 6.1%, in 1970, 8.1%, and by 1975, 14.4%. The advances in obstetric management have had a significant impact on the reduction of perinatal and maternal mortality.

The administration of Rho immune globulin to the Rh-negative woman following childbirth or a termination of pregnancy has resulted in a significant reduction of sensitized women and a concomitant reduction in the incidence of erythroblastosis fetalis.

Other developments (besides advances in obstetric management) which had an impact on maternal mortality were in the area of family planning. A moderate decline in maternal mortality was evident from 1965 to 1969, but nothing as spectacular as the decline from 1970 (when legalization of abortions occurred) to 1975. The single leading cause of death in pregnancy had been associated with the sequelae of "criminal" or "illegal" abortions (self-inflicted or by an unskilled nonmedical person) resulting in hemorrhage, sepsis, and shock. This was virtually eliminated as women desirous of terminating an unwanted pregnancy learned to secure an abortion under legally medical auspices. Whereas in 1965, 41 women in New York City died as a consequence of illegal abortions, the number dropped to 24 in 1969, 16 in 1970, to one by 1973, and to none from 1974 to the present. Death following legal abortions declined from an average of six for 1970 to 1973 to an average of one to two for 1974 to 1976. Most of the fatalities associated with legalized abortions have occurred with terminations induced in the second trimester of pregnancy.

Puerperal death associated with childbirth (excluding abortion-related deaths) also declined substantially from 63 in 1965 to 29 in 1973, 23 in 1975, and 31 in 1976.

When puerperal (including abortion-associated) deaths were analyzed by cause of death, among 122 which occurred from 1973 through 1976 (a four-year period), it was evident that abortions were no longer the single leading cause. Instead, the four leading causes in order of frequency for that period were:

Cause	No.	%
Pulmonary embolism	29	23.8
Toxemia	20	16.4
Anesthesia	17	13.9
Ruptured ectopic pregnancy	15	12.3

In 1976, the most recent year for which data are available, anesthesia assumed the lead in causes of death, with eight deaths attributed to complications following anesthesia, or 25% of all puerperal deaths. Of these, five were associated with cesarean sections, two with abortions, and one with vaginal delivery. Of the two abortions, one was a first-trimester termination and the second was associated with a D and C following a spontaneous incomplete abortion (data taken from Tables 15.1 to 15.12).

Despite the decline in maternal deaths, it would appear that these can be reduced further and that the irreducible minimum has yet to be achieved. The emergence of anesthesia as one of the leading causes is disturbing. Particularly in view of the trend for an increased proportion and number of cesarean sections, evident in New York City and nationally, the role of anesthesia in contributing to a safe or adverse outcome merits much more attention.

In 1974, the Commissioner of Health in New York City promulgated a recommendation endorsed by the Obstetric Advisory Committee with regard to obstetric anesthesia (5) (see Appendix, page 253).

The effort to establish regionalized perinatal care in New York City has already begun to take shape with the designation of tertiary units in hospitals which have the responsibility to care for the highest risk infants. Ultimately, the aim is to plan, wherever possible, to have women at high risk deliver at such hospitals rather than to transfer infants after birth. A significant number of women, estimated at 20% to 25%, who are not considered high risk prenatally will become high risk in the course of labor. Thus, the need for a special infant transport system will still exist.

The standards for modern-day obstetrics and neonatology are at such a level as to ordinarily preclude the feasibility of a hospital maintaining a service with less than 1000 deliveries a year. Current standards require an obstetric anesthesiologist and competent fetal monitoring staff, in addition to the medical, nursing, and social service and laboratory personnel. High quality care cannot be inexpensive. Therefore, resources must be marshalled and utilized efficiently and shared through a network of hospitals working together.

Conclusion

Recognition must be given to factors beyond medical control which contribute to the risks of maternal and infant mortality. Pregnancy among the unmarried teen-agers, women over 35 years of age, those with drug addiction, and of high parity, as well as neglect in seeking prenatal care are among such factors, serving as deterrents to further reducing maternal and perinatal mortality.

However, it can be anticipated that if optimal standards of care incorporating advances in obstetric and neonatal management are implemented in all maternity and newborn facilities, a further decline in maternal and perinatal mortality will be achieved. Such standards will have to include obstetric anesthesiology specifically.

Recommended Standards for Obstetric Anesthetic Care

The purpose of this outline is to define ideal standards for obstetric anesthetic care which are recommended to all hospitals or services in New York City engaged in rendering such care. It is the ultimate hope that the application of these standards will eventuate in the elevation and maintenance of the quality of obstetric anesthesia in New York City.

Personnel for Obstetric Anesthesia

Safety of obstetric anesthesia depends principally upon the skill of the anesthesiologist. The same level of competence of anesthesia personnel should be required for obstetric procedures as for surgical procedures.

Responsibility for obstetric anesthesia should rest with the Director or Chief of Obstetric Anesthesia Service, appointed by the Chairman of the Department of Anesthesiology. The Director or Chief of Obstetric Anesthesia should be a qualified anesthesiologist. He should be responsible for the technical medical policies and procedures for the conduct of the service and for the supervision of the service.

A qualified anesthesiologist is defined as having the following credentials:

a. A licensed physician who is a diplomate of the American Board of Anesthesiology or its equivalent or who submits evidence to the hospital department and the Department of Health that his training and experience qualify him for admission to the examination by such Board.
b. He should possess special training and knowledge of obstetric anesthesia including the management of maternal and perinatal complications.

The Director or Chief of Obstetric Anesthesia should establish guidelines approving those who are to administer or to supervise the administration of anesthesia to the obstetric patients. Those approved should be fully competent in all forms of inhalation, intravenous, and regional anesthesia as well as in the management of maternal and perinatal complications. At least one such qualified person should be on hospital premises in the vicinity of the delivery suite at all times and should have no other concomitant responsibilities.

The Director or Chief of Obstetric Anesthesia should ensure that senior consultant advice is available 24 hours a day.

Table 15.1   Number of Live Births in New York City by Age and Ethnic
Group of Mother, 1962–1975

Age of Mother	1962	1965	1966
White			
Under 15	28	39	64
15–19	6,161	6,300	6,733
20–24	33,122	31,676	31,083
25–29	31,475	28,938	27,543
30–34	19,650	16,152	14,816
35–39	9,433	8,067	7,318
40+	2,510	2,189	1,890
TOTAL	102,379	93,361	89,447
Nonwhite			
Under 15	169	216	267
15–19	6,216	7,482	8,040
20–24	13,573	14,713	13,612
25–29	9,130	9,764	9,534
30–34	5,368	5,340	5,278
35–39	2,736	2,702	2,504
40+	698	754	745
TOTAL	37,890	40,971	39,980
Puerto Rican			
Under 15	36	29	4,244
15–19	4,083	4,232	9,305
20–24	9,739	9,482	5,696
25–29	6,235	5,825	2,952
30–34	3,098	3,054	1,331
35–39	1,413	1,460	361
40+	371	401	23,907
TOTAL	24,975	24,483	18
All ethnic groups			
Under 15	233	284	19,017
15–19	16,460	18,014	54,000
20–24	56,434	55,871	42,773
25–29	46,840	44,527	23,046
30–34	28,116	24,546	11,153
35–39	13,582	12,229	2,996
40+	3,579	3,344	153,334
TOTAL	165,244	158,815	349

Obstetric Suite

The Obstetric Anesthesia Service should be a self-sufficient unit with its
own equipment and supplies. These should be of the same diversity and
quality as those used in the operating suite. Safe administration of obstetric

1969	1970	1971	1975
94	84	68	91
6,281	6,495	5,602	5,245
27,036	27,718	24,298	20,947
27,802	27,490	25,100	9,826
12,483	12,498	11,139	3,222
5,437	4,996	4,288	676
1,458	1,329	1,066	
80,591	80,610	71,561	56,587
355	340	259	254
9,012	9,280	7,895	
13,676	14,777	13,251	11,878
9,847	10,784	9,790	10,472
5,285	5,817	5,283	5,735
2,360	2,479	2,271	2,297
731	671	600	516
41,266	44,148	39,349	38,975
40	68	49	50
4,358	3,936	3,339	2,244
9,631	9,552	8,083	4,422
6,004	6,433	5,572	4,161
2,832	2,959	2,618	2,043
1,202	1,171	1,101	761
297	315	248	175
24,364	24,434	21,010	13,856
489	492	376	395
19,651	19,711	16,836	15,312
50,343	52,047	45,632	32,880
43,653	44,707	40,462	35,580
20,600	21,274	19,040	17,604
8,999	8,646	7,660	6,280
2,486	2,315	1,914	1,367
146,221	149,192	131,920	109,418

analgesia-anesthesia entails the ready availability of all essential equipment, drugs, and supplies. The labor-delivery suite should be stocked with syringes, needles, catheters, and other material necessary for intravenous infusions, blood transfusions, central venous pressure measurement, arterial

Table 15.2   United States Vital Statistics Data:
1960, 1965, 1970, 1975

	Fertility Rates		
Year	Total	White	Nonwhite
1960	118.0	113.2	153.6
1965	96.6	91.4	133.9
1970	87.9	84.1	113.0
1975	66.7	63.1	88.7

Table 15.3   Live Births by Weight and Ethnic Group in New York City:
1962–1975

Weight	1962	1965	1966
White			
Under 1001	443	436	388
1001–1500	510	498	479
1501–2000	1,302	1,111	1,186
2001–2500	5,428	5,037	4,972
Under 2501	7,683	7,082	7,025
2501 and over	94,696	86,279	82,422
TOTAL	102,379	93,361	89,447
Nonwhite			
Under 1001	603	663	613
1001–1500	525	626	570
1501–2000	1,112	1,234	1,193
2001–2500	3,498	3,898	3,990
Under 2501	5,738	6,421	6,366
2501 and over	32,152	34,550	33,614
TOTAL	37,890	40,971	39,980
Puerto Rican			
Under 1001	172	159	164
1001–1500	155	175	201
1501–2000	482	480	455
2001–2500	1,749	1,791	1,784
Under 2501	2,558	2,605	2,604
2501 and over	22,417	21,878	21,303
TOTAL	24,975	24,483	23,907
All ethnic groups			
Under 1001	1,218	1,258	1,165
1001–1500	1,190	1,299	1,250
1501–2000	2,896	2,825	2,834
2001–2500	10,675	10,726	10,746
Under 2501	15,979	16,108	15,995
2501 and over	149,265	142,707	137,339
TOTAL	165,244	158,815	153,334

blood sampling. Dextrose in water and electrolyte-containing solutions with and without dextrose as well as colloid should be available.

Labor Rooms

Labor rooms should permit easy rapid changes in body positions from head-up to head-down. A sphygmomanometer, an oxygen source, and a suction device should be provided at each bedside for the parturient woman, and a fetal monitor for the infant. A cart should be at hand containing the equipment and drugs necessary to establish and maintain the airway,

1969	1970	1971	1975
1,108	973	256	205
1,137	1,216	344	304
2,686	2,640	844	645
9,600	9,620	3,474	2,683
14,531	14,449	4,918	3,837
131,690	134,743	66,643	52,750
146,221	149,192	71,561	56,587
358	334	394	361
418	424	479	462
1,021	1,019	1,081	952
4,191	4,054	3,285	3,034
5,988	5,831	5,239	4,809
74,603	74,779	34,110	34,166
80,591	80,610	39,349	38,975
604	516	103	58
537	603	142	102
1,191	1,175	359	246
3,714	3,857	1,430	892
6,046	6,151	2,034	1,298
35,220	37,997	18,976	12,558
41,266	44,148	21,010	13,856
146	123	748	624
182	189	965	868
474	446	2,284	1,843
1,695	1,709	8,194	6,609
2,497	2,467	12,191	9,944
21,867	21,967	119,729	99,474
24,364	24,434	131,920	109,418

Table 15.4 Neonatal Mortality Rate* in New York City by Weight at Birth and Race† 1962–1971 and 1975

Weight at Birth (in grams)	1962	1963	1964	1965	1966	1967	1968	1969	1970	1971	1975
Under 1001	87.5	87.1	88.4	87.9	86.4	84.9	82.5	86.0	80.0	79.0	75.3
White	91.5	88.4	93.3	91.8	90.1	88.6	88.3	95.0	81.3	87.3	83.3
Nonwhite	83.6	85.8	83.9	84.5	83.3	82.1	77.4	78.8	78.8	71.8	69.7
1001–1500	45.0	44.3	43.8	40.8	36.6	35.9	34.5	39.0	33.4	33.8	31.2
White	50.5	49.8	52.6	48.0	40.9	43.2	38.9	47.5	38.4	42.8	36.8
Nonwhite	38.3	37.9	34.2	33.3	31.8	28.6	29.5	29.9	28.5	24.8	26.5
1501–2000	14.4	12.1	12.9	11.5	11.0	11.0	11.2	10.8	10.0	9.2	8.0
White	17.4	14.7	16.0	14.0	13.1	13.4	13.2	12.8	13.1	12.9	9.0
Nonwhite	9.9	8.6	8.9	8.4	8.2	7.7	8.4	8.4	6.3	5.8	7.1
2001–2500	3.2	2.8	2.8	2.6	2.4	2.2	2.3	2.6	2.3	2.5	1.7
White	3.5	3.2	3.1	3.1	2.8	2.5	2.9	2.9	2.7	3.2	2.2
Nonwhite	2.6	2.0	2.3	1.9	1.8	1.6	1.3	2.1	1.7	1.6	1.3
Under 2501	14.8	14.0	14.6	13.9	12.8	12.8	12.5	13.3	11.5	10.9	10.1
White	14.3	13.6	14.5	13.4	12.3	12.1	12.4	13.3	11.5	11.8	10.3
Nonwhite	15.7	14.6	14.9	14.7	13.5	13.8	12.7	13.3	11.6	9.8	9.9
2501+	0.5	0.5	0.5	0.4	0.5	0.4	0.4	0.4	0.4	0.4	0.4
White	0.5	0.4	0.4	0.4	0.4	0.4	0.4	0.4	0.4	0.3	0.4
Nonwhite	0.6	0.5	0.6	0.5	0.6	0.5	0.5	0.5	0.5	0.5	0.5
TOTAL	2.0	1.9	2.0	1.9	1.9	1.8	1.7	1.8	1.6	1.5	1.5
White	1.7	1.6	1.7	1.6	1.5	1.5	1.5	1.6	1.4	1.3	1.3
Nonwhite	3.0	2.8	3.0	2.9	2.8	2.7	2.3	2.4	2.2	1.9	1.7

* Per 100 live births
† Puerto Ricans are included in the white and nonwhite rates: 95% white, 5% nonwhite.

Table 15.5   Infant Mortality Rates* in New York City by Legitimacy and Ethnic Group: 1955–1971 and 1975 (Excluding 1968–1970, 1972–1974)

Ethnic Groups	In-Wedlock	Out-of-Wedlock	Ratio of Out-of-Wedlock to In-Wedlock	Total
		Infant Mortality		
	1955–1959			
White	20.1	35.0	1.7:1	20.4
Nonwhite	38.3	51.9	1.4:1	41.6
Puerto Rican	29.3	48.3	1.7:1	31.4
TOTAL	23.9	48.2	2.0:1	25.7
	1966–1967			
White	15.4	28.4	1.8:1	16.0
Nonwhite	30.7	41.1	1.3:1	34.5
Puerto Rican	22.3	32.7	1.5:1	24.4
TOTAL	19.4	37.1	1.9:1	22.2
	1971			
White	13.0	28.9	2.2:1	17.6
Nonwhite	21.6	35.3	1.6:1	27.4
Puerto Rican	16.9	25.1	1.5:1	19.7
TOTAL	15.4	31.7	2.1:1	20.9
	1975			
White	11.8	28.6	2.4:1	16.6
Nonwhite	16.9	27.7	1.6:1	23.7
Puerto Rican	16.4	19.3	1.2:1	17.7
TOTAL	13.5	26.3	2.1:1	19.3

* per 1000 live births

administer artificial respiration, and treat convulsions or severe hypotension.

Delivery Rooms

Each delivery room must contain its own well-functioning modern anesthesia machine, equipped with safety devices and precision vaporizers. Installation of scavenging devices for removal of waste anesthetic gases is desirable. Equipment for endotracheal intubation and drugs for routine and emergency use must be at hand. Means for left uterine displacement must be readily available. An oscilloscope for electrocardiographic monitoring and an anesthesia machine-ventilator, a respirometer, and a nerve stimulator should be at hand for selected cases. Nitrous oxide should be piped in. Oxygen and suction should be centrally supplied exclusively for anesthetic use and independently of surgical or neonatal requirements. If

Table 15.6   Infant Mortality Rates* in New York City by Age of Mothers and Birth Order: 1963–1975 (Excluding 1968–1970, 1972–1974)

Birth Order	Age of Mother						
	Under 20	20–24	25–29	30–34	35–39	40 and Older	All Ages
			1963–1965				
1	26.3	17.5	16.5	21.6	30.3	21.1	20.0
2	48.0	23.8	16.9	18.2	24.9	38.4	23.2
3	59.3	33.3	21.0	20.7	19.3	33.6	25.6
4	71.6	41.8	28.7	18.6	27.6	23.1	28.8
5+	93.8†	47.9	37.5	31.0	27.3	29.1	33.4
TOTAL	33.3	24.0	21.5	22.8	26.5	29.8	24.4
			1966–1967				
1	24.9	15.8	15.9	21.3	29.4	26.7	18.9
2	46.0	22.0	14.4	19.2	17.1	28.6	21.4
3	54.9	29.2	17.7	16.9	19.4	18.9	22.2
4	64.4	33.3	27.1	22.3	25.8	29.4	27.4
5+	63.5†	47.5	31.0	28.7	25.6	18.6	29.5
TOTAL	31.2	21.1	18.5	21.6	23.3	22.6	22.2
			1971				
1	26.7	13.7	13.3	16.3	18.6	10.6	17.0
2	41.8	15.7	13.3	14.0	18.3	21.3	17.0
3	54.5	28.1	16.1	15.5	21.5	31.9	21.0
4	42.6†	28.0	20.7	16.4	20.1	24.5	21.2
5+	71.4†	41.1	21.2	24.5	21.6	24.1	24.4
TOTAL	30.7	17.0	15.0	17.0	20.2	22.8	20.9
			1975				
1	22.3	14.5	11.7	18.1	17.5	‡	16.1
2	16.7	9.3	5.8	6.4	7.7	‡	8.2
3	‡	14.1	9.9	10.5	8.1	‡	10.9
4	‡	19.3	9.4	7.1	8.0	‡	11.0
5+	‡	‡	‡	‡	‡	‡	‡
TOTAL	24.8	18.3	13.3	15.9	17.5	‡	19.3

* Per 1000 live births
† Based upon less than 100 births
‡ Numbers too small to compute rates

explosive gases are utilized, the electric outlets and fixtures must comply with the recommendations of the National Fire Protection Association, and the floors of the delivery rooms, adjacent connecting areas, and corridors for at least 10 feet in any direction from the room entrance must be conductive.

Table 15.7   Perinatal Mortality Rates by Ethnic Group in New York City: 1960–1975

Year	Total	White	Nonwhite	Puerto Rican
1960	31.6	25.4	47.7	36.4
1961	31.1	25.3	43.4	38.0
1962	31.1	25.2	44.3	35.1
1963	31.2	25.4	43.2	35.4
1964	31.9	25.5	44.3	36.2
1965	29.9	24.6	41.3	31.0
1966	29.2	23.8	40.7	30.4
1967	28.7	23.5	38.4	31.4
1968	28.6	23.4	37.4	31.5
1969	29.0	25.2	37.0	27.8
1970	26.5	22.4	34.1	25.8
1971	24.7	22.4	29.0	24.8
1972	23.5	21.0	27.8	23.5
1973	22.2	20.0	26.0	21.7
1974	24.6	22.0	29.5	23.1
1975	22.8	20.6	26.3	22.2

Recovery Rooms

The recovery space, easily accessible from the delivery room areas, should be available for all postpartum patients for at least two hours. The obstetric recovery room must be as fully equipped as the surgical recovery room.

Pain Relief

There is no adequate, safe, routine analgesic or anesthetic technique universally applicable to all parturients. Patients differ in their response to labor and to medication. The need for sedation and analgesia must be

Table 15.8   Infant Mortality Rates for the United States in 1960, 1965, 1970, 1975

	Total			White			Nonwhite		
Year	Total	Neo- natal	Post- Neo- natal	Total	Neo- natal	Post- Neo- natal	Total	Neo- natal	Post- Neo- natal
1960	26.0	18.7	7.3	22.9	17.2	5.7	43.2	26.9	16.4
1965	24.7	17.7	7.0	21.5	16.1	5.4	40.3	25.4	14.9
1970	20.0	15.1	4.9	17.8	13.8	4.0	30.9	21.4	9.5
1975	16.1	11.7	4.3	14.4	10.7	3.7	22.9	15.8	7.1

Table 15.9   Infant Mortality by Cause and Age at Death in New York City: 1975

Cause of death	Under 7 Days	Total Under 28 Days	28 Days to 1 Year	Total Under 1 Year
Diarrhea	11	19	10	29
Other infectious diseases	6	13	14	27
Meningitis	3	4	9	13
Influenza and pneumonia	24	37	66	103
Other respiratory diseases	2	4	25	29
Congenital anomalies	173	229	121	350
Birth injuries	29	39	0	39
Hyaline membrane disease	146	170	9	179
Asphyxia of newborn	203	222	0	222
Immaturity	259	268	1	269
Other diseases of early infancy	465	523	7	530
Accidents	0	1	10	11
All other causes	31	57	252	309
TOTAL	1,352	1,586	524	2,110

Table 15.10   Maternal Mortality Rates for the United States: 1970, 1975

Year	Total	White	Nonwhite
1960	37.1	26.0	97.9
1965	31.6	21.0	83.7
1970	21.5	14.4	55.9
1975	12.8	9.1	29.0

Maternal Mortality Rates per 100,000

evaluated and the selection of drugs individualized. It is recommended that all patients be seen by an anesthesiologist on the eve of an elective procedure or upon their admission to the obstetric suite. All drugs used for pain during labor and delivery may adversely affect both mother and fetus. Therefore, continuous supervision by qualified personnel is mandatory.

Infant Resuscitation

Infant resuscitation should be the responsibility of the best qualified available member of the delivery room team.

Table 15.11   Maternal Mortality—Numbers and Rates per 100,000
in New York City: 1960–1976

	Maternal Deaths	
Year	Number	Rate per 100,000 Live Births
1960	115	69.2
1961	130	77.2
1962	121	73.2
1963	116	69.1
1964	74	44.7
1965	104	65.5
1966	80	52.2
1967	76	52.1
1968	66	46.5
1969	77	52.7
1970	68	45.6
1971	37	28.0
1972	54	46.1
1973	36	32.5
1974	28	25.3
1975	26	23.7
1976	32	29.1

Table 15.12   Maternal Deaths—Total and Due to Induced Abortions in
New York City: 1960–1976

Year	Total Maternal Deaths	Induced Abortions Illegal	Legal	Other Causes
1960	115	46	—	69
1961	130	55	—	75
1962	121	53	—	68
1963	116	42	—	74
1964	74	34	—	40
1965	104	41	—	63
1966	80	31	—	49
1967	76	20	—	56
1968	66	21	—	45
1969	77	24	—	53
1970	68	16	6	46
1971	37	4	8	25
1972	54	9	5	40
1973	36	1	6	29
1974	28	0	1	27
1975	26	0	3	23
1976	32	0	1	31

References

1. Daily, E., Nicholas, N.: A free pregnancy testing service. Fam. Plann. Perspect. **5**:6, 1973.
2. Glazier, R.A.: Census Bulletin No. 16. Research and Program Planning Information Department, Community Council of Greater New York, August 10, 1972.
3. Pakter, J., Nelson, F.: Factors in the unprecedented decline in infant mortality in New York City. Bull. N.Y. Acad. Med. **50**:829, 1974.
4. Program Briefs No. 4 (1977) N.Y. State Department of Social Service. Trends in Births in Family Public Assistance Cases in N.Y.C. 1964–June 1976. Bureau of Research.
5. Obstetric Advisory Committee to the Commissioner of Health, New York City Department of Health. Recommended Standards for Obstetric Anesthesia Care. July 25, 1974.

Index

ABO incompatibility, 202
Abortions
  age and, 245
  declining mortality rate and, 244
  legalized, and mortality rates, 251
  marital status and, 246
  parity and, 245
  ratio to out-of-wedlock births, 246
  socioeconomic status and, 247
Acid-base status of infant, 58, 60
Acidemia, 163
  hypoxemia and cardiac function and,
    164
Acidosis, metabolic
  acid-base regulatory mechanisms, 153–
    154
  alkalinizing agents for, see Alkalinizing
    agents
  asphyxia as cause of, see Asphyxia,
    perinatal
  blood transfusions and, 161–162, 174
    175
  buffering system and, 153–154
  cause of, 153
  consequences of, 163–166
    cardiac effects, 164
    central nervous system dysfunction,
      164
    combined hypoxemia and acidemia,
      165
    effects of pH on vascular tone, 165
    glycolysis inhibition, 164
    limited delivery of oxygen, 164
    pulmonary lecithin decrease, 165–166
    pulmonary vascular resistance
      changes, 165
  CSF (cerebrospinal fluid) and, 163–164
  exchange transfusion and, 210
  hypothermia and, 162–163

  maternal and fetal, in normal labor and
    delivery, 159
  neonatal limitations and, 154–155
  in normal labor and delivery, 155–159
    fetal oxygenation and, 156
    impairment of blood flow and, 156
    maternal pH and, 159
    postnatal pH adjustment of infant and,
      159
    renal excretory system and, 153–154
    second stage of labor and, 157–158
    respiratory distress syndrome and, 161,
      172–174
    treatment of, 166–175
      hypernatremia and renal damage
        after, 169
      sodium bicarbonate in, 166–169; see
        also Sodium bicarbonate
      THAM (trishydroxy methyl amino
        methane) in, 169–170
Acoustic perception, 51–52
Adaptive capacity of newborns, drugs
  and, 75
Addiction, drug
  maternal
    pregnancy and, 222–224
    supportive counseling and, 234
    withdrawal during birth, 225–226
  neonatal
    follow-up of passively-addicted in-
      fants, 235–236
    later complications of, 232–235
    parental behavior and, 234
Air embolism, 211
Air lung (neonatal lung), 117–131
  alveolar ventilation and, see Alveolar
    ventilation
  compliance of, see Compliance
  fetal hypercapnia, 120